History of Epidemics and Pandemics
Reverberations, Responses and Resilience

पितरौ वन्दे
Pitrau Vandé

श्रेश्चच प्रेयश्च मनुष्यमेतस्तौ संपरीत्य विविनक्ति धीरः ।
श्रेयो हि धीरोऽभि प्रेयसो वृणीते प्रेयो मन्दो योगक्षेमाद्वृणीते ॥2॥

(कठोपनिषद् 2/2)

History of Epidemics and Pandemics

Reverberations, Responses and Resilience

Edited by

Shreya Pathak

ANAMIKA PUBLISHERS & DISTRIBUTORS (P) LTD.
4697/3, 21A, Ansari Road, Daryaganj, New Delhi 110002
Phones: 011-23281655, 011-43708938
E-mail: anamikapublishers@yahoo.co.in

Edition 2026

ISBN 978-81-953814-6-3

PRINTED IN INDIA

Published by Anamika Publishers & Distributors (P) Ltd., 4697/3, 21A, Ansari Road, Daryaganj, New Delhi 110002. Typeset by Shivani Compuers, Delhi 110093 and Printed at Vikas Computer & Printers, Tronica City, Ghaziabad

FOREWORD

The commencement of the twenty-first century was marked by exhilaration and exuberance coated with amplified conviction and optimism free of any thought that in the ensuing years the entire world was going to witness the deadliest pandemic. Confoundedly soon the unthinkable became the harsh reality of life and the commencement of year 2020 left the most black scar on the world in the form of COVID 19 The edited book written by Dr. Shreya Pathak is a quintessence in this regard. The time of pandemic was one of those which was characterized by various academic activities like webinars and publications, and amongst all these constructive move, the endeavour of Dr. Shreya Pathak too is commendable, wherein the author has made a much productive contribution through her edited book **History of Epidemics and Pandemics: Reverberations, Responses and Resilience.**

As evident from the title itself, the thrust area of the book is entirely circumscribed to the history of pestilence and its related aspects. The book includes variety of research papers as well as conceptual papers covering the vast time horizon from ancient to medieval and modern era and study area includes World, Europe, Russia, India and also regional histories of India. Much emphasis has been given to the detailed study of epidemic, health policy and administration of the Governments and responses of the people during the epidemic times. The Book begins with chapters giving special focus on the indigenous medicine system in ancient India highlighting ancient Sanskrit texts, medicine systems, importance of *Ayurveda*, sense of health awareness and preventive measures in daily living that are still scientific and applicable with the same medical authenticity. It also focuses on regional study like States of Arunachal Pradesh, Bengal and Assam. The inclusion of women and pandemic coupled with the substance of gender dimension, migration, political dynamics and delving deep into the dimension of colonizing the indigenous renders to it the academic stature and eminence. The political, socio-economic, cultural, art, environmental and gender dimension of the book renders it a much academic repute. The exhaustive description made in the research paper magnifies the academic caliber and pertains into several issues with intricate detailing making it worth a read. It also discusses over the relevance of Gandhian ideology during and post epidemic times along with the environmental dynamics.

I congratulate Dr. Shreya Pathak for her academic accomplishment and her uphill endeavour to present such an enriching book with insightful and simulative articles hailing from different academicians. Comprehending and contemplating the incorporated research papers in the book will surely provide a sanguine approach for the future and leaves an etch on the mind.

Place: Ara

Date: 27. 6. 21

Prof. Devi Prasad Tewari
Vice-Chancellor
Veer Kunwar Singh University
Ara, Bihar

Acknowledgements

I express my heartfelt gratitude to the Divine and my father Late Sridhar Pathak (Retd. IPS) together as both are watching me from the heaven, guiding me, walking with my steps in tandem, lightening my way, holding my hands and showering their blessing for every venture that I take up in my life. My Pa, as I used to call him, would have been the happiest person to see this book in hands. His teachings covered with love will be there with me forever.

My sincere gratitude to the contributors, who are adept in the respective research fields. Their academic contributions are invaluable without which this book would have never been a reality. While the book was going through the process of publication, sudden lock-down in many states badly hampered the work progress, but the way all co-operated, showed patience and confidence in me, make me really feel obliged. I deeply express my gratitude to all of them for having undeterred confidence in my work. My special acknowledgement to Sri. Sameer Bannerjee, a renowned Gandhian scholar and writer, for his humble gesture and instant approval to include his paper as one of the chapter.

Any project that I take up cannot be accomplished without the unstinting support and love of the family. My Ma, for providing me the congenial environment and praying ardently with an incredible heart, and my sister, Dr. Shalini Pathak, for her never ending love, time, incessant support and her straight forward expert advices from time to time. They are my constant source of inspiration and are always there as an inseparable part of my life. I also avail this opportunity to extend my heartfelt obligation to my fervent admirer Sri. Manish Pandey, for infusing in me the most required encouragement and confidence without which I would have not made headway in this project.

I am grateful to the publisher Anamika Publishers and Distributors (P) Ltd., especially Sri. Pankaj Sharma and his team, for their endeavours in accomplishment of this project even at a time of crisis.

Varanasi, June, 2021 **Shreya Pathak**

Preface

History is one of the most fascinating subjects dealing with all aspects of human civilization since times immemorial. It is not simply collection of the information, knowledge, memories and experiences of the past, but what makes it indispensible is the way historians deal with those past collections. The main purpose of a historian is not to simply record the past events in a chronological manner, but to interpret and evaluate it logically and scientifically on the basis of genuine sources. Analyzing the past events by identifying the similarities and the differences, discovering the why and how behind what happened and also what did not happened, uncovering the potentialities and the consequences hidden in human action or historical events all these make history imperative for understanding the complexities of the present and the future both. E.H. Carr says historian job is not to love or emancipate from the past, but to master it as the key to understand the present.

The sudden outbreak of pandemic in the twenty-first century received attention of many from scholarly world as the last global experience was a century before in 1918 at the time when World War I was going on. The global lockdown made the academicians, particularly historians, to travel back in time and explore the different aspects of the unexpected changing world scenario. Here, I would like to quote historian Eric Hobsbawm, who states, "The future is systematically connected with the past, which in turn is not an arbitrary concatenation of circumstances and events. The structures of human societies, their processes and mechanism of reproduction, change and transformation, are such as to restrict the number of things that can happen, determine some of the things that will happen, and make it possible to assign greater or lesser probabilities to much of the rest". It is with these purposes in mind that I thought of working on a book focusing on various aspects of pandemic and epidemic in different nations and different times. There is an exigent need to revisit the past and explore things in light of the contemporary world. Though history doesn't simply give a straight forward formula for prognosis, but it surely enables us to throw light on urgent dimensions of the problems and the challenges being faced in the present and better possible way to be adopted for the future.

This is not the first pandemic situation that world is facing, but it is first of its kind in this technologically advanced era where all societies and economies are interconnected and shows domino effect. This forces all of us to be inquisitive of our developing ways, social framework, role of technology, health, hygiene, living habits and morals. Medical history is the new emerging branch of study since couple of decades and the recent pandemic compels historians and scholars to divert and focus their studies exploring various aspects of this. It was with these purposes that the idea of this book on a relevant theme came in my mind and I started working on it.

Other than straight factual history of various epidemics, the Book focuses on many other dimensions of pandemic starting right from its references in ancient Sanskrit texts, how to deal with epidemic according to *Ayurved,* hygiene, medical science, scientific precautions being practiced since centuries in India, public health policy, people's responses against ruling authorities during epidemic times, political and psycho-social models. It covers diverse contemporary issues like women's role and contribution, gender, environment, art, migration, role of museum, colonialism, regional history and Gandhian ideology. The Book delves into certain unexplored dimensions of epidemic history which will contribute significantly in fulfilling the research gaps and comprehending the present crisis. This historical introspection enables to derive observations from the previous pandemics that are relevant to combat and mitigate any future crisis through effective and immediate response, administrative interventions, strategies, planning and research. The Covid pandemic has forced all of us to ponder, revisit and re-explore our past to understand the present challenges and this book is an attempt in that direction.

Varanasi, June 2021 **Shreya Pathak**

List of Contributors

1. **Dr. Ashish Kumar,** Assistant Professor, Department of Sanskrit, NLS College, Jai Prakash University, Saran, Bihar.
2. **Dr. Jitesh Kumar Singh,** Department of Ancient Indian History and Archaeology, University of Lucknow, Lucknow.
3. **Dr. Mukesh Kumar Singh,** Assistant Professor, Department of Ancient Indian History, Culture and Archaeology, DAV PG College, Varanasi.
4. **Ms. Shivani Mishra,** Research Scholar, Department of Psychology, University of Allahabad, Prayagraj, U.P.
5. **Dr. Anurag Upadhayay,** Assistant Professor, Department of Psychology, Udai Pratap Autonomous College, Varanasi, U.P.
6. **Ms. Deepti Mishra,** Department of Psychology, University of Allahabad, Prayagraj, U.P.
7. **Dr. Amita Esther David,** Associate Professor, Department of History, Isabella Thoburn College, Lucknow.
8. **Dr. Amit Kumar Verma,** Department of Pharmacy, MJP Rohilkhand University, Bareilly, U.P.
9. **Dr. Somenath Ghosh,** Assistant Professor and Head, Department of Zoology, Co-ordinator, Department of Biotechnology, Rajendra College, Jai Prakash University, Chapra, Bihar.

10. **Dr. Rajkishor,** Assistant Professor, Department of History, Ramshray Baleshwar College, Samastipur (A Constituent Unit of Lalit Narayan Mithila University), Bihar.
11. **Dr. Aparna Pathak,** Assistant Professor, Department of Psychology, DAVPG College, Siwan, Bihar.
12. **Dr. Chandana John,** Freelance, Department of English (former), Gandhi Institute of Technology and Management (GTAM), Hyderabad.
13. **Dr. Paromita Das,** Professor, Department of History, Guwahati University, Assam.
14. **Mr. P.K. Yadav,** Research Scholar, Department of History, Banaras Hindu University, Varanasi.
15. **Ms. Anuradha Thakur,** Department of History, Vasanta College for Women (Admitted to the Privileges of Banaras Hindu University), Varanasi.
16. **Dr. Kamlesh Singh,** Professor, Department of Orthodontics and Dentofacial Orthopedics, Saraswati Dental College, Lucknow.
17. **Dr. Pranshu Mathur,** PG student, Department of Orthodontics and Dentofacial Orthopedics, Saraswati Dental College, Lucknow.
18. **Dr. Shreya Pathak,** Assistant Professor, Department of History, Vasanta College for Women (Admitted to the Privileges of Banaras Hindu University), Varanasi, U.P.
19. **Dr. Shalini Pathak,** Guest Faculty, Department of Western History, University of Lucknow, U.P.
20. **Dr. Moushumi Dutta Pathak,** Associate Professor, Department of History, Arya Vidyapeeth College, Guwahati, Assam.
21. **Dr. Punita Pathak,** Assistant Professor, Department of Sociology, Vasanta College for Women (Admitted to the Privileges of Banaras Hindu University), Varanasi, U.P.

22. **Dr. Tajen Dabi,** Assistant Professor, Department of History, Rajiv Gandhi University, Itanagar.
23. **Squadron Leader Ms. Toolika Rani (Retd.),** Research Scholar, Department of History, Babasaheb Bhimrao Ambedkar University, Lucknow.
24. **Ms. Jawa Madhur,** Museology Section, Department of AIHC and Archaeology, Faculty of Arts, BHU.
25. **Dr. Vibha Singh,** Assistant Professor, Department of Sociology, Vasanta College for Women (Admitted to the Privileges of Banaras Hindu University), Varanasi, U.P.
26. **Dr. Bhima Shankar M. Birajdar,** Assistant Professor, Department of History, Kisan Veer Mahavidyalaya, Wai, Satara, Maharashtra-412803.
27. **Shri Samir Banerjee,** Renowned Gandhian Scholar and Writer.

Contents

1
References of Pandemic and Epidemic in Ancient Sanskrit Texts

Ashish Kumar

ABSTRACT

Epidemic is defined as sudden widespread of a disease in a large population of a geographical region. The concept similar to epidemic is narrated by various scholars of Āyurveda in different names, i.e. Marakah (Suśhruta), Janpadodhwaṃa, Janapada Nāhaka (Caraka), Janamāra, Janapada Roga (Bhela), Āgantuja Vyādhī (Wāgbhaṭṭa) etc. The descriptions found in the ancient Sanskṛt texts viz. Veda, Purāna, Stotra literature, Āyurvedika texts etc. prove that our savant ancestors were not only acquainted to epidemic diseases but were also conscious about the preventive measures that could be taken to deal with such outbreaks by mitigating its severity and containing its further spread. This chapter is an attempt to understand the various references of such epidemic conditions in ancient times as mentioned in our ancient Sanskṛt texts.

Keywords: *Atharvaveda, Āyurveda, Bhela Samhitā, Caraka Samhitā,* Epidemic, Pandemic, *Purāna,* Sanskṛt text, *Suśrut Samhita, Veda.*

Disease has always been a part of human civilization in various phases of development since evolution. These diseases can be divided into two categories—communicable diseases and non-communicable diseases. Diseases which are caused by specific infectious toxic agents or products directly or indirectly, transmitted by infected person to person, animal to man, animal to animal or from environment to man can be categorized as communicable diseases. Polluted water, air and food are environmental causes for spread of diseases. Infectious disease is caused by micro-organism therefore it has potential to transfer to new individuals. All the communicable diseases are infectious but not all infectious diseases are communicable viz. tetanus is a disease caused by infection, but it can't spread from one person to another. Communicable disease is an infectious disease and has potential to be transmitted from one source to another by bacteria or viral organism. The risk factor for a communicable disease multiplies with lack of safe water, poor hygiene, poor living conditions and unsafe food and it becomes an outbreak after natural disasters *viz.* floods, drought, earthquakes or manmade war, industrial accidents etc. These communicable diseases can be divided into two categories: First, contagious diseases which usually spread through direct contact and the second is infectious disease which spread through physical, chemical and biological factors. These diseases do not require direct contact of infected person, but may spread by their physical discharge, cloths and other personal accessories etc.

Epidemic is sudden widespread of disease in a large population of a geographical region. The word 'Epidemic' has been originated from Greek words *Epi*= upon and *Demos*= people. It means an unusual occurrence of disease or change of health related behavior in a community or a geographical region. When the outbreak affects large proportion of population in a wide geographical area i.e. whole country or continent or whole world is known as pandemic. Along with communicable diseases many non-communicable diseases are also included in epidemic. Climate change, globalisation, urbanisation, uncontrolled incensement of population, malnutrition, poverty, lack of proper sanitisation, lack of good public health system, drugs addiction etc. are some major contributing factors that allow disease to transmit easily.

In traditional Indian contexts, it has been accepted that diseases are imbalance of body elements, generated due to various internal and external factors. All the endogenous diseases (*Nija Vyādhī*) occur due to the vitiation of *Vāta, Pitta* and *Kapha*. *Ācārya Caraka* explains that all the diseases are produced by disturbances in equilibrium in *Dhatu* and cannot occur without vitiation of *Vāta, Pitta* and *Kapha*—वायुः पित्तं कफश्चोक्तः शारीरो दोषसङ्ग्रहः। (Caraka, 1950, 1/57). The concept similar to epidemic is narrated by various scholars of *Āyurveda* with different names, i.e. *Marakah (Suśruta), Janpadodhwaṃsa, Janapada Nāśaka (Caraka), Janamāra, Janapada Roga (Bhela), Āgantuja Vyādhī (Wāgbhaṭṭa)* etc. The *Sanskṛt* synonym of epidemic is *Mahāmārī* which means great (*mahā*) destroyer (*mārī*). In *Śabdakalpadruma* the word *Mahāmārī* has been explained in two different ways "one who killed untamable demons is Mahāmārī"–*महतः दुर्दान्तान् दानवादीन् मारयती इति महामारी अर्थात् दुर्गा* (√मृङ्+णिच्+अण+ङीप्). According to *Mārkaṇya Purāṇa Devi Durgā* has been named as *Mahāmārī* (*Durgā Saptśatī, 12/38-39*) and the other *Mahāmārī* means great destroyer– म्रियन्ते प्राणिनो यस्या इति महती मारी (√मृङ्+घञ+ङीष्). In the tradition of *Sanskṛt* literature it isn't considered very good to describe epidemics. Therefore, written evidences or descriptions of such occurrence are not found. But in the prayers, veneration of epidemic goddesses and deities, we procure description of many diseases and fevers.

Vedic Literature

In the Vedic literature hymns are addressed to gods and goddesses, *viz. Agnī, Indra, Varuṇa, Savitra, Aśvinīkumāra, Rudra* etc. with a view to inducing them to grant the prayers for good health along with wealth, victory, long life and all happiness in this world. *Varuṇa* is mainly regarded as the God of water but many times been called the patron of medicines (*Bhiṣaka*) and prayed to save from fever *(Jvrra). Aśvinīkumāra,* the twin Gods, invoked in more than fifty hymns. They are worshiped as physician of God. They have been prayed to protect people from illness and safeguard health. *Rudra* is another important deity in *Ṛigveda* related to medicines and is the God of destruction. He kills people by thousands of arrows when he became angry. He is greatest physician–'भिषक्तमं त्वा भिषजां शृणोमि' (*Ṛigveda* 2/33/4). *Rudra* possess thousands of medicinal herbs. He is worshipped and offered prayers for his blessings to be merciful, to provide medicine and not to destroy the life and animals–'स्तुतस्त्व भेजषा रास्यस्मे' (*Ṛigveda* 2/33/12). Life saving medicinal herbs has been described as mother in *Veda*–

> औषधीरिति मातरस्तद्वो देवी रूप ब्रवे।
> सतेयमश्वं गाम् वास आत्मानं तव पूरुषे ॥ (*Ṛigveda 10/90/4*)
> या औषधीः सोमराज्ञीर्बह्वीः शतविचक्षणा ॥ (*Yajurveda* 12/92

As kings and warriors assemble to kill demons, medicinal herbs were used to cure diseases (*Yajurveda* 12/8)

> यत्रौषधीः समग्मत राजानः समितताविव।
> व्रिपः स उच्च्येत भिषग्रक्षोहामिवचातनः ॥

The term *Takma* or *Takmāna* is used for fever in *Veda. Takmanāshana Sūkta* of *Atharvaveda* (5/22) describes various kinds of fevers (*Jvra) viz.* malaria etc. These *jvra* took away the souls of men and make their life mournful—अयं हि विश्वान् हरितान् कृणोष्युच्छोचयन्नग्निरिवाभिदुन्वन् (*Atharvaveda*, 5/22/2). We regard *jvra* remove from the body–अधरोञ्चो प्रहिणोमि नमः कृत्वा तक्मने। (*Atharvaveda,* 5/22/4). The significance described here are similar to the concept of epidemics in contemporary era. Hymns of *vedas* also explain the causes of *jvra.* They strongly believed that *Kṛmi* or *Rākṣa.* Are the reasons of *jvra. Yātudhāna,*

Rākṣah, Niśācara etc. are another synonyms of *Rākṣah.* The characteristics of *Kṛmi* are much similar to the micro-organism of modern age *viz.* Bacteria or Viruses etc. *Kṛmi* are too small, they live in darkness and do not like sunlight, eat flesh and blood. They are mentioned as sorcerer for being able to change their characters. It recommends that people should live hygienically, cut hair and nails, wear white clean cloths, eat freshly prepared cooked foods to safeguard themselves from the attack of *Kṛmi. Kṛmighna Sūkta* (*Atharvaveda,* 5/23) of *Atharvaveda* describes the nature and prevention of micro-organism responsible for diseases. (*Atharvaveda,* 5/23/6)

उत् पुरस्तात् सूर्य एति विश्वदृष्टो अदृष्टहा।
दृष्टाञ्च घ्रन्नदृष्टाञ्श्च सर्वाञ्श्रच कृमीन् ॥

Fresh air and sunlight are natural remedies for prevention of outbreak of *kṛmi.* Hymns read as the prayer of sun says the rising sun kills the *kṛmi*—उद्यान्नादित्य कृमिन् हन्ति. Sun is soul of all living beings—सूर्य आत्मा जगतस्तस्थुषश्रच (*Ṛgveda, 2/33/1*), आदित्यो ह वै प्राणः (*Praśnopaniṣada.1/5*). The sunlight may never fall away from us—न सूर्यस्तय संदृशे मा युयोथा (*Ṛgveda, 1/115/1*). These descriptions of *kṛmi* or *rākṣah* show that our ancestors were well acquaintance about the concepts of micro-organism causes for diseases. This way we can say although the description of pandemic is not very clear in *Vedas* but there are undisputed notations of various kinds of diseases, causes of disease, fevers, outbreak of fever and other diseases and their treatment.

Paurāṇika Literature

Later in *Paurāṇika* literature *viz. Agnī Purāna, Garurda purāna, Viṣnu purāna* etc. we find exhaustive description related to the concepts of *Āyurveda. Agnī Purāna* has many chapters *viz. Siddhauṣadhāni, Sarvarogaharāni auṣadhāni, Nānārogaharāni auṣadhāni* etc. that include detail citations of ayurvedic medicines. *Garuda Purāna* also mentions in details various aspects related to ayurveda. A chapter named *Jvara Nidāna* has description of different types of *jvara,* their outbreak and treatment. According to a narration found in *Skaṇda Purāna, jvrra* is described as manifestation of *Rudra's* anger. *Devi Sati* (wife of *Śiva)* sacrificed her life in the sacred fire of his father's oblation because of the insult of *Śiva* by her father *Dakṣa.* This incident infuriated *Śiva* and he threw his tress on the hill, after which appeared redoubtable *Vīrabhadra, Mahākālī* and thousands of other ghosts. That time hundreds of fevers *(jvara)* also appeared from the hot inhalation of infuriated *Śiva*– (*Skaṇda Purāna, Kedār khaṇd 3/33-35*)

उद्धृत्यचजटारुद्रो लोकसंहारकारकः।
आस्फोटयामास रुषा पर्वतस्य शिरोपरि॥
ताडनाच्चसमद्भूतोवीरभद्रामहायशा।
तथा कालीसमुत्पन्नाभूतकोटिभिरावृता॥
कोपान्निः श्वसितेनैवरुद्रस्य च महात्मनः।
ज्ञातं ज्वराणांचशतसन्निपातास्ययोदश॥

Here we find the very first written evidence of epidemic. In the war between *Śivagana* and *devasenā, Indra* and his whole army were affected by the outbreak of various kinds of fevers and other diseases produced by the anger of Lord *Śiva.* That time *Aświnikumar* had taken cure them all (*Skaṇda Purāna, Kedār khaṇd, 3/65-68*)–

गणान्पराङ्मुखान्दृष्ट्वासर्वेतेभ्यो भृशम्।
रुद्रकोपात्समुद्रभूतादेवाश्रचा पिप्रदुद्रुव।
ज्वरैस्तु पीडितान्देवान्दृष्ट्वाविर्ष्णुसन्निवत।
जीवग्राहेण जग्राह देवांस्ताञ्श्रच पृथक् पृथक्॥
ज्वराश्चसन्निपाताश्च अन्येभूतद्रुदहस्तदा।
तान्सर्वान्निगृहीत्वाथ अश्विनौतौमुदन्वितौ॥

Later, in *Śiprā Mahātamya* in *Avantyakhaṇda* of *Skaṇda Purāna* river *Śiprā* has been called *Jvaraghnī*– वैकुण्ठे जायतेशिप्राज्वरघ्नीचसुरालये (*Skaṇda Purāna, Avantyakhaṇd, Shiprā Mahātmya- 9*). This means the one who cure fever. There is a story behind this name. Once the King of demons *Bānāsura,* a great devotee of *Śiva,* fought with *Shrīkṛṣna,* where *Kṛṣna* dismembered his thousand hands. After being defeated in the battle against *Kṛṣna, Bānāsura* took the shelter of *Śiva*. Looking his pathetic condition, *Śiva* became angry and went to the battlefield resulting in direct confrontation with *Kṛṣna*. This terrible battle between *Hari* and *Hara* produced two kinds of fever *Maheẓwara jvara* and *Vishnu jvara*. Whole universe was stricken by these *jvara*. Later both *jvara* went to *Śipra* to take a holy dip relieving the world from the outbreak of both the *jvaras* (*Skaṇda Purāna, Avantyakhaṇd, Shiprā Mahātmya, 40-42*)–

निमग्नश्चैवक्षिप्रायां ततः शान्तिंपरांययो। दृष्ट्वामाहेश्वरं शान्तं ज्वरंपरमकोपनम्।
वैष्णवोपिसमासाद्य तस्यामज्जनमाचरत्। तस्याः प्रभावान्नष्टौ ज्वरौ हरिहरिद्भवौ।
तस्मात्सर्वेष कालेषु ज्वरघ्नी सा भवत्क्षणात्।

Again in *Kāśī khanda* sacred water of *Gangā* is called *Bhiẓaka* for all diseases–सर्वस्व सर्वव्याधीनां भिषकश्रेष्ठयौ नमोस्तुते (*Skaṇda Purāna, Kāśī khaṇd,* 4/159). In *Śitalāṣṭkam* excerpt from *Skaṇda Purāna,* we found a detailed description of epidemic. *Śitalā Devi* is one of the important Goddess in Indian culture. She is regarded for the outbreak of fever (smallpox). In ancient text *Śitalā Devi* is featured as riding a donkey with broom in hand by which she sweeps away diseases. In *Śitalāṣṭkam* she is worshipped to safeguard from any outbreak of epidemics and her worship destroys the immense fear of fever and pox outbreak. Her name is regarded as a medicine for life of man who is suffering from fever. She is the only medicine (*amṛtavarṣiṇī)* that takes away the incurable diseases creeping over the body of men afflicted by pox disease. She is caretaking mother (*dhātrī*). *Śītalā Devi* has been described as mother of the world and only caretaker of the world (*Skanda Purāna, Maheshwar khaṇd/Śhitalāṣṭkam*) -

वन्देहहं शीतलां देवी सर्वेरोगभयापमहाम्।
यामासाद्य निवर्तेत विस्फटोभयं महत्।
शीतले शीतले चेति यो ब्रुयाद्दाहपीडितः।
विस्फोटभयं घोरं क्षिप्रं तस्य प्रणश्यति॥
शीतले तनुजान् रोगान् नृणां हरसि दुस्त्यान्।
विस्फोटविदीर्णानां त्वमेकामृवर्षिणी॥

In *Durgā Saptśatī* of *Mārkandeya Purāna* we find some signs of diseases and epidemics in the prayers of *Devi Durgā*– रोगानशेषानपहन्सि तुष्टा रुष्टा तु कामान् सकलानभिष्टान् (*Mārkaṇdeya Puāna, Durgā Saptśati, 11/29*). In the twelfth chapter *durgā* **has** been named as *Mahāmāri*. She became *Mahāmāri* at the time of devastation (*Mārkaṇdeya Purāna, Durgā Saptśati, 12/38-39*)– महाकाल्या महाकाले महामारीस्वरूपया। सैव काले महामारी सैव सृष्टिर्भवत्यजा॥ All types of epidemic outbreaks were destroyed by the grace of *Devi Durga*– उपसर्गानशेषांस्तु महामारीसमुद्भवान् (*Mārkaṇdeya Puāna, Durgā Saptśati, 12/8*). These are some examples from the *Paurāṇika* literature where we find descriptions of epidemic and pandemic.

Ayurvedic Literature

Āyurveda is an ancient Indian system of medicine with a rich collection of ancient text that deals with all aspects of life, including its adjoining environment. The patriarchs of *Āyurveda* have mentioned epidemics by various names in their creations. The first reference of pandemic has been found in *Suśruta Samhitā*. The period of *Āchārya Suśruta* is accepted about 700 BCE to 1000 BCE. He firstly mention epidemic as *Maraka*– शीतोष्णवर्षाणि खलुविपरीता-न्यौषधीर्व्यापादयन्ति। तासामुपयोगाद्विविधरोग प्रादुर्भावो मरको वा भवेदिति। (Sushrut, (1954) *Sutra sthanam/6/19*). *Suśrut* has mentioned the term *aupasargikā roga* for communicable diseases. The spread of these diseases were from man to man due to lack of proper hygiene cleanliness. *Kuṣṭh jvra, netrābhiṣyanda* (conjunctivitis) etc. are some examples of communicable diseases that can be transmitted through *prasanga* (contact), *gātrasansparśa* (touching), *nihśvāsa* (inhalation), *sahbhojana* (eating together), *sahśaiyā* (sharing bed) *āsana* (seating together), sharing cloths, ornaments etc. These *aupasargikā roga* or communicable diseases have potential to take a form of epidemic if not handled carefully. Here, we can see that above mentioned modes of prevention of epidemic are still relevant in present circumstances of Covid-19. At the same time, *Sushruta* mentioned that certain diseases like cough, fever, headache etc. affect a large number of people in certain area or country through polluted water, vitiated air or contaminated living place as mentioned in *Sushruta Samhita* (Sutra sthanam/6/21)

कदाचिदव्यापन्नेष्वप्यृतुष कृत्याभिशापरक्षक्रोधाधर्मैरुपध्यस्यन्ते जनपदाः। विषौषधिपुष्पगन्धेन वायुनोपनीतेनाक्राम्यते यो देशस्तत्र दोषप्रकृत्यविशेषेण कासश्वसवमथुप्रतिश्यायशिरोरुग्ज्वैरुपतप्यन्ते ग्रहनक्षत्रचरितैर्वा, गृहदारशयना-सनायनवाहन-मणिरत्नोपरकरणगर्हितलक्षण-निमित्तप्रादुर्भावैर्वा।

Another important text *Caraka Samhitā* of *Āyurveda* by *Ācārya Caraka*, gives a comprehensive description similar to the concept of epidemic under a broad heading *Janapadodhvṃsa*. The third chapter of *Vimānasthāna* in *Caraka Samhitā* has been named as *Janapadodhvṃsanīya Vimāna* (*Caraka Samhitā*, 1950). This term has two words—first *janapada* which means city or town and *udhvaṃsa* meaning destruction. So the meaning of *Janapadodhvsā* is disease affecting and causing destruction of a large population or a town. Air, (*vāyu*), water (*jala)*, habitat (*deśa*), season (*kāla*), sinful acts (*adharma*), war, curses (*abhiśāpa*) are major causes responsible for *Janapadodhvṃsa*– इमानेवं दोष- युक्ताञ्श्चतुरो भावान् जनपदोद्ध्वंसकरान् वदन्ति कुशलाः (*Caraka Samhitā. vimāna sthānam* 3/11). All types of pandemic and epidemic of the modern era are included under *Janapadodhvṃsavyādhī*. In this chapter *Ācārya Caraka* has elaborated not only the causes of epidemic but also the measures to control them (*Caraka Samhitā, Vimāna Sthānam* 3/12) विगुणेष्वपि तु खलवेतेषु जनपदाद्ध्वंसनकरेषु भेषजेनोपपाद्यमानानामभयं भवति रोगोभ्य इति।

In the same way later works of *Āyurveda viz. Aṣṭnga Saṃrah*, *Bhela Saṃhitā* and *Yoga Ratnākara* has mentioned epidemic in their own way. According to *Bhel Saṃhitā Janamāra* may occur due to diseases arising as a result of extreme variation in seasons (*Bhela Samhitā, Sutra Sthānam*, 13/8)–

मेघेवर्षतिवर्षासु हेमन्ते यत्र वर्षति।
ऋतुव्यापत्ति समये जनमारः प्रवर्तते॥

Aṣṭnga Saṃrah used the term *Sancārīroga* for communicable disease. The fourteenth chapter under *Nidāna Adhyāya, Ācārya Vāgbhaṭṭ* describes the preventive measures of *Sancāriroga viz* .eye infections, skin diseases, respiratory diseases, tuberculosis, cold etc. that can be spread from touching, eating together, sleeping together (Vagbhatt, 1951, *Nidan Sthanam* 14/44)

स्पर्शैकाहरश्य्यादिसेवनात्प्रायशे गदाः।
सर्वे सञ्चारिणे नेत्रत्वगिव्कारा विशेषतः॥

These are some references from the rich archive of ancient *Sanskṛt* texts. The list is very long. These are the evidences that prove our savant ancestors were not only acquainted to epidemics but also conscious about the prevention of their outbreak. This has been also justified that the role of micro-organism, knowledge of communicable diseases, epidemics and their preventive measures were invented by the scholars of *Āyurveda* in thousands of years ago and not the only contribution of western world.

REFERENCES

1. *Ṛigveda*
2. Agrawal, Deepali Jayesh and Swami, B. D. (2019). An Outline of Communicable and Infectious Diseases in Charak Samhita. *IAMJ*, 7(10), October. Retrieved on 22nd October 2020 from www.iamj.in
3. *Bhela Samhitā, Sutra Sthānam*
4. Caraka. (1950). *Caraka Samhitā* (Artideva Gupta, trans.). Varanasi: Bhargava Pustakalaya.

5. Dubey, Sushil Kumar, *et.al.* (2020). Preventive Measures for Communicable Diseases in *Ayurveda* and Ancient Indian Culture. *Annals of Ayurvedic Medicine*, 9(2) Apr.-Jun.
6. *Durgā Saptśatī.* Gorakhpur : Gita press.
7. *Mārkaṇdeya Purāna. Durgā Saptśati.* Gorakhpur : Gita press.
8. *Praṭnopaniẓada.* Gorakhpur : Gita Press.
9. Shukla, Nishant. Ayurvedic Approach to Communicable Disease: An Overview. Retrieved on 19th October 2020 from https://www.omicsonline.org/scientific-reports/srep122.php
10. *Skanda Purāna. Kedār khaṇd* Gorakhpur: Gita Press.
11. Shastri, Ambikadutta (ed.). (1954*) Sushruta Samhita.* Varanasi : Chaukhambha Sanskrit Series office.
12. Vagbhatt. (1951). *Aṣṭnga saṃrah* (Atrideva Gupta, trans.). Bombay : Nirnaysagar Press.
13. *Yajurveda*

2
Diseases in Ancient India: Spread, Preventions and Remedy in *Ayurveda*: An Analysis

Jitesh Kumar Singh

ABSTRACT

Men are facing many challenges since inception of the human evolution, mainly natural calamities, epidemics and pandemics. Diseases have been vital problems in every society since very beginning of the civilization. The sages and seers in ancient India through their inventions and experiences not only discovered the causes behind it, but also the preventions to stay safe and protected from these threats. Medicine with its theory of diseases has been developed in ancient India through a gradual progress in successive phases by our sages and seers. The ancient indigenous medical system of Ayurveda is a method of healing based on herbs, shrubs and a disciplined lifestyle as a medicine to maintain good health and long life and about 5000 years old and tested. This paper mainly deals with various causes of diseases as mentioned in ancient Sanskrit scriptures and analyse the preventive measures and remedy suggested in this ancient texts in context with the present pandemic times. Various principles of Ayurveda, written and compiled thousands of year back, has proved to be of perennial relevance and still go with the contemporary concepts of present times making it significant in enabling us to face the covid-19 pandemic.

Keywords: Ancient indigenous medical system, *Atharvaveda, Ayurveda,* Causes and prevention of diseases, *Charak Samhita, Susruta Samhita.*

Ayurveda is derived from two Sanskrit words *Ayur* means life and *Veda* means science. The ancient proponents of *Ayurveda* told that the smokes of *Yajnas* kill virus present in the environment. *Rigveda* also speaks about many diseases and how to stay safe from them. In a hymn of this *Veda,* deity is prayed to burn and destroy all kind of diseases in their flames and remove the effects of poisons. Ancient Indian scriptures mentions about *Yajnas* as a way to prevent the spread of contagious diseases. During the performance of *Havan* or *Havi,* an important element of *Yajnas,* mango woods are burned that produces Formic Aldehyde gas that kills the dangerous bacteria and other harmful microbes and purify the air and environment. This is now scientifically proved that *Agnihotra* ritual, frequently performed by Indian *Rishis,* remove the negative energy and kill virus in the environment. To stop the spread of contagious diseases, purification of environment is must and for the same *Agnihotra* and other *Vedic* rituals have been suggested by ancient sages and seers. (*Agnihotrena Pranude Saptnan*) This hymn of *Atharvaveda* says that through the *Agnihotra* enemies like diseases can be thrown away. In a place in *Atharvaveda* it is said that "*Samiddho Agnih Supuna Punati*" which means the flames of *Yajnas* purifies the environment (*Atharvaveda,* 12.2.11).

We can have several descriptions of epidemics and pandemics in ancient Indian scriptures in different phases from Indus Valley Civilization to modern era. Pondering over causes behind the decline of Indus Civilization, the spread of epidemics are counted as a responsible factor by some scholars. In the *Vedic* period extracts and fluid of several vegetations were used as *Rasayan* (chemical) to cure the diseases and as preventives. Later, in *Vedic* texts too, several verses and hymns are composed to be protected from these epidemics and pandemics.

The ancient Indian literature in one or another form suggested adopting *Ayurveda* as a *mantra* to keep these diseases away and live a happy and healthy life of hundred years. The main objectives behind *Ayurvedic* treatment is "*Ayurveda* deals with happy and unhappy life." It talks about what is good and what is inappropriate in context of health and life as well as it measures life expectancy and quality of life. According to this theory of medical science the human body is the network of seven principal tissues—*Rasa, Rakta, Mansa, Meda, Asthi, Majja* and *Shukra*. *Ayurveda* says, "The first pleasure is healthy body". It further believes that most of the diseases are born in our mind. *Atharvaveda* describes about many herbs and shrubs being effectively used to destroy the harmful microbes present in environment and causes diseases in human. In a *Sukta* of same *Veda* we get the descriptions of tiny and poisonous microbes which die in sun light. The main concepts of *Ayurveda* are based on interconnections among the people, the bodily constituents, health and the universe. *Ayurveda* prescribe individualized treatments according to the causes and nature of the diseases which includes herbs, diet, exercise and a recommended lifestyle. According to ancient seers the nature has secret and remedy of all evils which pose a threat to human life and existence and thus advised to follow *Ayurveda*.

Evolution and Development of *Ayurveda* (Indian Medical Science)

According to *Atharvaveda* gods inflicts diseases as punishment for sins of human being. *Rudra, Soma, Varuna, Aditya, Maruta* etc. are gods who have powers to cause diseases. *Jalodara* (*Atharvaveda*) Atharvaveda, I, 25.3, vi, 96.2 (Ascites) is a disease caused by *Varuna* and *Takman* (fever) caused by his son. Lord *Brahma* is the chief profounder of the art of healing and medicine. He handed over this art and other healing virtues to *Surya* (Sun) to relief the mankind from sufferings. Thus, Sun God is regarded as father or source of medical knowledge and energy in ancient India. The twin sons of Sun (*Ashwin Kumars*) became the first to receive the knowledge of medicine from the God father. They worked as surgeons in wars between gods and demons and healed the wounds and injuries of the deities during war. They taught the *Ayurveda* to *Indra,* who delivered this knowledge to his two worthy disciples Dhanvantri and Aitreya. Dhanvantri is regarded as divine father of ancient Indian and Hindu medicine. According to *Atharvaveda, Rudra* is the best physician and possess healing remedies. He is the first physician who can cause the diseases as well as cure them. Thus, the foundation of medical science was laid down in India. Further, this knowledge was developed and enriched by Charaka and Susruta. During the epic age and even thereafter, the progress of *Ayurveda* continued with additional masterpiece of expertise in this field. According to descriptions available, there were renowned physicians employed in the royal courts with the duties assigned to take care of the health of king and members of the royal family and officials in court. *Jivaka* was another prominent medical expert of ancient India associated to the court of Magadha King Bimbisaara. The medical achievements of Indians were highly recognized and appreciated by Arabs as the works of Charaka, Susruta and other Sanskrit literary texts were translated under the patronage of Caliphs.

The *Atharvaveda* is famous for the medical tradition of ancient India. Types of diseases, their prevention and treatment are one of the prime subject and concern of *Atharvaveda*. The medical science in ancient India is known as *Ayurveda*. Besides *Atharvaveda,* many other Vedic literatures such as *Brahamanas, Upanishads* and *Sutras,* directly or indirectly, describes about ancient Indian medical traditions. The Indians in ancient times were very well aware about the medicinal virtues and values of mineral, metal chemicals (acid, base, ashes, salts) along with herbs and shrubs and thus they developed magical expertise in the field of medicines (Pathak, 2012, 400). Our ancient sages and seers through their research found that one who consumes minimum five leaves of bitter taste *Neem* in the month of *Chaitra,* will be protected from several kinds of bacteria and other diseases. The each and every part of this plant such as roots, leaves, flowers, barks, seeds are having immunity and medicinal virtues that can be used against almost all diseases in one or other way and that why it is said *Sarv Roghari Nimbah* (means *Neem* tree is the remedy which can remove all diseases). *Ayurveda,* as the science of life has been most ancient discovery of medical theory of human civilization. The importance and relevance of *Ayurveda* can be understood by the fact that the basic principles mentioned here, are still recognized by the modern medical science. In *Charaka Samhita, Ayurveda* is described as perpetual that shows the everlasting nature and existence of its remedies. *Acharya* Charaka had delved deeply into the research study about anatomy, diabetes, tuberculosis and cardiac diseases etc. He gives remedies and details about all these diseases in his book *Charaka Samhita*. According to *Ayurveda,* lord *Rudra* invented these drugs for the welfare of mankind. Though the *Ayurveda* did not develop any specific branch of epidemiology, but its principles described unsystematically can be compiled to interpret modern theories of epidemiology. Even the current scenario of Covid-19 as a pandemic the various principles of *Ayurveda* have been proved significant. *Ayurveda* speaks about lifestyle free from all kind of pain and diseases.

Ayurveda as the science of life is most ancient and significant medical doctrine of human evolution and a precious gift to mankind from ancient Indian seers and scientists. It's a boon of nature to mankind to keep healthy and enjoy the pleasure of life. *Ayurveda,* not only describes the remedy of diseases and epidemics, but also talks about the causes and origin of these so that one can understand the sources of threats and keep themselves away from them and protected. The sages and seers in ancient India were well aware about the concept of keeping the patient of contaminated diseases isolated from others in family which is in modern medical science called "quarantine" (Samal, 2013). In the hymns of *Atharvaveda* sages and seers have directly prayed to the medicines that they may bring back the isolated patients and enable them to contact people again while being recovered and healthy. They understood well the role of will power and spirituality in recovery from diseases and thus they opine that prayer and hymns always increases the will power and soul power that helps in growing immunity against diseases. In a *Sukta* of *Atharvaveda* it has been described that Goddess Earth, remain the power of hearing, God Sun, the strength of vision and God *Agni,* the brightness and shinning. They all keep us safe. The principal concept of *Ayurveda* is *Tridosa* or the three humeral theories of *Vata* (wind), *Pita* (bile) and *Kapha* (phlegm). The entire concept of physical, physiological process along with pathological causes of all diseases are discussed in terms of these three *Dosas.* Any imbalance or disproportion in these main and elementary standards of the body causes disease (Lad, 2002, 25-29). The *Ayurveda* gives detail description of kind of micro-organism such as bacteria, virus, fungi and other microbes which causes diseases in human and other creatures. The presence of these micro-organisms is mandatory, but not sufficient to cause the diseases as several physical and chemical factors too are required to spread the diseases. These organisms and factors are called agents of diseases (School of Public Health). The interrelation of agents, host and environmental factors in a very complex ways cause diseases in human being (U.S. Deptt. of Health and Human Services, 2006). Daksha, Ashwin Kumars, Atreya, Dhanvantari, *Acharya* Susrut, Charaka, *Rishi* Chyavana, Patanjali etc. are the proponents of *Ayurveda,* noteworthy for their contribution in field of diseases and their cure from *Ayurveda.*

Method of Diagnosis, Preventions and Treatment

Ayurveda is primarily and a foremost preventive medicine that deals with patient in a holistic way focusing the environment (*Desha*), the body (*Prasanna*), the senses (*Indriya*), the mind (*Manah*) and the soul (*Atma*). These are gradually representing the five soul ingredients of body—earth, air, water, fire and ether. According to *sanatan* system, the human body is composed of five elements—wind, fire, water, earth and ether and each of them are having their respective and specific qualities of dryness, sharpness, fluidity, heaviness and lightness. The proper balance and harmonious action of these elements and their qualities constitute good health and immunity. The classical *Ayurvedic* texts throws light on various components of occurring diseases. Charaka has mentioned above three components behind the diseases in human. He said that agents and environmental factors jointly as *Niyata hetu* and *Aniyata hetu* affect the man and its community causing diseases. *Susruta* too has same opinion that micro-organism causes diseases in human. Agents in interaction with microbes caused diseases (Susruta, 24.7). *Ayurveda* gives different phases of disease formation in its specific ways called *Kriyakala* (Acharya, 1992). It is also known as *Shatkriyakala* (A concept of *Ayurveda*). *Shatkriyakala* is significant from public health diagnosis approach and moreover to keep a control over diseases. This principle and process enable to prevent the disease at each and every stage through the appropriate measures. It can be termed as similar to the concept of disease cycle of natural history of disease in modern medical science. There are several intervention measures suggested in *Ayurveda* at different stages of disease such as *Dincharya* (daily health promotional activities), *Ritucharya* (seasonal health promotional activities), *Ahara* (healthy diets), *Vyayama* (exercise) etc. as the aim to maintain good health and keep diseases away while increasing the immunity level. The physicians in ancient India had a detailed procedure of diagnosis of the diseases. They examine the patient through eyes, tongue, skin, voice and urine etc. To clinically diagnose the disease *Nadi Pariksha* (examination of pulse), *Darshana* (inspection), *Sparshana* (palpation) and *Prashna* (interrogation) etc. while *Shaman* (alleviation) and *Shodhna* (purification) has been described at several occasion in *Ayurveda*. *Panchkarma Chikitsa* (five modalities of treatment) was one of the very prominent methods of treatment under this system.

Causes and Diseases

We get the descriptions of several diseases in ancient Indian texts mainly in *Vedic* and *Sanskrit* literature. *Janapadodhwans* is described in *Ayurveda* which can be compared with many variants of epidemics. It occurs due to vitiation of *Vayu*, *Jala*, *Desha* and *Kala*. These variants can be compared well with different aspects of environmental pollution (Acharya, 2000). Even today the environmental pollution is one of the main and most dominating factors causing several diseases. In the *Susruta Samhita*, there are three categories of diseases—*Adhyatmika*, *Adhibhautika*, *Adhidaibika* and these are further classified into subcategories (Susruta, 24.7). Susruta has described different modes of contaminated diseases in his classical composition of *Susruta Samhita*. These are—*Gatrasansparsat* (physical contact), *Nihsavasat* (expired air), *Saha Bhojanat* (eating with other mainly one who is suffering from a kind of disease), *Sahasayyasanaccapi* (sharing a bed), *Vastmalynulepanat* (using clothes, garland etc.) to spread the infectious diseases from one person to another and it is noteworthy that these are relevant and accepted even today in terms of communicable diseases. Mention of some communicable diseases through these modes have been given here such as—*Sosha* (Pulmonary Tuberculosis), *Netrabhisyanda* (Conjunctivitis), *Jvra* (Pyrexia), *Kushtha* (skin disease) etc. (*Susruta*, 5.33.34). These aforesaid descriptions of communicable diseases remain relevant in later phases and even today, accepted by medical science. In the Vedas we get several herbs and shrubs that can be used to cure many diseases such as a *Sukta* of *Atharvaveda* mention a medicine *Varuna* used in curing Tuberculosis, insomnia etc (*Atharvaveda*, 10.3). At another place in the same text, description is given to cure the *Kushtha* (leprosy) (*Atharvaveda*, 5.4). *Kushtha* is considered one of the highly contagious diseases. *Susruta* said the disease can be transmitted from the sick to a healthy man by touch or breathe of patient or using any article of patient anyhow. In *Atharvaveda*, there is mention of a herb which cures the pale and white patches of *Kushtha* and completely disappeared (*Atharvaveda*, 22.23). Tuberculosis is described in Indian Sanskrit texts as *Sosha*. The Moon God was the first victim of *Sosha* disease, hence it is also known as *Rajyakshma* or king's disease. Vichitravirya, the ancestor of Kauravas and Pandavas of *Mahabharata*, supposed to be killed by tuberculosis. Another contaminated disease of the ancient period was plague. As per *Susruta*, it causes fever, burning like fire feeling and kills the patient within 15 days. It is called *Agairohini* and an incurable disease. We also find description of different types of human viruses in *Rigveda* and other ancient Indian Sanskrit texts. References of Smallpox are also found in *Rigveda* (Sharma, 1991, 769). Even today, smallpox is attributed to the displeasure of goddess *Shitlamata* by most communities in India substantiate the conjecture. *Ayurveda* speaks about the treatments of smallpox through the paste of barks of herbs and other spices. According to *Charaka*, to keep ourselves healthy and disease free what one has to do is only *Dharma* (*Charak*, 8.23). *Ayurveda* did not develop any specific branch of epidemiology, but its principles can be compiled to interpret modern theories of epidemiology

Conclusion

A very unique and high quality of medical expertise was prevalent in India since very early period of civilization. The evidences discovered from excavations of various sites to *Harappans* shows their high sense of sanitation and hygiene. The analysis of *Vedas* speaks about references regarding different aspects of health, diseases and medicines. *Atharvaveda* is even regarded as encyclopedia of ancient Indian medicines as *Ayurveda* is termed as *Upa Veda* (supplementary subject) of this *Veda*. The history of ancient Indian medical science can be traced back to the period of early Antiquities. The ancient Indian medical system is as old as their civilization and helped others to lay the foundation of their medical system and principles. The hymns of *Rigveda* mention the herbs and shrubs with medicinal virtues along with hygienic properties of water, air and vegetables. The juice of *Soma* is praised as *Amrita* in many hymns and *Suktas* and was being used as medicine for sick ones. *Ayurveda* tells us to coordinate with our lifestyle and natural changes that affect health issues. Healthy diet, balanced routine along with natural environment one can keep himself fit and healthy. The *Ayurvedic* strategies described in *Shatkriyakala* to prevent the diseases, stand important and relevant even today. The analysis of *Ayurveda* and concept of modern medical science if taken together, can be very significant in fighting against many diseases and even epidemics. Even the modern medical science has boldly advocated the several aspects of *Ayurveda* as the only and complete remedy of many diseases. Due to the changed circumstances and increased level of pollution day by day its very correct time to adopt the golden *mantra* and healthy lifestyle as mentioned in *Ayurveda* as it builds up a strong immunity system and increases the resistance power against all types of virus and bacteria. Research in the field of *Ayurveda* in recent few decades through different platform has given much recognition and higher expectations to this system. Due to tradition acceptance, usefulness, easy accessibility, socio-economic advantages etc. *Ayurvedic* medicines have become more popular and globally accepted. *Ayurvedic* medicines have become so acceptable that nowadays these are available in forms of tablets and capsules too along with its natural forms. We are required to look back to the past and our *Vedic* and traditional medical system to face the medical challenges and health issues faced by world today. The modern and extensive researches have proven the quality, safety, stability and efficiency of *Ayurvedic* medicines as well as the importance of this system.

REFERENCES

1. Acharya, Y.T. (Ed.). (2000). *Charak Samhita*, VI. 3.6. Varanasi: Chaukhambha Surbharati.
2. Acharya, Y.T. (Ed.). (1992). *Susruta Samhita of Susruta with Dalhana Tika.* 21.36.37. Varanasi: Chaukhambha Orientalia.
3. *Atharvaveda.*
4. *Charaka Samhita.*
5. Lad, V.S. (2002). *Fundamental Principle of Ayurveda*, Albuquerque, New Mexico: The *Ayurvedic* Press.
6. Pathak, M. (2012) *Vaidika Gyanvigyan Kosha*. New Delhi: Rajpal and Sons. (Rajpal Publishing).
7. Samal, J. (2013). The Concept of Public Health in Ayurveda. *International Ayurvedic Medical Journal*, 1(2), March-April, 1-5.
8. School of Public Health. *Introduction to Epidemiology*. Chicago: University of Illinois Retrieved from https//www.uic.edu/sph/pepare/courses/ph 490/resources/epilesson01.pdf
9. Sharma, G. S. (1991). *Rigveda.* New Delhi: Sanskrit Sahitya Prakashan.
10. Susruta. (1941). *Susruta Samhita*. Mumbai: Niryansagar Publication.
11. U.S Department of Health and Human Services. (2006). Principles of Epidemiology in Public Health Practice, 3 edn. Centre for Disease Control and Prevention (CDC): Atlanta Georgia.

3

The Sense of Health Awareness in Ancient India: Integrated Approach of Mind, Body and Environment

Mukesh Kumar Singh

ABSTRACT

Health is the key component of the life journey of a human being. Every culture and nation has specific ideas about their health and sanitation. Cultural health heritage comprises several things like the medical system, mental health ideology, sanitation practices, environmental awareness, and food choices. India has a great cultural heritage with several dimensions. Holistic health ideology is an important aspect of ancient Indian cultural heritage. Ayurveda is an important line of medical therapy discovered by ancient Indians. Body purification and environmental cleanliness are key aspects of ancient Indian society. A healthy body and a clean environment have a crucial role in human health at the level of the individual as well as society. Several types of superstitions and miracle related ideas were also prevailed in health ideology in ancient India. Divine intervention was necessary for some types of cures to illness. State and intellectuals have expressed their view on health and sanitation from time to time in ancient India. The ancient Indians identified humans as an integral part of nature and stressed the importance of maintaining complete harmony with all the living and non-living components of earth. Mind-body relation was also an important point of contemplation for ancient Indians concerning the healthy development of the human being. In this article, I will try to identify the key health awareness legacies of ancient India.

Keywords : Ancient India, *Ayurveda,* Cultural heritage, Health system, Holistic health, Mind-body relation, Sanitation

Health plays an important role in the growth of an individual as well as of society. The well-being of society is scaled by the health system of a particular society. Since ancient times in most of the cultures health is probably understood as the "absence of disease". Although, it is generally accepted that the concept of a universal health system has been developed in the last century in India, its basic roots are in the early Indian civilization. The approach of the ancient Indian health system was a holistic nature, which cares about all aspects of human health and disease. Some key aspects of healthcare are medical system, mental health status, sanitation practices, environmental concerns, and food habits.

Evidence for the medicinal ideas and practices of ancient India can be derived from accounts of the contemporary Greek visitors to India, Buddhist texts, and Chanakya's *Arthashastra* and archaeological sources. For *Ayurvedic* theory, the *Charaka-Samhita* and *Sushruta-Samhita* are the key ancient sources. The people of India from the very beginning of their civilization were conscious and concerned about their health. The excavations at Harappan sites bear ample examples of the proficiency reached by the people of the Indus valley civilization in matters of health and sanitation. It appears that Harappan cities were built after careful planning. Houses were provided with modern amenities like baths, lavatories, drains, fresh-water tanks, courtyards, and bedrooms. The main drains could be cleared by lifting a specially made cover of bricks. The whole concept of town-planning shows remarkable concern for sanitation and public life that was, perhaps, without parallel in those days (Allchin *et.al.*, 1982; Zysk, 1998).

The Vedic literature provides some glimpses of health-related traditions in contemporary times. During the *vedic* times, a separate medicinal branch of medical science *Ayurveda* evolved and practiced. The *Rigveda* contains many hymns related to the desire for a long life. According to *Rigveda,* a good physician concentrates on herbs (*Rig-Veda,* X.97.6). Many *Rigvedic* divinities were healers of good health. *Rudra, Varuna, Asvin* brothers were the main healers of Rigvedic times. The *Asvin* brothers were capable of rejuvenating the old, ensuring the safe delivery of children, and providing the injured with an artificial limb, if there was a loss of limb. The roots of *Ayurveda* lay in the *Atharvaveda* in its observation on the medicinal value of plants and other matters. However, *Ayurveda* emerged as a fully developed rational theory of health and disease, purposefully shifting away from magico-religious to empirical thinking. *Atharvaveda* has ample references to health and diseases. Prayer for long life and health, immunity from all diseases, securing perfect health, fever, worms in children, etc. are various issues, which are incorporated in *Atharvaveda*. The concept of food contamination is also discussed in the *Atharvaveda* (Winternitz, 1985).

The ideas of *Ayurveda* and surgical knowledge that was propagated by Charaka and Susruta shows evidences of our ancient tradition in the scientific healthcare of people (Sharma, 1983; Singhal, 2018). The *Charaka Samhita* sought to teach the physician the foundational ideas of logic so that diagnosis and treatment could be based on valid observations and reasoning. *Ayurvedic* medicinal therapy based on *tridosa* theory of *Vayu, Pitta,* and *Kapha,* and all physical, physiological processes, as well as the pathological causation of disease, are explained in terms of the three *dosas*. Equilibrium of the three *dosas* manifested as health whereas the disequilibrium of these three resulted in disease. The ancient Indian *Ayurvedic* texts describe various kinds of diseases and diagnostic practises. Some of their diagnostic practices are very relevant in the time of pandemic also. *Kriyakala,* also known as *Shatkriyakala,* is a unique concept of *Ayurveda.* It describes various stages of the disease with a very careful method. This concept is comparable to the natural history of disease studied by modern medicine. *Kriyakala* provides a scope to stop the disease early or at the stage when the disease identified. The stage of *Sancaya* and *Prakopa* is comparable with the stage of susceptibility. If we care and study appropriately, we can stop the progression of the disease at that level (Samal, 2016). Sanitation and hygiene practices are also a key component in the *Ayurvedic* way of health management. It is clear that the ultimate goal of *Ayurveda* is to ensure complete and comprehensive health of human beings and it can be an effective and safe way in managing even infectious diseases.

We find various examples of healers and medicine practices through text and archaeology in ancient India. Jivaka was a renowned medical practitioner at the time of Buddha. His study was completed in Taxila. He treated many renowned people of his time like Buddha, Bimbisara, and King of Pradyot of Ujjayini. He was an expert in medicine and surgery. The medicine prepared by him belongs to roots, leaves, fruits, gums of tree; various types of oils, and some types of clays (Majumdar, 1968).The Mauryan ruler Ashoka also made arrangements for the health of his people. From the second rock edict, we get information about the medical arrangement for human beings and animals. Ashoka further claims to have planted trees that could have included herbs and plants endowed with medicinal properties (Sircar, 1965).

We also find hospitals for specific diseases in ancient India. The excavations conducted at Nagarjunakonda led to the discovery of a hospital attached to a monastic complex in the early centuries of the Common Era. An inscription found in this place refers to a principal Buddhist monastery *(viharamukhya)* within which was situated a healing house (*vigatajvaralaya*). The term *vigatajvaralaya* can be explained as a building or structure (*Alaya)* meant for the termination (*vigata*) of fever (*jvara)* (Chakravarti and Ray, 2011). In *Ayurveda* fever has been given the highest importance. Another example of a hospital in ancient India found in Kumrahar (Patna, ancient Pataliputra) excavations. A seal found from this place dateable between 3rd and 4th century A.D., speaks of the congregation and monastery of Buddhist monks (*bhikshu-samghasya*) and a hospital (Chakravarti and Ray, 2011).

Fa-Hien, a Chinese traveller who visited India during the times of Chandragupta II of the Gupta dynasty, provides us details about the charitable dispensaries in Pataliputra. According to Fa-Hien, the heads of the *Vaisyas* families established city houses for dispensing charity and medicines. All the poor and destitute in the country, orphans, widowers, and childless men, maimed people and cripples, and all who are diseased go to houses. They are provided with every kind of help and doctors examine their diseases. After inspecting their diseases the physicians treated them and when cured, they departed at their convenience (Legge, 1886).

Hiuen-Tsang, another Chinese traveller contemporary of Emperor Harsha, also provides a description of the health and sanitation practices of that time. According to him, they were very careful about their personal cleanliness. They wash before eating and they never use that has been leftover. After eating they clean their teeth and wash their hands and mouth (Watters, 2018). He also describes some healthy practices about their health. Everyone who falls sick fasts for seven days. Many sick persons recovered in this period, but if the sickness continued then they took medicines (Watters, 2018). An Inscription located in Saidapur (District—Nalgonda, Telangana) refers to the eulogy of the royal physician

Aggalayya. The inscription expresses light of the helpful nature of Jain physician Aggalayya. He is always helpful to good people. He practiced his profession very efficiently and also cured very difficult cases (Jawaharlal, 1994).

A healthy body and a healthy mind are both vital for the proper development of the human being. Ancient Indians have keenly explored proper mind-body balanced functioning for a healthy life. The *yoga* system has made great contributions towards mental health and physical health in ancient India. The *yoga* system in India was systematized by Patanjali. The primary objective of *yoga* psychology is to prepare the process of thinking in its ethical aspect of progress towards self-illumination, which is identical to salvation. It is the highest goal of *yoga* philosophy, but the journey of this path is not an easy task. The first and foremost requirement of this journey is a concentrated mind, which is also a difficult goal. The obstacles to concentration are classified under different heads. A healthy body is the first requirement for a concentrated mind. If any type of sickness persist in the body, the mind is unable to concentrate on anything. Idleness is also a distraction for concentration. A person may fail for a lack of drive just as he may fail for a lack of energy. Extra engagement in worldly affairs also creates a lot of hurdles in concentration. A human must control his feelings as well as his thoughts and actions. The desire to enjoy the life is the main enemy of concentration of the mind. The *yoga* system provides a clear roadmap for a healthy mind. The first thing necessary for concentration is the cleanliness of the body. Body fitness is the second important thing for a healthy mind. In this regard, different types of *asanas* are prescribed in the *yoga* system, but merely bodily control is not enough to ensure concentration and transformation of the mind. Controlling the sense organs is also an important task to achieve a healthy mental status. The *yoga* system derived the methods to become master of their sensory desires (Bhattacharya, 1975).

Buddhism and Jainism have also made significant contribution to the mental health of Ancient Indians. Buddhism finds that the purity of mind and continuous moral practices are the paths of a healthy mind. It rejects the claims of those who believe that religious purity and liberty can be achieved through ritual practices. The study of mental concentration is at the centre of the Buddhist system of knowledge. To understand the nature and function of mind are the main goal of all sects of Buddhism. Buddhism meditation techniques are based on disconnection from the sense-objects, which engaged it in pleasure-seeking activities. According to Buddhism, only self-effort can transform and purify the mind. This is made possible by the practice of mindfulness (Prasad, 2007).

Jainism is also very careful about mental health of human being. Jainism believes that the soul has infinite perception, infinite knowledge, infinite vigour, and is non-attached in his original form, but the soul in its worldly form is unable to realize these features, because it is covered with the wrong notion of actions or *karmas*. The *karmas* are mainly motivated by four passions; anger, ego, deceit, and ego. *Tirthankars* have described many ways to liberate ourselves from these four passions and attain salvation. One of the ways is the practice of six essential rites. By practicing these six essential rites with true feelings, one will be able to free him/her-self of passions that will ultimately help in spiritual progress. These six essential rites to be practiced daily, are as follow: the practice of equanimity (meditation); reciting verses in praise of the twenty-four *Tirthankars*; reverence for the mendicant teachers; atonement; abandonment of the body and renunciation (of certain foods, indulgences or activities, for a specified period) (Stevenson, 1915). Therefore, it is clear that mental health is also a very important aspect of health and ancient Indians especially recognized this in several ways.

There were some irrational ideas that prevailed in the

health-related matter in ancient times in India. Some people believed that super-human and malefic elements being the cause of diseases. Ailments classed under this category are recognized as *adhidaivika*. *Bhutavidya* was a specific category of ailments which were believed in supernatural origin. Mental illness like insanity, epilepsy, etc. was believed by the influence of demons and other evil powers, but these ideas were not very popular in the general medical stream and this line of thinking was ignored by later medical practitioners (Bose *et.al.*, 1971).

Environmental factors play a key role in human health. Occasionally environment alone exerts sufficient to impact health. Many type of diseases triggered by environmental causes in humans. In these circumstances, ancient Indians have extended a lot of honour to natural bodies. The Vedic hymn to the earth, the *Prithvi Sukta* in *Atharvaveda* is the most beautiful song in honour of mother earth. The Vedic seer declares a lot of caring and nourishing quality of mother earth in the hymn: '*Mata Bhumih Putroham Prithivyah*: Earth is my mother; I am her son.' Mother earth is revered for all her natural gifts and especially for her herbs and vegetation. Her blessings are sought for prosperity in all endeavours and fulfilment of all righteous aspirations (Vatsyayan, 2012). Many verses in the *Rigveda* and *Atharvaveda* have been devoted to the praise of Lord *Surya* (sun), *Vayu Devta* (Lord of the winds), *Agni Devta* (God of fire), *Varuna Devta* (God of water), *Prithvi Mata* (Mother Earth), *Vanya Devi* (Goddess of forests), etc. Therefore, cutting of trees, polluting air, water, and land were regarded as sins. Charaka and Sushruta, the two ancient masters of medicine also emphasized that the geographical environment, climate, water, and quality of air have a great impact on human health. Charaka refers that the air which is not in accordance with the season, excessively moist, harsh, speedy, cold, hot, rough or blocking, terribly sounding, excessively comedies with each other, whistling, unsuitable smell, or contaminated with particles from poisonous flowers (pollens), gravels, dust or smoke, etc. are unwholesome and not conducive to good health and are responsible for diseases and epidemics. The ancient masters have recognized the importance of pure water in the maintenance of good health. Water has been recognized not only as making a positive contribution to human's health and well-being in assisting him to create a clean and healthy environment but also as a potential hazard when acting as a vehicle for waterborne and water-related diseases. We find that many types of diseases spread through poor quality of water were included in the great ancient *ayurvedic* works like *Charaka Samhita*, and *Susruta Samhita*.

Food habits have also great impact on human health. Right food choices ensure good health and long life in human being. Every country and every region has its specific food traditions. India has very rich food tradition heritage which comprises lots of regional diversities. Every regional food heritage is influenced by lots of values and beliefs. Religion is also influenced by food choices of human being. Ancient Indians are too much concerned about the purity of food. Upanishadic literature emphasised that good memory and mind concentration depends upon the purity of foods (Prakash, 2005). The sages of ancient India believed that the mental setup of a child revolve around the type of food which a mother took during the pregnancy (Sen, 2014).

We have lots of evidences about the food choices of Harappan inhabitants. Wheat and barley were main crops of that time. People also grew peas, chickpeas, sesame, mustard, linseed, and lentils. They also ate fruits such as melons, dates, coconuts, pomegranates, and bananas. Some popular non-vegetarian foods were fish and domestic foul. Vedic people were also very careful about their food choices. Barley was the primary staple of early Vedic people. Later, they use wheat, lentils, millet, sugarcane, and rice etc. (Prakash, 1961).

Ancient Indian chief health system, *Ayurveda*, has great understanding about the material and biological qualities of foods. Proper food is essential base of healthy life. Charaka provides detail list of incompatible foods for humans. The *Ayurvedic* literatures describe twenty basic properties of physical materials, which are also found in foods and drugs. Heavy, light, dry, oily, dense, liquid, hot, cold, sharp, soft etc. are chief properties of foods. According to *Ayurvedic* concept our body has a great quality of self-healing. Proper food habits are decisive in the self-healing process. A physician should always respect the self-healing mechanism of the human body. *Ayurveda* has also emphasised the proper processing of foods. Charaka and Susruta describe various principles of processing of foods. Natural qualities, combination, quality, habitat and climate, temporal quality etc. are main components of processing of food. Fasting was also an important aspect of food management in ancient India. Ancient Indian literature contains ample references to fasting as a source of mind-body purity. Fasting provides energy for rejuvenation of body. Fasting facilitate cleaning and detoxification to body. Fasting can be done with various ways. Short fasting may be administrated by water or lime water, but fast for long time should be done with combination of water, fruit juice and vegetable juice (Rastogi, 2014).

From above mentioned discussion, we can say that ancient Indians have holistic thinking about health practices. They have thought about the health and well-being of the whole body, rather than focusing on illness or specific parts of the body. It takes into account how an individual interacts with its environment and emphasizes the connection between mind, body, and natural environment. The holistic approach further encourages people to accept responsibility for their health and integrate with the social setup. They developed a medicine system, which were based on overall improvement of human health. They were also aware about the key aspects of mental health. Food choices, sanitation and environmental awareness were also key areas, where they tried to make balance between natural environment and human health. The subsequent development of Indian life was enriched by several legacies of the ancient Indian health system. Therefore, we can say that the legacy of health awareness is unique cultural heritage of ancient India.

REFERENCES

1. Allchin, B. G., Allchin, B., & Allchin, R. (1982). *The Rise of Civilization in India and Pakistan*. Cambridge University Press.
2. Bhattacharya, H. (1975). *The Cultural Heritage of India: Vol III: The Philosophies*. Calcutta: The Ramakrishna Mission Institute of Culture.
3. Bose, D. M., Sen, S. N., & Subbarayappa, B. V. (1971). *A Concise History of Science in India*. New Delhi: The Indian National Science Academy.
4. Chakravarti, R. & Ray, K. (2011). *Healing and Healers Inscribed: Epigraphic Bearing on Healing-Houses in Early India*. Kolkata: Institute of Development Studies.
5. Jawaharlal, G. Saidapur Jain Inscription of Jagadekamalla I Saka 956. In *Epigraphia Andhrica* vol. VI, edited by N. R. V. Prasad, Hyderabad: The Government of Andhra Pradesh,1994, pp. 37-42
6. Legge, J. (1886). *A Record of Buddhistic Kingdoms: Being An Account by the Chinese Monk Fa-hien of his travels in India and Ceylon (AD 399-414) in search of the Buddhist Books of Discipline*. Clarendon Press.
7. Majumdar, R. C. (1968). *The Age of Imperial Unity* (Vol. 2). Bombay: Bharatiya Vidya Bhavan.
8. Prakash, O. (1961). *Food and Drinks in Ancient India*. New Delhi: Munshiram Manoharlal Publishers.
9. Prakash, O. (2005). *Cultural History of India*. New Age International.
10. Prasad, H. S. (2007). *The Centrality of Ethics in Buddhism*. Motilal Banarsidas Publishers.
11. Rastogi, S. (2014). *Ayurvedic Science of Food and Nutrition*. Springer.
12. Samal, J. (2016). Fundamental Tenets of Epidemiology in Ayurveda and their Contemporary Relevance. *Indian Journal of Health Sciences and Biomedical Research (KLEU)*, *9*(1), 20.
13. Sharma P.V. (ed). (1983). *Caraka (700 BC) Caraka Samhita*. Varanasi: Chaukhambha Orientalia.
14. Sen, C. T. (2014). *Feasts and Fasts: A History of Food in India*. Reaktion Books.
15. Singhal, GD, *et. al.* (eds.). (2018). *Susuruta (600BC) Susuruta Samhita*.

Varanasi: Chaukhambha Surabharti.

16. Sircar, D. (1965). *Select Inscriptions Bearing on Indian History and Civilization* (Vol. 1). Calcutta: University of Calcutta.
17. Stevenson, M.S. (1915). *The Heart of Jainism*. New Delhi: Munshiram Manoharlal.
18. Watters, T. (2018). *On Yuan Chwang's Travels in India (AD 629-645)*. New Delhi: Munshiram Manoharlal Publishers (1973).
19. Vatsyayan, Kapila, (Ed.) (2012), "Bhumi ko Devatav Pradan", in *Vasudev Sharan Agrawal Rachna Sanchayan*, New Delhi: Sahitya Akadami.
20. Winternitz, M. (1985). *History of Indian Literature*. New Delhi: Motilal Banarsidass Publishers.
21. Zysk, K. G. (1998). *Asceticism and Healing in Ancient India: Medicine in the Buddhist Monastery* (Vol. 2). New Delhi: Motilal Banarsidass Publisher.

4
History of Pandemic and its Consequences

Shivani Mishra, Anurag Upadhyay and Deepti Mishra

ABSTRACT

Pandemics are a serious threat and it has affected millions of people, causing widespread serious illness in a large population and thousands of deaths. The nature of a disease becomes more terrible when it turns into an epidemic or pandemics. To cope with such a crisis in such a situation, it is imperative that the person starts changing his behavior and this change tries to enable the person to deal with such an emergency situation on the one hand, on the other hand it also puts a psychological burden. The depleting psychological crisis in developed countries is a legal proof of this fact. If we look at the related events of the past, the historical scenario in the past enables us to develop some new ideas towards such problems, by which we are able to handle the immediate situation. Even in the context of the present pandemic (Covid-19), this is not wrong. Thus, the purpose of this present research paper is to understand the nature and symptoms of all the major pandemics that took place in human history and their origin places as well as their morbidity and mortality rate over a wide geographic area is also highlighted. It has been found that pandemics have a vast impact on our social aspects (such as decreased quality of life, school closure, restriction in transport and tourism, limited social interaction), cultural aspects (such as literature, art and customs are shaped by pandemics), health (such as negative impact on psychological and physical health) and economic aspects (such as decreased GDP rate, job loss, low income, changes in work environment). Moreover, the final aim of this article is also to discuss significant economic, social, cultural, health and political disruption caused by pandemics.

Keywords: Cultural, Health, Psychological, Social and Economic Aspects, Pandemic.

The world has changed a lot in the last few epochs. Thousands of people lost their lives. Millions of people are sick. A new pandemic has wrecked havoc on all of them and those who survived this outbreak have also changed completely. A number of significant pandemics have been recorded in human history, including smallpox, cholera, plague, dengue, AIDS, influenza, severe acute respiratory syndrome (SARS), west nile disease and tuberculosis. These pandemics are unpredictable that can have severe consequences on societies over worldwide area. After the outbreak of this pandemic, everything in the world has been reversed. Now, the first question that strikes the mind—what is Pandemic?

What is Pandemic?

When a new disease spread in all over the world then it is called pandemic. The word "Pandemic" originates from the Greek word *pan* and *demos* and its meaning is "all" and "the people or population". It can be said that almost all of the people or population is affected by a pandemic. Pandemic is different from epidemic as it spread across a wider geographical range and it is generally used to refer to a worldwide epidemic of a contagious disease. A very well-known and internationally accepted definition of pandemic given in the *Dictionary of Epidemiology* (Last, *et al.*, 2001) is significant to quote here when an epidemic affecting worldwide, or over a large area, crossing international boundaries and taking a large number of people in its grip, is called pandemic. An epidemic converts into a pandemic only when it spread beyond a country's borders and is not limited only to a single continent. There are some key features of a pandemic, including wide geographic extension, disease movement, novelty, severity, high attack rates and explosiveness, minimal population immunity, infectiousness and contagiousness, which help us to understand the concept better. When an epidemic spreads beyond a country's borders that's when the disease officially becomes a pandemic.

History of Pandemic

In the past, world has witnessed outbreaks of many significant diseases that became pandemic, for example Spanish Flu, Hong Kong Flu, SARS, H7N9, Ebola, Zika (Rewar, *et al.*, 2015; Maurice, 2016). These pandemics and their nature will be discussed below in detail.

In history, earliest pandemic occurred during Peloponnesian War (430 B.C) in Athens (Cartwright, 1972). This disease included symptoms of fever, thirst, bloody throat and tongue, red skin and lesions. It spread through Libya, Ethiopia and Egypt and crossed the Athenian walls as well. In 165 A.D., Antonine Plague occurred among Huns and then infected Germans and Romans empire (Cartwright, 1972). This disease was considered possibly an early appearance of smallpox that included symptoms of fever, sore throat, diarrhea and pus-filled sores. Duration of Antonine Plague in the history was from 165 A.D. to 180 A.D.

In 250 A.D., a new pandemic came into light and its name was Cyprian Plague. Its first victim was the Christian Bishop of Carthage and its major symptoms were fever and gangrenous hands and feet, diarrhea, vomiting, throat ulcers.

Ethiopia was the origin point of this pandemic from where it gradually covered Northern Africa, into Rome, then onto Egypt and northward area also. The most disaster thing about this disease was that it appeared again and again over the next three centuries. In 541 A.D., Justinian Plague came into light with its origin in Egypt and then it affected the area of Palestine and the Byzantine empire and then the Mediterranean. In 1520 A.D., smallpox infection took Aztec empire into grip. Many people were killed from this disease and incapacitated others. The years 1665 and 1666, London witnessed many deaths during Great Plague pandemic (Cartwright, 1972). As the death rate increased, many cats and dogs were slaughtered as the susceptible cause for this disease and the disease spread through ports along the Thames.

After that, over the next 150 years, seven cholera pandemics appeared in history. First cholera pandemic appeared in Russia in 1817. It is a small intestine infection that spread through feces-infected water and food. In India millions people died because of this disease. Besides, British empire and its navy, cholera spread across Spain, Africa, Indonesia, China, Japan, Italy, Germany and America and led to death of 150,000. In 1855, Bubonic plague appeared in China with its further spread in India and Hong Kong. This disease was spread by fleas in Yunnan initially (Cartwright, 1972). It sparked revolt against British as this disease was used as an excuse for repressive policies of British government. This disease is also considered as a major factor in the Parthay rebellion and Taiping rebellion. In 1875 pandemic of Fiji measles came into light (Cartwright, 1972). During measles outbreak, Royal party of British empire visited Australia and brought the disease to their island. In 1889, Russian flu pandemic started in Siberia and Kazakhstan travelled to Moscow, further it spread to Finland and then Poland (Cartwright, 1972). In the subsequent year, it spread to the rest of Europe and crossed the ocean into North America and Africa. There were 360,000 deaths by the end of 1890 because of this pandemic. It was considered as one of the first significant flu pandemic.

In 1918, an avianborne flu appeared in Europe, Spanish flu, led to deaths of 50 million people. It effected United States and parts of Asia and then around the world. Situations became worsen because of lack of effective drugs and vaccines to treat the Spanish flu. The avian-borne flu that resulted in 50 million deaths worldwide, the 1918 flu was first observed in Europe, the United States and parts of Asia before it swiftly spread around the world. At that time, there were no effective drugs or vaccines to treat this killer flu strain. Wire service reports of a flu outbreak in Madrid in the spring of 1918 led to the pandemic being called the "Spanish flu". This influenza pandemic of 1918-1919 is cited as the most devastating epidemic in recorded world history. During this pandemic, there was crisis of body storage scarcity as many Americans died. After some time, flu threat disappeared in the summer of 1919. Reason for its disappearance was that many infected people either boosted their immunity level or died. Influenza pandemic is considered to be the most devastating epidemic, recorded in human history as it killed more than 20 million people.

In 1957, Asian flu that occurred in Hong Kong and spread to China, United States and England caused deaths of 14,000 people (Cartwright, 1972). In early 1958, second wave of the flu started, resulting in estimated deaths of about 1.1 million. Later an effective vaccine was developed to control this pandemic. In 1981, human immune deficiency virus/ acquired immune deficiency syndrome (HIV/AIDS) disease came into light in American gay communities. It is believed that in the 1920s this disease developed from a chimpanzee virus from West Africa. HIV destroys human body's immune system to fight with pathogens. Consequently, victim becomes weak and easily infected by disease. People with HIV disease suffer from fever, headache, and enlarged lymph nodes. This disease, attack on t-cells also. In 2003, a new disease severe acute respiratory syndrome (SARS) appeared. This disease possibly started from bats and spread in cats and then to humans in China. It spread to 26 other countries, led to 774 deaths. Lessons from the pandemic were used to control other diseases such as H1N1, Ebola and Zika. So, health professionals saw SARS disease as a wake-up call to improve the outbreak responses.

And now in this present time, world is facing negative impact of covid-19 pandemic on very large scale that emerged in Wuhan, China in December 2019, a new severe respiratory illness and it spread all over the world. Novel corona virus, now called SARSCoV-2 is responsible for the disease Covid-19. It is a matter of grave concern as COVID-19 has extraordinary contagious properties and it leads to high rates of both morbidity and mortality (Lipsitch, *et al.*, 2020). Till May 2020, it entered almost all countries worldwide. Deadly severity of this pandemic can be imagined by the confirmed cases of 43,94,660 in the world (MoHFW, WHO 13 May 2020). This virus can be transferred from one person to another. This virus transmitted through respiratory tract secretions and touch or contact (surface or person to person) (Lai, *et al.*, 2020). The World Health Organization had declared COVID-19 as a pandemic on March 11, 2020.

Impact and Consequences of Pandemic

There are several impacts of pandemic including influence on cultural, social, political, economic as well as psychological aspects of life.

Cultural Consequences of Pandemic

Epidemic and pandemic affect and change the society in which it occurs and due to pandemic outbreak work of artists and intellectuals have been changed. Politics is also shaped by disease. Disease outbreaks has entrenched racial and social discrimination. There are several incidences that show that pandemic influenced our cultural and political aspect of life. It shapes history and revolutions. It has been observed that sometimes significant changes take place in history due to pandemic. Pandemic has also determined the outcomes of wars and sometimes, it plays a major role in starting a war. In 1832, when cholera disease spread in Paris, 19,000 Parisians died (Snowden, 2019). Then rumors of conspiracy theory spread that the unpopular government under King Louis Philippe was poisoning wells with arsenic to spread the disease that resulted in violence. Another example of shaping history can be observed in Napoleon Bonaparte's nineteenth-century imperial expansion westwards across Atlantic Ocean during yellow fever pandemic. Yellow fever also entered his army in France's Caribbean colony of Saint-Domingue (now Haiti) (Snowden, 2019). Dysentery and typhus were obstruction in materializing his eastern ambitions. Major contribution of yellow fever pandemic in the success of the Haitian rebellion and Toussaint Louverture cannot be ignored (Snowden, 2019). In the same way during World War I, Spanish influenza pandemic occurred that led to an estimated deaths between 50 million and 100 million people. Pandemic as Bubonic plague caused death of half of the population of the whole continent, it had a significant effect on the onset of industrial revolution, on slavery and serfdom. Social and political stability has also been affected by the pandemic.

Impact of pandemic can be observed in literature, philosophy of life and art also. During pandemic, positive aspects of humanity also can be seen. For example, in literature, Italian novelist Alessandro Manzoni's great plague novel *The Betrothed*, first published in 1827, shows how an archbishop of Milan was willing to lay down his life to look after the poorest and most unwell people. There are some major changes in previous rigid belief system such as when people saw deaths, sufferings and plight of human being because of pandemic, they start to raise question on existence of God (Snowden, 2019). When plague outbreak emerged, people's relationship with God as well supreme authority of God was questioned. Even many people started to doubt about the omniscient divinity and all–knowing God. Pandemic attacked on our health system as well as previous rigid belief system and philosophy. Artist's response to plague can be seen in their creations whose main themes were temporary and provisional nature of life. In the artistic genre allegory, the *danse macabre* where everyone was swept away shows theme of suddenness of death. It is allegory of the Late Middle Ages. Several art, painting and literature were inspired by this philosophy.

Pandemic widens inequality, and high mortality can lead to loss of human resources that in turn can promote some ill practices. Tradition of slavery system was promoted during late middle ages. Consequences of pandemic can be seen in the Harriet Beecher Stowe's novel *Uncle Tom's Cabin* in 1852. It shows bitter truth of slavery system and romanticizing tuberculosis disease and cholera epidemic. During tuberculosis epidemic, artists, poets glorified this disease as disease of beauty and elite. During this period, Toulouse-Lautrec painting, an anorexic-looking woman with her face covered with to give her a pale look like tuberculosis people can be seen. It can be said that pandemic influenced previous belief system and shaped our history, tradition and literature and philosophy.

Pandemic Impact on Physical and Psychological Health

Pandemic has also an impact on physical and psychological health. Pandemic and contagious disease caused high morbidity and mortality rate in the world. In developing countries situation become more worsen as the pandemic and contagious disease have the potential to claim many lives. According to World Health Organization, high fatality rate with estimated range between 250,000-500,000 deaths each year was caused by influenza and it can be transmitted from one person to another very rapidly and easily. In the history of Latin America, 2015-2016 dengue epidemic was the worst experience. In May 2015, the first case came into light and very soon up to December 2015 it reached more than 1.5 million cases. Gradually, it took more than 34 countries in its grip up to March 2016.

Adverse impact on mental health has been observed during pandemic and this adverse impact still remains for the longer times even when it was over. In recent researches, it has been found that during COVID-19 pandemic, there are increased symptoms of depression, anxiety, and stress related to pandemic because of psychosocial stressor such as fear of illness and fear of negative economic effects (Li, *et al.*, 2020, Mukhtar, 2020). Another research showed that after one year of Ebola response, participants have symptoms of PTSD and anxiety-depression (Jalloh, *et al.*, 2015).

Pandemic Economic Impact

Pandemics also have an effect on the economy, it depresses economy system, and takes years to recover the loss. For example influenza pandemic was a serious threat not only to the population of the world but also to the economy. It is resulted in instability of the economy. The Global Health Risk Framework for the Future (GHRF) Commission reported that every year infectious disease outbreaks direct cost the world about USD 60 billion (Maurice, 2016). Annual GDP of China was decreased by 1% in 2003 due to SARS pandemic and GDP of Southeast Asia also decreased by 0.5%. Lee and McKibbin (2004) reported that due to SARS outbreak in 2003, approximate income loss ranges from USD 12.3—28.4 billion for East and Southeast Asia.

Pandemic Social Impact

Social impacts can also be seen due to the pandemic. During the pandemic it is observed that travel was strictly limited and schools were closed, markets and sporting were closed, any kind of large gatherings were prohibited. Chen, *et, al.* (2011) suggested that timely school closure and prohibition of public gatherings was significantly correlated with the decreased mortality related to the 1918 influenza epidemic in United States. Quality of work life, life qualities of communities and families were disrupted by Ebola pandemic in 2013 and 2015. It has been reported that essential fundamental services such as education, transport and tourism were adversely affected by Ebola pandemic in West Africa and beyond in other countries (Nabarro & Wannous, 2016). In 2009, negative impact of H1N1 can be seen not only in mortality, but also in the area of transport, education, and in financial sector. A pandemic event threatens all aspects of the economic and social fabric (Drake, *et al.*, 2012).

Pandemic in Present Context

If we observes pandemic in present context then it is notable that now world is facing COVID-19 pandemic, this pandemic spread globally and influenced major part of our social, economic, psychological, physical aspect of our life. Some guidelines related to health measures such as 'social distancing', 'self-isolating' or 'in quarantine' and 'work from home' may contribute to negative emotions such as anxiety and fear. These guidelines are inspired by previous pandemic such as Spanish flu. WHO has issued guidelines not only to control COVID-19 but also express concerns for mental health during pandemic (WHO, 2020). Governments of almost all countries have imposed lockdown quickly and issued guidelines to control the situation. Promotion of work from home strategy can be very demanding for some person.

Current pandemic COVID-19 disrupts many aspects of life, for example, in some countries tourism is significant source of their income. Because of COVID-19, potential loss of 850 million to 1.1 billion international tourists and potential loss of $910 billion to $1.2 trillion in export revenues from tourism have been reported (UNWTO, 7 May 2020). During this pandemic, estimated 100 and 120 million jobs are reported at risk. Escalation of job losses can lead to almost half of global workforce at risk of losing livelihoods. It has been reported that 60 per cent of the income was lost by 1.6 billion informal workers, now they have very little or no saving (ILO, April 2020). Large number of people are facing food insecurity and crises. It has been reported that about 265 million people in low and middle-income countries are at risk of acute food insecurity by the end of 2020 (FSIN, 2020). Global trade values fell 3 per cent in the first quarter of 2020 (UNCTAD, 2020). So, during this pandemic people face many problems such as low income and job loss, remittances flow reduction, decline in global trade, fallen commodity prices, increase in food insecurity, and dramatic fall in tourism.

In human history, many pandemics have been recorded. On the basis of above discussion, it can be concluded that pandemics influence major part of human's life for a longer time. It takes many years to recover the loss and reach the end stage of the outbreak. Sound understanding of previous pandemics enables us to develop effective policies to control and manage the negative impact of present and future pandemic. The implication of this research paper is that it would be helpful to develop the good strategy to handle the adverse impact of pandemic. Negative consequences of the contemporary pandemic can be controlled by analyzing the social, economic, health consequences of previous pandemic situation and adverse impact of a pandemic can be controlled by an effective and efficient emergency response.

REFERENCES

1. Cartwright, F. F. (1972). *Disease and history*. New York: Crowell.
2. Chen, W.C., *et.al.* H.S. (2011). Social and Economic Impact of School Closure resulting from Pandemic influenza A/H1N1. *Journal of Infection, 62*(3), 200-203.
3. Drake, T. L., Chalabi, Z., & Coker, R. (2012). Cost-effectiveness analysis of Pandemic Influenza Preparedness: What's missing? *Bull World Health Organ*, 90(12), 940-941. doi: 10.2471/BLT.12.109025.
4. Food Security Information Network (2020). Global Report on Food Crises 2020. https://www.fsinplatform.org/global-report-food-crises-2020.
5. International Labour Organization. (2020). As job losses escalate, nearly half of global workforce at risk of losing livelihoods. https://www.ilo.org/global/about-the-ilo/newsroom/news/WCMS_743036/lang—en/index.htm
6. Jalloh, M. et al., (2018). Impact of Ebola experiences and risk perceptions on mental health in Sierra Leone, July 2015. *BMJ Global Health*, 3(2), e000471. doi: 10.1136/bmigh-2017-000471.
7. Lai, C. C., Shih, T. P., & Ko, W. C. (2020). Severe Acute Respiratory Syndrome Coronavirus 2 (SARS-Cov-2) And Corona Virus Disease-2019 (COVID-19): The Epidemic And The Challenges. *International Journal of Antimicrobial Agents*, 55(3), 69-74.
8. Last, J. M. (2001). *A Dictionary of Epidemiology*. Oxford: Oxford University Press.
9. Lee, J. & McKibbin, W., (2004). Globalization and Disease: The Case of SARS. *Asian Economic Papers*, 3(1), 113-131. doi: 10.1162/1535351041747932.
10. Li, J. *et al.* (2020). Anxiety and Depression among General Population in China at the peak of the COVID-19 Epidemic. *World Psychiatry*, 19(2), 249-250. doi: 10.1002/wps.20758.
11. Lipsitch, M., Swerdlow, D. L., & Finelli, L. (2020). Defining the Epidemiology of Covid- 19 Studies Needed. *New England Journal of Medicine*, 382, 1194-1196.
12. Maurice, J. (2016). Cost of Protection against Pandemics is Small. *The Lancet*, 387 (10016), 12.
13. Mukhtar, S. (2020). Psychological Health during the Corona Virus Disease 2019 Pandemic Outbreak." *International Journal of Social Psychiatry*, 66(5), 512-516. doi: 10.1177 /00 20764020925835
14. Nabarro, D., & Wannous, C. (2016). The Links between Public and Ecosystem Health in Light of the Recent Ebola Outbreaks and Pandemic Emergence. *Eco Health*, 1(3). doi: 10.1007/s10393-016-1123-y
15. Rewar, S., Mirdha, D., & Rewar, P. (2015). Treatment and Prevention of

Pandemic H1N1 Influenza. *Annals of Global Health*, 81(5), 645-653. doi:http://dx.doi.org/10 .1016/j.aogh.2015.08.014

16. Snowden, F. (2019). *Epidemics and Society: From the Black Death to the Present*. New Haven, London: Yale University Press.
17. United Nations Conference on Trade and Development. (2020). COVID-19 triggers Marked Decline in Global Trade, new data shows. Retrieved from https:// unctad.org/en/pages/newsdetails. aspx? Original Version ID=2369.
18. United Nations World Tourism Organization. (2020). International Tourist Numbers Could Fall 60-80% in 2020, UNWTO Report. Retrieved from https://www.unwto.org/news/covid-19- international tourist -numbers-could-fall-60-80-in-2020
19. World Health Organization. (2020). Mental health and Psychosocial Considerations during the COVID-19 Outbreak. WHO reference number: WHO/2019-nCoV/Mental Health/2020.1.https://www.who.int/docs/default-source/coronaviruse/mental-health considerations.pdf

5
A History of Major Epidemics and Peoples' Responses

Amita Esther David

ABSTRACT

We are living and experiencing an extraordinary period in human history. The Covid-19 pandemic has taken the entire world by storm and surprise. The entire world is going through a new phase of life called 'lockdown' courtesy novel corona virus. While there are several accounts of pandemics in the past, living through one, offers us many first-hand experiences. This chapter attempts to trace the history of past major pandemics and epidemics. It also attempts to analyse the similarities our century has to offer and differences that have been experienced over various pandemics; the religious and superstitious connections attached to and emanating from this experience over centuries, if any; the ways and means used to try to contain the spread of the disease, over centuries by royalty and common people alike. This chapter also attempts to draw a conclusion on what lessons mankind has learnt from the past, if at all.

Keywords: Beliefs, Contagion, Infection, Pandemic, Peoples' Response, Pestilence, Plague, Precautions, Quarantine.

> *"So all a man could win in the conflict between plague and life was knowledge and memories."*
>
> **Albert Camus, *The Plague***

It is interesting to note that everytime mankind is faced with a calamity of enormous proportions we delve into the past to find answers. One cannot help but be reminded of E. H. Carr's (1961, 29) definition of history *"being an unending dialogue between the present and the past and the chief function of historians is to master and understand the past as a key to the understanding of the present."* The Corona virus or Covid-19 offers us a chance to actually live through a new and unique experience in human history. It gives us an opportunity to delve through the annals of history to figure out how we have dealt with pandemics in the past in an attempt to make sense of the present watch-word of the century - *'lockdown'*. There have been three great world pandemics of plagues recorded in history, in 541, in 1347 and in 1894 CE, causing innumerable deaths of humans and animals across the globe.

Definition of a Pandemic

It is imperative to understand the origin and meaning of the word pandemic before we meander into the by-lanes of history trying to trace and analyse the patterns of different pandemic occurrences and how mankind persevered to deal with each new form of the disease. The term 'Pandemic' originates from two Greek words *pan* meaning 'all' and *demos* meaning 'people'. A pandemic is defined as *"an epidemic occurring worldwide, or even a very widespread area, crossing international boundaries and usually affecting a large number of people"* (Last, 2001). Thus, pandemics may be said to occur annually in each of the temperate southern and northern hemispheres given that seasonal epidemics cross international boundaries and affect a large number of people. But seasonal epidemics will be different from pandemics.

Origin of Pandemics through the Ages

Ever since man's hunter-gathering days, there is evidence of deadly epidemics but the change from a nomadic existence to an agrarian lifestyle and the formation of communities contributed significantly to the possible spread of deadly diseases. Before the invention of soaps, people scrubbed sand to clean their skin and washed it off with water. With the advent of agriculture, farmers began to grow enough food to sustain life in towns and cities. It brought them in contact with each other, close enough to transmit infection. New cities attracted a steady stream of immigrants from the countryside, bringing a new supply of possible victims' every-time. Animals were domesticated and precious livestock was kept near or within the homes, which led to many animal diseases mutating to infect humans for example, tuberculosis and probably smallpox came from cows, influenza from pigs and ducks, common cold from horses, measles from cows or dogs, whooping cough from pigs or dogs etc. Infection also passed from animals to humans through bug-bites that lived on livestock or in stored food (Love & Drake, 2013, 17-18).

Some of the deadly epidemics that surfaced early in human history include malaria, tuberculosis, influenza, smallpox, and leprosy, followed by cholera, plague, dengue, Auto–Immune Deficiency Syndrome (AIDS), Severe Acute Respiratory Syndrome (SARS) and the West Nile disease. Of all of these, the deadliest are the plague and influenza. The origin of epidemics has mostly been in the East Asia. The first epidemic originated in Egypt and travelled to Constantinople (541 CE), spreading to the Middle East and Mediterranean Europe until 767 CE. The Black Death was the most devastating plague epidemic that swept across the Europe and the Middle East (1347–1352) and then repeatedly struck from three hundred to five hundred years (1347–1842) is regarded as the second pandemic. The third pandemic originated in Hong Kong and

Canton in 1894 and spread via steamships to India, Africa, South and North America and continued at least until an outbreak in 1994, in Surat, India (Rosenwald, 2020).

Factors affecting the spread of Contagion

Climate is also known to affect the spread of contagion. For instance, the plague prevalence among the great *gerbils* in Kazakhstan is known to be strongly positively affected by the warm springs and wet summers. In Europe, the climate and the order of the seasons seem to be inverted (Hecker, 1844). The maritime import of plague plays an important part in the reintroduction of plague in Europe as seen in the continent during the second wave, i.e. Black Death. Ships were isolated before isolating their cargo, giving rise to concept of quarantine.

Justinian's Plague 541–542 CE

The plague (*Yersinia Pestis)* arrived in Constantinople in 542 CE, almost a year after skirting the outer provinces of the Byzantine Empire. It continued to sweep across the Mediterranean region for 225 years before disappearing in 750 CE. It is said to have originated in China and carried to Africa via land and sea routes, through black rats (Ratlus ratlus) which travelled on grain ships and carts, sent to Constantinople as tribute to Emperor Justinian. Procopius records that unusual climate changes occurring in southern Italy with fall of snow and frost in mid-summer, resulted in spoilt harvests, leading to food shortages, people afflicted with cold and they migrate in search of food. These migrants unknowingly became carriers of plague infected rats. He talks of a "sudden fever" that would take a person by surprise, followed by a "bubonic swelling" either "inside the armpit" or "in some cases also beside the ears, and at different points on the thighs". People either went into a "deep coma" or suffered from "violent delirium". The victims had difficulty in eating food as they could not swallow. Many died due to hunger or lack of care or committed suicide by throwing themselves from a height. Even the physicians were perplexed with the symptoms and "decided to investigate the bodies of the dead. And upon opening some of the swellings, they found a strange sort of carbuncle that had grown inside them (Procopius, 2005, 11-17). Depending upon their immunity, people could suffer for days or die almost immediately from the pestilence.

It was the duty of the emperor to make provisions. He *"detailed the soldiers from the palace and distributed money"* and made Theodorus in-charge of the task. After the tombs were filled with corpses, trenches were dug and once those were filled, people *"mounted the towers of the fortifications of Sycae"*, tore off the roofs and threw bodies into the towers until they were filled and then covered them with roofs again. Bodies were dumped into the sea. All customary rites of burial were overlooked. Even animals perished in the plague. The city dwellers suffered most due to starvation (Procopius, 2005, 11-17).

> *"And work of every description ceased, and all the trades were abandoned by the artisans and all other work as well ..."*

Leprosy

Leprosy finds mention in the Bible, but it is not Hansen's disease or leprosy as we know today. The term leprosy has been referred in the Hebrew language as *'Tzaraat'* (*zara'at*) which may refer to a skin infliction or disease, for example,. psoriasis, seborrheic dermatitis, atopic dermatitis, scabies, scarlet fever etc. *Tzara'at* comes from a word meaning 'to smite'. In Jewish tradition a leper is smitten by God. Leprosy and biblical leprosy became entwined due to two inaccurate translations: the first was in the 6th century when the Hebrew word *Tzaraat* was defined as leprosy and then in the 9th century when it was translated as 'lepra' in Arabic (Grzybowski and Malgorzata, 2016). Leprosy was curable and there are many stories regarding the same in the *Old* and *New Testament*. Some of the famous people who were cured of their skin inflictions included Moses, Naaman and Simon. The disease was seen as a punishment from God for disobeying His Word.

Biblical references to the skin disease are found in the Book of Leviticus in the *Old Testament*, which gives a very detailed description. It is the story of priestly class of Levites who performed certain religious duties for the Israelites and were teachers of Torah and judges. Chapter 13 and 14 mentions a leprous disease that must be shown to the priest, who examines the person, his garment and even the home, very patiently. The book explains the entire quarantine process under the watchful eyes of the priest.

> *"As for the leper who has the infection, his clothes shall be torn, and the hair of his head shall be uncovered, and he shall cover his moustache and cry, 'Unclean! Unclean! He shall remain unclean all the days during which he has the infection; he is unclean. He shall live alone; his dwelling shall be outside the camp"* (Leviticus 13:45-46 KJV)
>
> *"And the priest shall examine the disease, and shut up that which has the disease for seven days; then he shall examine the disease on the seventh day." (Leviticus 13 : 50-51a RSV).*
>
> *"If the disease has spread in the garment, in warp or woof, or in the skin, whatever be the use of the skin, the disease is a malignant leprosy; it is unclean. And he shall burn the garment, whether diseased in warp or woof, woollen or linen, or anything of skin, for it is a malignant leprosy; it shall be burned in* the fire." (Leviticus 13 : 51b-52 RSV)

In case the disease had not spread in the garment, whether linen or woollen, then it had to be washed and 'shut up' for seven days after which the priest would re-examine it. The priest also examines a person who might be suffering from leprosy, as well as, the dwelling place. If the priest found the house infected then all the belongings were removed and the walls of the house had to be scrapped clean and the dust thrown outside the village. Then the house walls had to be re-plastered.

Leprosy since Medieval Times

The earliest known case of leprosy was found 4000 years ago in a skeleton, in India. Historians believe that a virulent strain was carried back to the Middle East with Alexander's army in 324 BC from where it slowly spread to Europe with the movement of the Roman armies and the Crusades. Leprosy has been around since the 10th century in Europe. The earliest known endowed hospital St. Peter's and St. Leonard's hospital York was founded in 936 AD by the King Athelstan. In 1101, Matilda, Queen of Henry I founded a leper hospital of St. Giles in the fields. It was later known as Matilda's Hospital. Another endowed leper house was a hospital of St. James, in the Fields beyond Westminster. Older leper hospitals (about 5-6) were on the outskirts of London. Ireland and Scotland too, had leper houses. England's charitable foundations before the dissolution of the monasteries numbered 509 in the index of Bishop Tanner's *Notitia Monastica* (Creighton, 1891, 87).

In India, it was rampant during the 19th and 20th century. William Carey was the first missionary to set up the first modern Protestant Mission – Serampore Mission—near Calcutta on January 10, 1800 (Mangalwadi, 1999) and was the first to fight against the inhumane treatment of lepers. He was supported in this cause by Raja Ram Mohan Roy, who spearheaded the campaign. He provided medicines for them and established a hospital (Haldar, 2015). Earlier lepers were often buried or burned alive because of the belief that a violent death purified the body on its way to reincarnation into a new healthy existence (Allen, 2011). There were many medical missions sent to India. In 1835, General Sir H. Ramsay founded a Leper hospital in Almora, which was transferred to the London Missionary Society in 1851 and later supported by the Mission to Lepers (later the Leprosy Mission). Wellesley Bailey, an Irish missionary attracted public attention through his pamphlet 'Lepers in India' and soon a society 'Leprosy Mission in India' was founded at Ambala in 1874 (Kakar, 1996). By 1878, it became a proper Missionary Society with Lady Dufferin, Vicereine of India, as its patroness and Archbishop of Dublin as its president. Asylums were set up in different parts of the country with both sexes being kept separately except in case of married couples and separate homes were established for untainted children of these couples (David, 2006, 90-91).

By 1898, the Leper Act was passed. Nearly 60 per cent of the world's leprosy patients live in India (The Hindu, 2016). However, according to WHO report released in September 2019, 208,619 new cases, including more than 16,000 children—from 127 countries worldwide were registered in 2018. Leprosy is primarily affecting those living in poverty and, according to the report, India, Indonesia, and Brazil account for 79.6 per cent of new cases globally (The Lancet, 2019).

The Black Death 1348

The Black Death first appeared in China in 1333. It was identified by inflammatory boils on the arms and thighs, tumours in the glands, chest infections and breathing problems. Black spots appeared on the skin giving it the name Black Death in Germany and the northern kingdoms and in Italy it was called *la Mortalega Grande* or The Great Mortality (Hecker, 1844). 'The issue of blood from the nose was a manifest sign of inevitable death'. The symptoms began 'in both, men and women alike' by the emergence of certain tumours in the armpits and groin and their size varied from an egg to an apple. The common people called it *'gavaccioli'*. It passed from the infected to the healthy by mere touch of cloth or any item or object touched by the infected person. A single symptom could be fatal for one, while another with multiple symptoms could get cured. No drink could quench the thirst of victims and their tongue would turn black. It affected the poor chiefly in the first wave but was prevalent among the affluent classes in 1360 AD.

The Black Death entered England via a port of Dorsetshire in early August 1348, and spread through Dorset, Devon and Somerset almost killing everyone. It spread to Gloucester, Oxford and then to London by All Saint's Day - 1st November, according to chroniclers. The severity of the plague caused Parliament to be prorogued on 1st January, 1349, and then again on 10th March 1349, before spreading its tentacles to Wales and Scotland between 1349–1350. The description of the disease is the same as Boccaccio's. It affected the common man, the clergy and the cleric class the most. Everyone was fearful of coming close to the sick and dead bodies were shunned. In a single day 20, 40, 60 or more corpses were buried in the same trench. According to Avesbury's account, more than 200 a day were buried. London's mortality is estimated higher than 20,000 or 30,000. The population reduced greatly and the prices of cattle fell. When the harvest of 1349 had to be gathered, the price of labour rose enormously. The threshing rates were unparalleled as scarcity of working hands led to doubling of wages of labour (Gough, 1977, 241).

Florentine writer, poet and Petrarch's student Giovanni Boccaccio (1313–1375) gives an eye-witness account of the infestations and fatality in Florence. The disease spread from men to animals via touch. He saw two hogs, who sniffed and touched the rags of a dead man being removed from the way. The two hogs then turn round and round, "as if they had taken poison" and then fell on those very same rags (Boccaccio, 1348). He was inspired to write his literary masterpiece *The Decameron*. The story revolves around a group of ten – three men and seven women – who fled to a country villa from Florence, where the Black Death was raging, and, proceeded to entertain themselves by telling a story a day for ten days.

The Practice of Quarantine

The practice of quarantine began in the 14th century, in Ragusa, present day Dubrovnik in 1377 with thirty days quarantine. Among the well-known figures to undergo lockdown, either self-imposed or compulsory were Pope Clement VI (1291–1352), who self-isolated himself in a room at Avignon. He had two enormous fires burning day and night to keep the Black Death at bay. He got medical men and astrologers to study the plague and decreed that all those who died of the plague were granted remission of sins. He consecrated the RhÙne river so that bodies could be dumped in it, and condemned all those who blamed the Jews for the pestilence, saying that it was killing both Jews and Christians alike (Dinkins). He supervised care for the sick and burial of the dead in the town, while nearly between a quarter and a third of his own staff and cardinals succumbed to the plague.

In Florence, there were officials appointed to supervise the cleaning of the city; all people with any kind of illness were denied entry into the city. Merchants practised renunciation of goods and bestowed their wealthy belongings to churches and monasteries. The monks shut their gates but they cast them over the convent walls. Some people affirmed that there was no better medicine for the disease than flight. This prescription was followed by a multitude of men and women, who chose to care only for themselves. Thus, cities wore a deserted look. People left their homes, their estates, their belongings and even their relatives and entered into a self-imposed quarantine or migrated to other parts of the country.

People's Response to the Black Death

During the Middle Ages, the cause of the plague was unknown and was attributed to supernatural forces and, primarily, the will or wrath of God. The people banked on religious belief, folklore and superstition, and medical knowledge, all of which were informed by Catholic Church in the West and Islam in the Near East. The perceived failure of God to answer these prayers contributed to the decline of the Church's power and the eventual split leading to the formation of Protestant Church. In the East, Islam remained intact, more or less, owing to its insistence on the plague as a gift which bestowed martyrdom on the victims and transported them instantly to paradise as well as the view of the disease as simply another trial to endure such as famine or flood (Mark, 2020). Jews were soft targets of persecution by the rest of the people during the 14th century plague, as the seeds of enmity go back to the Biblical times of Queen Esther. It was their religious customs that caused misunderstandings among the people. There was a notion that Jews were responsible for plague originated in southern France and Spain (Dinkins). Although the Spanish Inquisition did not begin with the Black Death, the plague may have increased the Inquisition's fury by spreading fear and prejudice against non-Christians throughout Europe (Doherty).

Boccaccio observes that people avoided each other; neighbours were scarcely seen asking about each others' welfare and 'never met'. He continues to write that the plague instilled such "terror in the hearts of men and women that brothers abandoned brothers, uncles their nephews, sisters their brothers and in many cases wives deserted their husbands". Even worse was the fact that *"fathers and mothers refused to visit or tend to their very children, as they had not been theirs"* (Hecker, 1844). If bodies were accompanied by people to church, they were usually the 'pick man', who performed the task for a price. The 'pick man' would carry the body, *"not to that church which the dead man had chosen before his death"*, but most often to the nearest church or burial site available and *"thrust him into whichever grave they found unoccupied"* without a proper formal service. As consecrated ground was not sufficient for the vast multitude of corpses, they dug trenches to lay the corpses, *"pilling them as merchandise.......tier upon tier"* until the trench could hold no more and covered it with earth (Boccaccio, 1348).

The famous Moroccan traveller Ibn Batuta was in China during 1342-1346. In the summer of 1348 he undertook a journey from China to Damascus, Aleppo and Cairo in 1348 via the East–Indian sea-route to the Persian Gulf. He too was an eye-witness to the ravages of the Black Death at each of these places, but he is silent on the origin of the plague. While at Granada, Spain, in 1350, he spent some time among his countrymen. He mentions four of them in his journal but does not mention the most famous – Ibn-ul-Khatib - while discussing on all topics with the most eminent Moors of Granada. It is Ibn-ul-Khatib, in an account of the Black Death at Granada, who quotes the report of Ibn Batuta that *"the pestilence arose in China from the corruption of unburied corpses"* (Creighton, 1891, 147). The plague devoured the population of the coastal towns in the first instance. It reached the northern European kingdoms, e. g. Poland, probably via Germany by 1348-1349 and appeared in Russia in 1351 (Lazarus, 2014). Europe in the first half of the fourteenth century was visited by five to six plagues. Gabriele de' Mussis provides us with the most informative account of the Black Death, which he believes to be universal and reckons it with the Christian perception of the end times.

> *"The scale of the mortality and the form that which it took persuaded those who lived, weeping and lamenting, through the bitter events of 1346 to 1348 – the Chinese, Indians, Persians, Medes, Kurks, Armenians, Cicilians, Georgians, Mesopotamians,*

> *Nubians, Ethiopians, Turks, Egyptians, Arabs, Saracens and Greeks (for almost all of East had been affected) – that the last Judgement had come."* ('Gabriele de' Mussis, 1994, 18)

Royal Responses to the Epidemic during the Tudors and Stuart Age

The reign of the Tudors and Stuarts was plagued with frequent epidemic outbreaks forcing monarchs to leave the capital for safety. The Sweating Sickness, also known as 'the English Sweat' because it originated in England before spreading to the European continent. The first outbreak was in 1485 when the Tudors came to power and then in 1551, when it suddenly declined, killing tens of thousands with each occurrence (Byrne, 2020). But it was not always fatal. In 1517, Henry VIII escaped the Sweating Sickness by leaving London with a small entourage and moving from place to place. His entourage ran out of food but he was refused to take from any other food supplier for fear of contagion spreading. He moved again in 1528 during another epidemic outburst. "This disease is the easiest in the world to die of", reported the French ambassador, Cardinal du Bellay, from London in June 1528.

"You have a slight pain in the head and ache in the heart; all at once you begin to sweat. There is no need for a physician you are taken off without languishing."

> *"About two thousand only have been attacked by it in London"*, reported du Bellay. *"Twelve years ago, when the same thing happened, ten thousand persons died in ten or twelve days, it is said: but it was not so sharp as it is now beginning to be Everybody is terribly alarmed."* (Letter of Monsieur du Bellay to the Marshal of France)

When Henry heard of his beloved Ann Boleyn afflicted with the sickness, he refused to visit her, though he sent her a love letter with one of his second-best physicians, William Butts.

Henry VIII was the greatest hypochondriacs ever to sit on the English throne (Byrne, 2020). Many well-known individuals of the Tudor Court contracted the Sweating Sickness, including Anne Boleyn's brother and father, George and Thomas, along with Cardinal Wolsey. The Sweating Sickness killed numerous nobles and courtiers, including two of the Duke of Suffolk's sons, Henry and Charles, and Mary Boleyn's first husband, William Carey (History Extra). Henry VIII's daughter Elizabeth survived a small bout of smallpox early in her reign. When she moved to Windsor to avoid an outbreak, gallows were erected outside to deter people from entering.

Isaac Newton was studying at Cambridge when the university closed in August 1665 because of the Great Plague, forcing him to retreat to his house in Lincolnshire and study privately. Between 1665 and the spring of 1667, during the Stuart period, when he returned to Cambridge, he had an astonishing burst of energy and insights that formed the basis of most of his later career, including work on calculus and optics.

The Plague in Mughal Times

At the start of the 17th century in India, Jehangir, the fourth Mughal emperor (1605–1627) travelled to Ahmedabad to escape the plague that was raging in Agra. He continued to listen to people's grievances until he himself got afflicted with the plague on 15th June, 1618, and regrets having come there. He calls Ahmadabad *'Bimaristan'* (abode of sickness), *'Zaqqum'* (the thorn-bed) or *'Jahannamabad'* (the house of hell). Even his son Shah Jahan contracted the illness (Jahangir). Fortunately, both father and son recovered after a brief bout but others perhaps were not so lucky.

The Bubonic Plague in British India

The years 1896–1898 were the most unfortunate period in the

history of British rule in India, especially Bombay, due to the outbreak of the Bubonic Plague. It came via a steamship from Hong Kong. It was co-found by a Franco—Swiss scientist Alexandre Yersin (1894) and was name, *Yersinia pestis* in his honour (Lazarus, 2014). The government had no firsthand experience of the plague to deal with it nor there were any special laws regarding plague during its onset. Although the plague spread from Bombay to other commercial centres, there is a likelyhood of the plague reaching Bengal in 1896. When the first suspected case of plague was reported, Sir Alexander Mackenzie, Lieutenant-Governor of Bengal, issued a resolution to appoint a Medical Board headed by Mr. H. H. Risley, Secretary to the Bengal Government, which was formed on 10th October, 1896, to prevent the spread of the disease (Chatterjee, 2006). The plague in Bombay broke out among the Lohanas – men mostly employed on board steamers trading with China. A bundle of infected clothing is quite sufficient to have caused the outbreak in Bombay (The British Medical Journal Report, 1896, 1252). Rats were dying in huge numbers even before the news of the plague reached the masses.

Experiments on the Plague

According to the report of the epidemic of plague, the smaller and domesticated animals most susceptible to plague were mice, rabbits, guinea-pigs, rats and monkeys. It could spread through clothing worn by the patient. A washerman at a plague hospital at Hong Kong died in 1896. Laboratory experiments in India proved that the power of the infection on clothing lost after 10 days. Grain would get affected naturally. Mr. Hankin in India experimented on artificially infected grains and found that grain lost its infecting power in less than eight days (Lowson, 1897).

So great was the mortality that children used to amuse themselves by throwing dead rats into the gullies and frightening and chasing each other in the streets with the carcasses of the rats they found (The British Medical Journal Report, 1896, 1254). The merchants who lived in Mandvi were violently opposed to all killing and especially those of rats (Deshmukh, 1988, 478). The disease was present in the merchant class or *'Banias'*. Among the preventive measures used, the most effective was "complete evacuation" which helped check the crescent epidemic, lessened plague mortality and shortened the duration of the epidemic. The British had scant regard for the religious sentiments of the people. There were forced medical inspections of sensitive parts like armpits and groin of men, women and children (Deshmukh, 1988, 478). Clothes, grains and other belongings infected were burnt and patients were forcibly taken to hospitals. Other measures adopted were burning, disinfection, house-to-house visitations by plague medical officer; corpse inspection, village inspections, railway inspections, segregation camps and segregation at hospital level and the making of grants under 'Discretional Relief Fund'.

The Epidemics Disease Act of 1897 was introduced by the British authorities to deal with the outbreak of the plague in Pune, India. This Act was effective in controlling the spread of the epidemic but Bal Gangadhar Tilak, one of the leaders of India's freedom movement, criticised the heavy-handedness of the administration in his newspaper. After the assassination of a British officer, Tilak was convicted for sedition, but, upon release, he was hailed as a hero. However, these draconian rules were not acceptable to people as they did not believe it to be infectious (Deshmukh, 1988, 478) and riots broke out in Bombay. The police came to the rescue of the Municipal team. The bubonic plague resulted in mass exodus of people thereby increasing the danger of the plague spreading to the rest of the Presidency and other parts of India too. It affected the family life as parents fled from their children and abandoned each other (*The British Medical Journal*, 1896).

Influenza

The Influenza epidemic cost many lives both in India and other British colonies. The city of Sheraz in Persia, lost 10,000 of its 50,000 population. From 1905 to 1911, Bahrain was visited by plague every second year (Persian Gulf Pilot, 1920). There were outbreaks of the bubonic plague in 1910, followed by the cholera epidemic in 1910 and 1911. All ships arriving from India in 'good condition' had to undergo a five day quarantine period, in addition to 'disinfection and destruction of rats'. Ships carrying passengers had separate regulations. Quarantine regulations were strictly followed. In Washington (September, 1918), the sanitation division issued an advisory to all to keep surroundings clean; remain in fresh and sunny environs; avoid being sprayed by throat and nose secretions of others; keep out of crowded places like cinema halls; avoid rail travel until absolutely necessary; eat healthy and nutritious food and drink plenty of water; avoid constipation and sleep for seven hours at least etc.

Typhoid

Another classic case is that of Mary Mallon (1869- 1938) which brings forth another aspect of plague – the 'carrier'. A cook by profession, who migrated from Ireland to the US in 1884, was a healthy carrier of *Salmonella typhi*, which earned her the social stigma 'Typhoid Mary'. She was in and out of the hospital and continued to work as a cook and infect people, until 1915 when she was quarantined for life. This case brings to light the following - prejudice provoked by the Health Care system; the problematic nature of the subject and the need for enhancing medical and legal social treatment model aimed at improving the status of the disease carrier and limiting their impact on society (*Annals of Gastroenterology*, 2013, 132-34). At the turn of the 20th century, Waldemar Haffkine, a Jewish doctor worked on finding a vaccine for cholera in

Bombay, while Robert Koch had already found the vaccine for anthrax disease cycle (1876), bacteria responsible for tuberculosis (1882) and cholera (1883).

Smallpox

Smallpox plagued the world from the 5th to the 7th century, then during the middle ages and again in the 18th century until Edward Jenner (1749–1843) found the vaccine for immunization and its ultimate eradication. On May 8, 1980, the World Health Assembly announced that the world was free of smallpox and recommended that all countries cease vaccination: "The world and all its people have won freedom from smallpox, which was the most devastating disease sweeping in epidemic form through many countries since earliest times, leaving death, blindness and disfigurement in its wake" (WHO Report, 1980).

The People's Response to Plagues through Art and Literature

There is a sizeable amount of literature on the plague available written mostly during self-quarantine. Boccaccio wrote The Decameron while in quarantine. Shakespeare, who lived during the 16th century, wrote his most famous works during the period of plague outbreaks. He manages to avoid writing about the plague in all his writings except in Romeo and Juliet:

> *'Going to find a barefoot brother out,*
> *One of our order, to associate me,*
> *Here in this city visiting the sick,*
> *And finding him, the searchers of the town,*
> *Suspecting that we both were in a house*
> *Where the infectious pestilence did reign,*
> *Sealed up the doors and would not let us forth.'*
>
> (Romeo and Juliet Act 5 Sc 2)

Daniel Defoe, while recounting his experience of the Great

Plague of London in 1665, says that there were no newspapers "to spread rumours and spread of things, and to improve them by the invention of men" (Defoe, 9). Rose Tremain's *Restoration*, Geraldine Brook's *Year of Wonders* and Alessandro Manzoni's Italian classic *The Bethroned* and Edgar Allen Poe described impact of the Yellow Fever and Cholera epidemics in the US saying that "no pestilence had ever been so fatal, or so hideous" and that "the very air seemed... redolent with death" in *Masque of the Red Death* and *The Sphinx* respectively (Byrne, 2020). Mary Shelley's apocalyptic *The Last Man* was in conflict with Christian thought as it seemed to be a frightening prophecy for the future. Albert Camus' *La Peste* in 1947 is a story based on a Cholera epidemic in Oran in 1899. Edvard Munch (1863-1944), who was troubled throughout his life by mental health issues painted many self-portraits. He caught the Spanish Flu, which infected millions, at the end of the World War I in 1918. His *Self-Portrait with the Spanish Flu* is a haunting depiction of a lonely figure. It is the only famous work of art to come out of a global pandemic.

Conclusion

The pandemic brought their share of mourning and grief to one and all. In Europe, many grand palaces and stately homes which once brimmed with social gatherings and a retinue of servants, now withstood the ravages of the pandemic abandoned. In most cases, there was no claimant to the ancestral wealth and domain. People abandoned their near and dear ones for fear of contagion and quarantined themselves. However, there was another lot of people who continued to 'eat, drink and be merry' as if the plague did not exist. Many believed the plague to be affliction, sent from God, and other prejudices grew rife. Vaccines took longer to be invented and complete eradication of a disease was a herculean task. There was also a risk of the infection being passed on by asymptomatic carriers to vulnerable people. The

Epidemic Diseases Act of 1897, introduced by the British, was again enforced by the government to treat the outbreak of Swine Flu in 2009 in Pune. The same Act with Amendments is being used to control the Covid-19 pandemic in 2020. In the past, European clerics fell victim to plagues and other epidemics as they were the care-givers and thus exposed to the disease. In present times, the medical staff and ambulance drivers are at risk. The attitude of people towards the health risks involved has not changed. Many believe the pandemic is over and will not affect them. In China, a web-user mused in November 2019, "Bird flu in the year of the rooster...swine flu in the year of the pig. Next year is the year of the rat...the plague is coming" (Brophy, 2020). Was he/she far from the truth?

REFERENCES

1. Allen, Scott. (Sep-Oct 2011). William Carey: A Missionary Who Transformed a Nation. *Mission Frontiers*, issue: Making Disciples. Retrieved from *https://www.missionfrontiers.org/issue/article/william-carey*
2. Avesbury, Robertus de. (1720). *Historia de Mirabilibus Gestis Regis Ed. III.*, Oxon. Also in the Rolls series. Edited by E. Maunde Thompson, 122.
3. Boccaccio, Giovanni, *The Decameron*, translated by J. M. Rigg. E-book Gutenberg Project, 8 – 28.
4. Byrne, Eugene (2020). How did people cope with 'lockdowns' of the past? *BBC History Magazine*: History Extra, April 9.
5. Carr, E. H. (1961). *What is History?* New York: Vintage Books.
6. Chatterjee, S. (2005). Plague and Politics in Bengal 1896 to 1898. *Proceedings of the Indian History Congress*, 66, 1194-1201. Retrieved from http://www.jstor.org/stable/44145931
7. Creighton, Charles. (1891). *A History of Epidemics in Britain*. Cambridge: Cambridge University Press.
8. David, Amita Esther. (2005). Socio-Cultural Advancement, Nationalism and the Christian Missionaries in the 20th century with Special Reference to Uttar Pradesh (1858 – 1900). Ph.D. Thesis (unpublished).
9. Deshmukh, C. (1988). The Bombay Plague (1896-1897). *Proceedings of the Indian History Congress*, 49, 478-483. Retrieved from http://www.jstor.org/stable/44148433
10. Dinkins, Courtney Pariera. Persecution of the Jews during the Great Plagues of the 14th Century. Persecution of the Jews - Insects, Disease, and History,

Montana State University. Retrieved from www.montana. edu/historybug/yersiniaessays/pariera-dinkins.html.

11. Doherty, Melissa. Plague's Contribution to the Spanish Inquisition. *Contribution to the Spanish Inquisition - Insects, Disease, and History*, Montana State University. Retrieved from https://www.montana.edu/historybug/yersiniaessays/doherty.html.
12. EClinical Medicine. (November 2019). Forgotten but not gone: the threat of Leprosy. *The Lancet*, 16, 1.
13. Gabriele de' Mussi. (1994). The Arrival of the Plague (Historia de Morbo). In Rosemary Horrox (Ed.). *The Black Death*. Manchester, U.K.: Manchester University Press.
14. Gough, Richard. (1789) *Camden's Britannia, Surrey and Sussex*, Hutchinson, 1977.
15. Grzybowski, Andrezej and Malgorzata, Nite. (2016). Leprosy in the Bible. *Clinics in Dermatology*, 34(1), 3-7. Retrieved from https://doi.org/10.1016/j.clindermatol.2016.03.001
16. Haldar, Dipankar. (2015). *William Carey the Shoemaker and His Christian Ethics in India*, 6. Retrieved from https://www.wmcarey.edu/carey/legacy/dh/
17. Hecker, Justus Friedrich Carl. *The Epidemics of the Middle Ages*. B. G. Babington, (Trans.) Project Gutenberg eBook. (London: George Woodfall & Sons, 1844). Retrieved from The Epidemics of the Middle Ages, by J. F. C. Hecker, M.D.—A Project Gutenberg eBook
18. Hecker, Justus Friedrich Carl. (2007). *The Black Death and The Dancing Mania*. B. G. Babington, (Trans.) Project Gutenberg eBook. Cassell & Company. Ltd. 1888. Retrieved from https://www.gutenberg.org/files/1739/1739-h/1739-h.htm#startoftext
19. Jehangir *Tuzuk-i-Jehangir*. (Alexander Roger, Henry Beveridge and Nuru-d-din Jehangir (Trans.) *Royal Asiatic Society*, Vol. II, 1914, 12, 15.
20. Kakar, Sanjeev. (1996). Leprosy in British India 1860–1940: Colonial Politics and Missionary Medicine. *Medical History*, 40, 218. Retrieved from https://core.ac.uk/download/pdf/206314543.pdf
21. Khan, Inayatullah. (2013). Visitations of the Plague in Mughal India. *Proceedings of the Indian History Congress*, 74, 2013, 307.
22. Last, J.M. (Ed.). (2001). *A Dictionary of Epidemiology*. 4th edn. New York: Oxford University Press.
23. Lazarus Sarah. (2014). When death came calling: How the plague swept through Hong Kong. *Post Magazine*, 21st June. Retrieved from https://www.scmp.com/magazines/post-magazine/article/1535499/when-death-came-calling-plague-hong-kong
24. Letters of Monsieur du Bellay Bishop of Bayonne, to the Grand Master and Marshal of France. Retrieved from http://www.luminarium.org/

encyclopedia/dubellaysweat.htm

25. Love, Ann, and Drake, Jane. (2013). *Pandemic Survival: It's Why you're Alive*. Tundra Books.
26. Lowson, James A. (1897). *Report of the Epidemic of Plague from 22nd Feb – 16th July*, 1897. https://archive.org/details/b24974511/page/10/mode/2up
27. Mangalwadi, Ruth and Vishal. (1999). *The Legacy of William Carey: A Model for the Transformation of a Culture*. Wheaton, IL: Crossway Books, VX.
28. Marineli, Filio. (2013). Mary Mallon (1869-1938) and the history of typhoid fever. *Annals of Gastroenterology*, 6(2), 132 – 134. Retrieved from https://www.ncbi.nlm.nih.gov/pmc/articles/PMC3959940/
29. Mark, Joshua J. (2020). Religious responses to the Black Death. Retrieved from https://www.ancient.eu/article/1541/religious-responses-to-the-black-death/
30. *Persian Gulf Pilot comprising The Persian Gulf, The Gulf of Oman and The Makran Coast*, Washington, Government Printing Office, 1920, 134. Retrieved from https://www.wdl.org/en/item/17261/view/1/7/#q=Bubonic%20plague
31. Procopius *History of Wars*, Book II, Chapter XXII. http://www.gutenberg.org/files/16764/16764-h/16764-h.htm#BOOK_II
32. Pune Mirror e-paper (2009, August 6). *How the Epidemic Act plagued Pune in 1897*, e-paper/ articleshow/32543504.cms
33. Rosenwald, Michael S. (2020, April 7). Washington Post.
34. Sarkar, Natasha. (2001). Plague in Bombay: Response of Britain's Indian Subjects to Colonial Intervention. *Proceedings of the Indian History Congress*. 62, 445.
35. *The British Medical Journal* Report. (1896). *The Plague in India*, October 24, 1252, 1254
36. The British Medical Journal. (1900). Vol 2, No. 2078, October 27, 1250.
37. WHO. (1980). The Global Eradication of Small Pox. Final Report of the Global Commission for the Certification of Small Pox Eradication. Geneva: WHO.

6

History of Influenza Based Pandemic

Amit Kumar Verma

ABSTRACT

Pandemic influenza is often thought of as a thunderstorm or hurricane—a sudden disaster that comes with little warning signs and devastates socially and economically in a relatively short time. An influenza epidemic occurs within few years causing an increase in the annual number of deaths past the average with 10,000 to 15,000 additional deaths. Researchers believe that the globe stands on the verge of an influenza pandemic. Greek sculpture of 412 BC explains about what today is known as 'Influenza outbreak'. According to epidemiologist, the pandemic of 1580 is the earliest known pandemic. Influenza pandemic occurred at least three times in the eighteenth century in 1729-30, 1732-33 and 1781-82. In nineteenth century pandemic occurred in 1832-33 and 1890. Pandemic influenza viruses have emerged three times in twentieth century: in 1918 ("Spanish" influenza, H1N1), in 1957 ("Asian" influenza, H2N2), and in 1968 ("Hong Kong" influenza, H3N2). The influenza pandemic of 1918 was exceptional in both breadth and depth. Total mortality accounted to 1918 pandemic was approximately around 40 million. In twenty first century Swine flu took tool and still persisting. The lesson of the history of pandemics appears to be that at least the initial attack may sometimes occur with gentleness and thus, may afford a substantial background space for the planning and use of vaccine and drugs.

Keywords: Asain Flu, Bird flu, China, Pandemic, Russia, Spanish influenza,

About 6,000 years ago human disease came into existence. Influenza viruses are named for the Latin word *influentia* or Influenza (Broxmeyer, 2006). Influenza term was coined by an Italian during 1700s to designate the disease arising from bad air (*miasma*) Influenza can be classified into two type pattern - Pandemic influenza and Seasonal influenza. Emergence of new influenza virus for which no immunity found in masses give rise to Pandemic Influenza whereas Seasonal Influenza generally caused by influenza A or B virus occurring each year during favourite time of the year. Influenza was discovered as a direct observation on animal diseases. A veterinarian in 1918 established the similarity between the disease in pig and Spanish influenza. In 1928 N. McBryde conducted an experiment to transmit influenza from pig to pig, by taking filtered mucus from respiratory tract of the pigs, while Robert Shope in the same year, repeated the same experiment with unfiltered material, thus it was evidenced that influenza was caused by a virus. In 1933 Wilson Smith, Patrick Laidrow and Christopher Andrews first identified the virus that caused influenza in humans. It is an observation that pandemic occurs at ten to fifty years interval with changing magnitude of severity and social–economic impact. Greek sculptor of 412 BC describes about what today is known as influenza outbreak (Kuszewski and Brydak, 2000; Potter, 1998). In 1357, in Florence people called it epidemic, Italy Influenza **di freddo,** i.e. cold influenza —a disease possible cause (Potter, 2001; Daly *et. al.* 2007). In 1414 French people described epidemic that affected upto one lakh people in Paris. They said it originated from *vent puant et tout plein de froidure* or a smelly and cold wind.

Pandemic of 1580

According to epidemiologist, this pandemic is the earliest known pandemic that started in Asia during summer that spread to Africa, European continent and further to North America (Pyle, 1986). The actual figure of the deaths is not known, but estimated deaths were around 8000 in Rome only. The disease spread from Malta to Sicily in July 1580. Philip II ruled the Iberian Peninsula, southern Italy and several North American parts. The early July outbreak in Spain and Netherlands was most likely caused by the troops sent by Philip II to fight against the Dutch. Influenza pandemic occurred at least three times in the eighteenth century: first occurred in 1729-30, second in 1732-33 and third in 1781-1782. In addition to this, there were two major epidemics that could possibly be considered pandemic in 1761-62 and 1789.

Pandemic of Russia, 1729

In 1729 Pandemic occurred in Russia, Europe and engulfed whole continent within six months of its origin [Pyle, 1986; Hirsh, 1883; Finkler, 1899). King Louis XV was infected and explained that the diseases spread like foolish little girl or follette in France, Moscow and Astrakhan, on the Caspian Sea in April 1929. In September, it spread to Sweden, in October it get spread to Vienna, in November it spread to Hungary and Poland and finally to London and Ireland. On the basis of evidences, pandemic causes sickness, morbidity with generally low mortality, but in North Italy fatality rate was at serious pace, where vulnerable population like elderly and the pregnant woman's were worst affected.

Pandemic of China, 1781

Four years later, in 1781, pandemic occurred in China and it spread to Russia and then further engulfed Europe and North America over the next year. At the peak of its severity, it infected 30,000 people each day in St. Petersburg and affected two-thirds of the Rome population. In India outbreak occurred in British occupied territories during autumn of 1781, the pandemic spread to westward in 1782. Transport was one of the factors for its rapid spread.

Pandemic of 1832-33

This pandemic began in China and through sea route transportation via ships it spread to other nations like Philippine, India, Indonesia and finally across Russia and to the interior of Europe. Outbreak occurred in North America in 1831-32 and affected 20-25% of the world population.

Pandemic of 1890

It began in the late 1889 and spread after several months throughout the world showing its peak in North Europe and USA. In the spring of 1891 (over a year after first wave) second wave peaked and a third wave in the early 1892 (Jordan, 1927).

Pandemic of 1918

The influenza pandemic of 1918 was landmark in the health history of the human civilization. The disaster is called as the "Greatest Medical Holocaust in History". The effect of this pandemic was reflected by three distinct ways: a) The Spring of 1918, b) The Fall of 1918, c) The winter of 1918-19 (Humphries, 2013; Johnson and Mueller, 2002)

Out of these three distinct waves, the second wave was disastrous, killing more than tens of millions people. One-third of the world population may have been clinically infected during pandemic (Frost, 1920; Burnet and Lark, 1942) with mortality rate of more than 2.5% while 0.1% mortality in other influenza epidemic (Marks and Beatty, 1976; Roseanau and Last, 1980). This in total mortality was probably around forty million (Crosby, 1989; Johnson and Mueller, 2002; Patterson and Pyle, 1991). The unique feature of 1918 pandemic was three extensive outbreaks happened within one year. Intra pandemic influenza outbreak generally occurs in a single annual wave in the late winter season. Due to the absence of antibiotics many individual died during the pandemic because of the bacterial pneumonia secondary infection. However, deaths occurred after the onset of symptoms with massive acute pulmonary hemorrhage or pulmonary edema (LeCount, 2020; 1920). On considering age group most death occurred among young adults (usually low death rate from disease). Influenza and pneumonia death rate for 15 to 34 year old were twenty times higher in 1918 than in previous years (Linder and Grove, 1943).

In the observation it was found that people less than 65 years old contributed for more than 99 per cent of all excess influenza related deaths in 1918-19 (Simonsen, *et. al.*, 1998), On the other hand, same age group contributed for only 36 per cent of all excess influenza related mortality in 1957 H2N2 pandemic and 48 per cent in 1968 H3N3 pandemic. In 1918, virus strain contained a hemagglutinin gene encoding, why history contains a novel sub-type for which the population did not have protective immunity (Kilbourne, 1997; Reid and Taubenberger, 1999). The other dominant surface protein NA also would have been replaced by antigenic shift before the start of 1918 influenza (Reid and Taubenberger, 1999; Taubenberger, *et.al.*, 2000) and gene encoding two surface proteins were derived from an avian like Influenza virus shortly before the start of the 1918 disease. It was the public health system unpreparedness that increased or compounded the 1918 pandemic potential. Many clinical doctors still believed that the influenza was caused by the bacillus influenza bacterium. However, physician did not find any bacillus during the autopsies (Van Epps, 2006). Doctor misdiagnosed the influenza as a common cold, chloera or bubonic plague. Influenza disease was not a part of regulation under the reportable disease in those countries. Vaccines to counter influenza and antibiotics to treat secondary bacterial infection were not known. Mixture of the water, salt, topical cream and coal oil (USDHHS) was given to patients. Non-pharmaceutical remedies such as a face mask, quarantine, banning social gathering were used (Markel, *et. al.*, 2006). However, the closure of the schools and the social gatherings has positive impact in terms of the reduction of the influenza cases.

Pandemic of 1957-58 (Asian Flu)

A new influenza strain H2N2 was originated in the Yunnan province of China in February 1957 (Jordan, 1927). The spread of virus can be traced from China to Hong Kong in April, then to Singapore, Taiwan and Japan (Fukumi, 1959). It became pandemic spreading to twenty countries (Dunn, 1958). The spread diffusion of the disease could be attributed to the land and sea route. It spread to Russia to Scandinavia and Eastern Europe and also at an international conference held in Iowa (Langmuir, 1961; Payne, 1958). The pandemic was followed by successive wave, second wave being more severe than the first wave. The period witnessed clinical attack rate in the school of 40 to 60% (Henderson, *et. al.*, 2009). It was comparatively mild influenza pandemic with a maximum case fatality rate estimated to be about 0.67% and caused death worldwide of one to two million (Guan, 2010; Rogers; Henderson, *et. al.*, 2009; Viboud *et. al.*, 2016). During the pandemic disease global surveillance system was established, vaccine was there to counter the disease.

Pandemic of 1968-70 (Hong Kong Flu)

Ten years after Asian flu, the Asian flu strain, undergoes antigenic shift to H3N2 causing a new pandemic called Hong Kong flu. It was milder compared to Asian flu. The virus was first traced in July 1968. The major cause of virus spread was due to army mobility where soldiers stationed in Vietnam were returning to USA (Cockburn, *et. al.*, 1969; Sharrat, 1969). Other than military activities, virus spread was also due to extensive air travel. Children were the most affected group of population (Norris, 2009). The striking feature of this pandemic was the mortality rate reported in USA was 70% and in Canada it was 54 per cent during first wave of pandemic while Asia and Europe experienced 70 per cent of mortality rate during the second wave of pandemic. Hong Kong flu estimated death toll was between five lakh to two millions worldwide (Guan *et. al*, 2010; Reperant, *et. al.*, 2016). Pre-existing immunity to neuraminidase antigen (N2) was the reason behind the low mortality rate.

H5N1 Avian Influenza Pandemic (Bird Flu)

H5N1 Avian influenza virus is highly pathogenic causes poultry disease. Its outbreak in China and seven other East Asian countries in late 2003 and early 2004 was another challenge for Asia in the history of epidemics and pandemics. However, the virus was fatal to humans mainly in Thailand and Vietnam (WHO, 2004) and killed forty humans. Research indicates that virus receptor specificity didn't prevent the direct transmission of Avian Influenza to humans.

Pandemic of 2009-10 (Swine Flu)

PH1N1/09 virus was also called the swine flu outbreak in Mexico April 2009 (Bijl and Schellekens, 2011). On 11th June 2009 WHO declared it as an influenza pandemic (WHO). The emergence of this global disease was the result of triple viral reassortment between the two influenza lineages that were in pig for years (Smith, *et. al.*, 2009). This pandemic exhibited wave behavior and almost three wave profiles were exhibited by Mexico in different season: spring, summer and fall wave (Chowell, *et al*, 2011). Two wave profile occurred in the USA (spring, summer, fall wave). India experienced three wave peaks in quick frequency in September 09, December 09 and August 10 (Mishra, 2015). Estimates of economic loss range from 0.5 per cent to 1.5 per cent of GDP in affected countries (Polycom, 2011; Smith, *et. al.*, 2009). Maintaining health hygiene and voluntary isolation of symptomatic individuals were the important non pharmaceutical measures taken (*Cantey, et. al.*, 2013). This pandemic marked the combined use of the vaccine and antiviral.

Conclusion

Presently in China a new H1N1 swine influenza strain, containing the European avian and other constituents is Found indicating the emergence of new pandemic soon. Emergence of the reassortant viral strain containing the mixture of the animal and a human influenza genetic composition causes pandemic to re-emerge. Swine are considered as one of the major source of the reassortant strains as they are susceptible to infection with the avian, swine and the human influenza A viruses. According to the major warning by Chinese researches novel swine influenza virus SIV A H1N1 has become prevalent in pigs and has potential to spread pandemic spread potential. So let's keep watch on it.

REFERENCES

1. Bijl, D., Schellekens, H. (2011). The Sponsored Pandemic of the Mexican Flu. *Int. J. Risk Saf. Med.*, 23, 73–79.
2. Broxmeyer, L. (2006). Bird Flu, Influenza and 1918: The Case for Mutant Avian Tuberculosis. *Med. Hypotheses*, 67, 1006–1015.
3. Bults, M. *et al.* (2010). Mexican Flu: Risk Perception in the General Public, Precautionary Measures and Trust in Information provided by the Government. *Ned. Tijdschr. Geneeskd.*, 154, A1686.
4. Burnet, F. and Clark, E. (1942). *Influenza: A Survey of the Last 50 Years in the Light of Modern Work on the Virus of Epidemic Influenza*. Melbourne, Macmillan.
5. Cantey, P.T., *et al.* (2013). Public Health Emergency Preparedness: Lessons Learned about Monitoring of Interventions from the National Association of County and City Health Official's Survey of Nonpharmaceutical

Interventions for Pandemic H1N1. *J. Public Health Manag. Pract.*, 19, 70–76.

6. Chowell, G. *et al.* (2011). Characterizing the Epidemiology of the 2009 Influenza H1N1 Pandemic in Mexico. *PLoS Med.*, 8, e1000436.
7. Cockburn, W.C., Delon, P.J. and Ferreira,W. (1969). Origin and Progress of the 1968–69 Hong Kong Influenza Epidemic. *Bull. World Health Organ.* 1969, 41, 345–348.
8. Crosby, A. (1989). *America's Forgotten Pandemic.* Cambridge, Cambridge University Press.
9. Daly, P., Gustafson, R. and Kendall, P. (2007). Introduction to Pandemic Influenza. *BC Med. J.*, 49, 240–244.
10. Dunn, F.L. (1958). Pandemic Influenza in 1957: Review of International Spread of new Asian Strain. *JAMA*, 166, 1140–1148.
11. Finkler, D. (1899). Influenza in twentieth century practice. In Shipman, T.L. (Ed). *An International Encyclopaedia of Modern Medical Science.* London, Sampson Law & Marston.
12. Frost W. (1920). Statistics of Influenza Morbidity. *Pub Health Rep.* 35, 584–597.
13. Fukumi, H. (1959). Summary Report of the Asian Influenza Epidemic in Japan, 1957. *Bull. World Health Organ.* 1959, 20, 187–198.
14. Guan, Y. (2010). The Emergence of Pandemic Influenza Viruses. *Protein Cell.* 1, 9–13.
15. Henderson, D. *et al.* (2009). Public Health and Medical Responses to the 1957–58 Influenza Pandemic. *Biosecur. Bioterror.* 7, 265–273.
16. Hirsh. (1883). *Handbook of Geographic and Historical Pathology.* London: New Sydenham Society.
17. Humphries, M. (2013). Paths of Infection: The First World War and the Origins of the 1918 Influenza Pandemic. *War Hist.*, 21, 55–81.
18. Johnson, N. and Mueller, J. (2002). Updating the Accounts: Global Mortality of the 1918–1920 "Spanish" Influenza Pandemic. *Bull. Hist. Med.*, 76, 105–115.
19. Jordan E. (1927). *Epidemic Influenza: A Survey.* Chicago: American Medical Association.
20. Jordan, E.O. (1927). *Epidemic Influenza: A Survey.* Chicago, : American Medical Association.
21. Kilbourne, E.D. (1997). Perspectives on Pandemics: A Research Agenda. *J Infect Dis* 176 (Suppl 1), S29–S31
22. Kuszewski, K. and Brydak, L. (2000). The Epidemiology and History of Influenza. *Biomed. Pharmac other.* 54, 188–195.
23. Langmuir, A.D. (1961). Epidemiology of Asian Influenza. *Am. Rev. Respir. Dis.* 1961, 83, 2–18.
24. LeCount, E.R. (1919). The Pathologic Anatomy of Influenza

Bronchopneumonia. *JAMA*, 72, 650–652.

25. Linder, F.E., Grove, R.D. (1943). *Vital Statistics Rates in the United States: 1900–1940*. Washington, DC: National Office of Vital Statistics. Government Printing Office.
26. Markel, H. *et al.* (2006). Jr. Nonpharmaceutical Influenza Mitigation Strategies: US Communities, 1918–1920 Pandemic. *Emerg. Infect. Dis.*12, 1961–1964.
27. Marks, G. and Beatty, W.K. (1976). *Epidemics*. New York: Scribner.
28. Mishra, B. (2015). Resurgence of Influenza (H1N1) : Smoldering Pandemic in India?. *J. Glob. Infect. Dis.*, 7, 56–59.
29. Norris, S. (2009). *Influenza Pandemic*. Ottawa, ON, Canada: Library of Parliament, Social Affairs Division.
30. Patterson, K.D. (1987). *Pandemic Influenza 1700–1900: A Study in Historical Epidemiology*. NJ, : Rowan & Littlefield.
31. Patterson, K.D. and Pyle, G.F. (1991). The Geography and Mortality of the 1918 Influenza Pandemic. *Bull Hist Med*, 65, 4–21.
32. Payne, A.M. (1958). Symposium on the Asian Influenza Epidemic. *Proc. R. Soc. Med.* 51, 1009–1015.
33. Polycom. (2011). *A Swine Flu Vaccine for Businesses: Ensuring Operational Continuity Amid a Global Pandemic*. CA, Polycom.
34. Potter, C. (1998). Chronicle of Influenza Pandemics. In Nicholson, K.G., Webster, R.F., Hay, A.J. (Eds.). *Textbook of Influenza*. Oxford, Blackwell Science LTD.
35. Potter, C. (2001). A History of Influenza. *J. Appl. Microbiol*, 91, 572–579.
36. Pyle, G.F. (1986). *The Diffusion of Influenza: Patterns and Paradigms*. NJ, Rowan and Littlefield.
37. Reid, A.H. and Taubenberger, J.K. (1999). The 1918 Flu and other Influenza Pandemics: Over there and Back Again. *Lab Invest* 79, 95–101.
38. Reperant, L.; Moesker, F.M.; Osterhaus, A.D. (2016). Influenza: From Zoonosis to Pandemic. *Eur. Respir. Soc. J.*, 2, 1–4.
39. Rogers, K. *Asian Flu of 1957*. Retrieved on 11th March, 2016 from http://www.britannica.com/event/Asian-flu-of-1957
40. Rosenau, M.J. and Last, J.M. (1980). *Maxcy-Rosenau Preventative Medicine and Public Health*. New York: Appleton-Century-Crofts.
41. Sharrat, R.G. (1969). National Influenza Experience in the USA. *Bull. World Health Organ.*, 41, 361–366.
42. Simonsen, L. *et.al.* (1998). Pandemic versus Epidemic Influenza Mortality: A Pattern of Changing Age Distribution. *J Infect Dis*, 178, 53–60.
43. Smith, G.J. *et al.* (2009). Origins and Evolutionary Genomics of the 2009 Swine-origin H1N1 Influenza Epidemic. *Nat. Med.*, 459, 1122–1125.
44. Smith, R.D. *et al.* (2009). The Economy-wide Impact of Pandemic Influenza on the UK: A Computable General Equilibrium Modelling Experiment.

BMJ, 339, b4571.

45. Taubenberger, *et.al.* (2000). The 1918 Influenza Virus: A Killer comes into View. *Virology*, 274, 241–245.
46. USDHHS. *The Great Pandemic: The United States in 1918–1919*. Retrieved on 9th March, 2016 from http://www.flu.gov/ pandemic/history/1918/ index.html.
47. VanEpps, H.L. (2006). Influenza: Exposing the True Killer. *J. Exp. Med.*, 203, 803.
48. Viboud, C. *et. al.* (2016). Global Mortality Impact of the 1957–1959 Influenza Pandemic. *J. Infect. Dis.*, 213, 738–745.
49. WHO. 2004. Avian Influenza A (H7) Human Infections in Canada. Retrieved on 17th December, 2004 from http:// www.who.int/csr/don/ 2004_04_05/en/
50. WHO. *World Now at the Start of 2009 Influenza Pandemic*. Retrieved on 23rd March, 2016 from http://www.who.int/mediacentre/news/statements/ 2009/h1n1_pandemic_phase6_20090611/en/
51. Winternitz, M.C., Wason, I.M. and McNamara, F.P. (1920). *The Pathology of Influenza*. New Haven, CT: Yale University Press.
52. Wolbach, S.B. (1919). Comments on the Pathology and Bacteriology of Fatal Influenza Cases, as observed at Camp Devens, Mass. *Johns Hopkins Hospital Bulletin* 30, 104.

7
Prevention of Pandemic in India: Past and Present

Somenath Ghosh

ABSTRACT

Covid-19 has made many changes in our daily livelihood. The present generation, has witnessed a pandemic in our lifetimes. In this context it is very much relevant to get an idea about any kind of remedial procedures, discussed or mentioned in literature down the ancient history of India. India is mother of ancient civilization. There are various discoveries made by Indian scientists in ancient times and now these are recognized by modern science. Amongst them most important is Ayurveda. In recent years, the herbal ameliorating role of Ayurveda in various kinds of diseases is accepted by the modern scientific and/medical personnel. In this context, The research has done some survey of literature (both online and off line). Based upon the available information the present review is designed and the study is divided in two parts. In the beginning, we will look into the occurrence of pandemics in ancient India. Second, throws some light regarding the remedial procedures and measures taken to contain the spread of pandemic mentioned in Ayurveda. In this regard, I have got very interesting results. I noted occurrence of pandemic in India times back to B.C.E and this was prevalent in 19th century as well. For prevention of this pandemic number of measures are mentioned in ayurveda including quarantine, isolation, home isolation etc. As part of remedial measures, boosting up of immunity, reframing and refreshing of metabolic systems of body, different tests and methods for enhancing lung capacity, physical mobility (in forms of yoga and meditation) are prescribed as non-invasive methods. Thus, present study will encompass the rich cultural as well as scientific heritage of ancient India.

Keywords: Ancient India, *Ayurveda*, pandemic, prevention, occurrence.

When the globe was heading towards conquering Artificial Intelligence as an inherent tool for virtually doing everything in 2020, the dream line trajectory was deviated by a virus. Originating from China in December 2019 the novel Corona virus reached to about 19 countries by the end of January when the WHO declared it a Public Health Emergency of International Concern (WHO, PHEIC, 2020). The prevention and control guidelines were released by the WHO on 29th March, 2020 on its website and Ministry of Health & Family Welfare (MoHFW), Govt. of India. The simple good personal hygiene measures and physical distancing were declared as most effective protections for the Covid-19 (CDC). Age old traditions and customs have been the core of Indian culture. The Indian way of living - *Sanatan Sanskriti*—has many scientific principles inherited in it, to prevent infectious diseases (*Yathartha Sandesh*, 2017). We follow them traditionally sometimes not even realizing the rationale behind it. This article tries to explore the correlation between preventive measures and traditional practices of *Sanatan* principles of life. These principles were capable of preventing infectious diseases, major killers in ancient times. Many measures are coherent with the modern public health approaches of handling infections and there is a need to realize this reality.

Role of Customs, Culture and Traditions of "*Sanatan* way of life" in Disease Prevention

India is the most ancient civilization and has its own way of living; the scriptures mention it as *Sanatan* way of living. It has customs, traditions and culture which define the different codes of ethics, behaviour, lifestyle and every aspect of human life. It talks about one's daily routine, type of diet, *Yoga-asana*, and rituals. It is not a religion but rather a way of living. It is based on the tenets of achieving *Moksha* or salvation and thus, restricts to its followers to speak truth and follow the right path. The *Sanatan Sanskriti* is above the religion and based on experiences rather than blind teachings. This *Sanatan* way of living is much ancient to Hinduism, which was the religion being practiced by majority of people in this geographical area. The principles of *Sanatan Sanskriti* were central to Hinduism. The *Sanatan Sanskriti*, *Yoga* and *Ayurveda* are invaluable gifts of India's ancient tradition. *Sanatan Sanskriti* defines how to live a life; *Yoga* unites mind, body and soul for attainment of physical, mental and spiritual health. *Ayurveda* deals with preventing diseases and promoting positive health (*Patanjali Yogasutra*; Sadguru, 2018). All these are known to increase immunity and our defense mechanism essentially needed to fight all diseases including Covid 19. Our lifestyle, behaviour and nutrition are the key factors to fight from diseases. The *Sanatan* way of living has stressed on these tenets for living a healthy life and numerous scriptures are available in support of that. The *Sanatan* practices have many of the preventive measures essentially required to fight Covid-19. We shall see how these ancient measures are capable of preventing pandemic and are in coherence with our modern epidemiological and scientific knowledge.

Hand Washing

The concept of cleanliness ("*Shaucha*" in Sanskrit) is vital in

Sanatan traditions. The cleanliness or purity of anything decides if it is usable or not. The importance given to hand washing, cleaning of body, surroundings and objects to be used is such that your work will be fruitful only if everything is clean. The use of unclean object was rather a sin in ancient traditions. In *Sanatan* concept it is essential to wash hands before eating and performing any ritual. It was also essential to wash hand with water and fly ash or clay or *Lona* (having detergent properties) after use of toilets. To prevent infection there was a concept of separate slippers made of wood, for outdoor and indoor work. Bringing outdoor slippers inside the rooms and vice-versa was strictly prohibited. People following these rules of *Sanatan* way of life requests visitors to remove sandal, shoes or slippers outside the house to prevent any probable spread of infection. The description of cleanliness, hygiene and purity are mentioned by *Patanjali* in *Yogasutras*, here *Shaucha* is described as—

शौचात्स्वाङ्गजुगुप्सा परैरसंसगगः ॥ (2.41)
सत्त्वशुद्धिसौमन्यैकाग्र्येन्द्रियजयात्समदशगनयोग्यत्सवानन च ॥ (2.41

Shaucha is that from which there arises dislike i.e., dispassion towards one's body and detachment towards contact with others. *Shaucha* gives rise to purity of mind, contentment, one-pointedness, conquest of the senses and competency to attain *Atma-Darshana* (Self-Realization). *Manusmriti* also describes *Shaucha* as one of the four *Niyamas* or duties (Sridhar, 2020).

अहिंसा सत्सयम् अ्तेयं शौचम् इन्द्रियननग्रः ।
एतं सामानसकं धमं चातुवगर्ण्ये अब्रवीन् मनुः ॥ (10.63)

Non-violence, truth, non-stealing, cleanliness/purity and sense-control are the duties that are common for all four classes, so declares Manu. Hence, cleanliness is a prime duty as per *Sanatan* traditions. Violation of cleanliness of body, mind or soul was considered as sin. Quite similar to these during Covid-19 times where not washing hand is a sin and every celebrity, sportsperson and others are requesting to wash hands with soap or sanitizer regularly.

No Spitting in Public

The *Sanatan* philosophy further stresses on cleanliness of environment. *Atharvaveda* mentions the Earth as a Mother, a Living force. The *Manusmriti* says that no one should throw filthy substances like urine, faeces, saliva, cloths infected by impure substances, blood and other poisonous things. Thus, at that timeour culture also cared for water pollution, soil pollution and bio-medical waste. It also emphasizes on about hygienic disposal of faeces and urine and suggested covering them in deep ground with sticks, grass, leaves, clod etc. for natural decomposition. Thus, *Sanatan* culture was following hygienic practices and environmental friendly methods of waste disposal to sustain healthy life, environment and development much before the world thought of the concept of hygiene, waste disposal and sustainable development (*Manusmriti*).

Yoga and *Ayurveda*

Yoga uses various postures, breathing exercises, and meditation to improve overall health. *Yoga* was developed in India as a spiritual practice thousands of years ago. Today, many western nations have adopted *yoga* for exercise and to reduce stress. *Yoga* is one of the best ways available for stress management. It emphasizes on unifying mind with body and soul to promote mental, spiritual and physical wellbeing. Vedic literature says, one has to clean all the body secretions to avoid various infections and allergies. This includes nasal mucus secretions, ear wax, phlegm, tears, rheum of the eyes and sweat. Even in the times of Covid-19, *Yoga* will not only improve lung capacity but also stabilize mental health to overcome the stress and depression associated with pandemic.

Ayurveda originated in India more than 5,000 years ago and is often called the "Mother of All Healing." In *Sanskrit* it means "The Science of Life". Here emphasis is on prevention and encourages the maintenance of health through close attention to balance in one's life, right thinking, diet, lifestyle and the use of herbs (Bihar Yoga; U.S. National Library of Medicine; Lad).

Namaste—The Indian Welcome starts with *Namaskar*

The Indian way of greeting one another has become global now as it does not require touching or coming close. Many famous international personalities have adopted Indian *Namaskar* for greeting others instead of handshake. Now its importance is being realized for implementing the social distancing. *Namaskar* means "I bow to the divine in you" and is a way of saying 'May our minds meet', indicated by the folded palms placed before the chest. This is an evidence of India's rich cultural heritage being in line with modern scientific rationale.

Social Distancing—Social Stratification in Ancient India

Social distancing is being followed to prevent the spread of Corona virus. The idea is to avoid being too close to contact the aerosols from infected person. Public is advised to stay out of crowded places and avoid going out. (CDC, Social Distancing). But people in essential services like doctors, health care workers and others called Corona Warriors— have to go out and are unfortunately getting infected. The occupational risk of getting infected is highest amongst doctors and staff of hospitals. This has given rise to social stigma and some people see these frontline workers as agents of infection. Probably the public has to realize that in this Covid-19 era we have to follow physical distancing, but not any kind of hatred with Corona warriors as they are the real fighters.

When we look at ancient Indian system of social stratification, i.e., the *Varna Vyayastha,* it was based on occupation or *Karma* and main principle behind was probably the risk of transmission of infectious agents. As mentioned in *Manusmriti,* the society was stratified into four categories (*varnas*) - *Brahmins, Kshatriyas, Vaishyas* and the *Shudras. Brahmins* were mainly priests, teachers and intellectuals. *Kshatriyas,* were the administrator, warriors and rulers, *Vaishyas* were the artists, farmers, merchants and traders. *Shudras* were manual laborers. It is understandable that due to different occupational nature of *varnas,* their risk of transmitting infections were different. The *dalits,* truly the warriors of keeping public safe, were involved in cleaning of wastes, streets and drains. They definitely had the highest risk of transmitting infection to others, while the *Brahmins* had minimal risk of transmission to other *varnas* due to their nature of work. Such type of stratification must have been carefully thought and used at those times to prevent spread of infectious diseases from one section to the other. However, unfortunately with time, the work-based concept of *varna* system converted to birth-based caste system in the society. Though, today the caste system has many more implications in our society, the original concept of *varna* system might have been to prevent disease by maintaining the Social Distancing (US History, 2021).

Protection from Mask: Our Traditional Gamchha

The MoHFW, Govt. of India has recommended the use of mask in public places for protection from COVID-19. Earlier, its use was limited to those with symptoms and healthcare workers, but expert opinion has changed because of asymptomatic carriers (CDC, Atlanta). Then queries raised on type of mask and its availability for 1.3 billion Indians.

The homemade mask of cotton cloth was declared to be good enough for the public by MoHFW (Government of India Advisory, 2020).

Indian *gamchha* is a traditional thin cotton cloth used very commonly in many rural parts. This works well as a mask considering its availability. Traditionally, it is used to dry the body after bathing or wiping sweat and worn on one side of the shoulder. Its appearance and name varies from region to region and is produced as a handicraft. It serves an excellent purpose of protecting public from contracting disease. It can be easily used by anyone as compared to the surgical mask, which is costly, short of supply and has a specific way to use (CDC Atlanta, Use Masks).

Indian Vegetarian Food: *Sanatan Dharma's Satvik Bhojan*

Our traditional food is mainly vegetarian; in fact, globally India has maximum number of vegetarians. Even in the diverse range of cuisines the basic tenets are the same, use of vegetable, fruits and spices are essential. *Mnasollsa* (The Delight of Mind), written in 12th century, describes the need to change cuisine and food with seasons (Live History India, 2018). Utilization of local foods was promoted in *Satvik Bhojan* for staying healthy and fit. Indian philosophy of non-violence (*ahimsa*) keeps us away from animal chain of infective diseases. Rather we have the concept of worshipping animals, as cow is regarded the symbol of fortune and wealth. Non-vegetarian diet is a taboo in *Sanatan Sanskriti*. This is the best example of disease prevention in Indian philosophy. As we all know the suspicious, but official origin of this SARS-CoV2 is animal market of Wuhan, China. The relation of food and health was well known as reflected in this quote from the *Bhagavad Gita* (*Bhaktivedanta Vedabase*).

"Foods dear to those in the mode of goodness, increase

the duration of life, purify one's existence and give strength, health, happiness and satisfaction. Such foods are juicy, fatty, wholesome, and pleasing to the heart. Foods that are too bitter, too sour, salty, hot, pungent, dry and burning are dear to those in the mode of passion. Such foods cause distress, misery and disease. Food prepared more than three hours before being eaten, food that is tasteless, decomposed and putrid, and food consisting of remnants and untouchable things is dear to those in the mode of darkness." (*Lord Krishna, Bhagavad-Gita 17.8-10*)

Intake of Vitamin D

We all know that vitamin D plays a significant role in our immunity system. The studies on COVID-19 are showing that low level of Vitamin D is associated with high mortality especially in elderly population of developed countries (Morris, 2020). Vitamin D supplementation is now recommended to prevent these deaths (Ilie, Stefanescu and Smith, 2020). Vitamin D synthesis occurs naturally in our skin cells on exposure to sunlight. Daily exposure to early morning sunlight is required. It is advised to get exposure to sunlight, sunbath for 30-40 minutes in a week with about 40% uncovered body (Nair and Maseeh, 2012). The *Sanatan* way of living had a concept of offering water to the sun just after taking bath in the morning in minimal clothes. This early morning exposure to the sunlight if done regularly for seven days serves the modern scientific recommendation. We need to realize the science behind our culture and follow it. (Chandwani, 2018).

Disposal of Dead Dodies of Covid-19 Patients

The Covid-19 infected bodies have to be treated with utmost precautions, and guidelines were issued for the same to avoid spread of infection to person performing last rites. In *Sanatan* system, dead bodies are cremated by burning to ashes, a complete mechanism of killing or destruction of disease causing agents as compared to the process of burial, which might transmit infection through worms. These worms could be eaten by birds or bats; and might again be eaten by humans to get infected. In *Sanatan* system during these rituals the person, who perform last rites, has to discard all his clothes, remove hairs and take bath many times and remain almost in quarantine for at least thirteen days. Probably these thirteen days, compulsory quarantine would have been made equal to the duration of incubation period of infectious diseases. During this period he has to stay alone, keep physical distancing with other family and community members, and only one person gives him food and other essential things. The *Sanatan* traditions of removing hair and staying separate were probably to reduce the chance of spreading infection. Thus, we understand that *Sanatan* cultural practices were scientific, evidence based and quite efficient in prevention of infectious diseases.

Conclusion

Most of us today are inclined towards modern and advanced culture of the West without even exploring or realizing what all we have in *Sanatan* culture. Indian civilization has been one of the most ancient and biggest one. This was the place of learning for scholars all around the world. *Sanatan Sanskriti* has many preventive measures essentially required to fight Covid-19. Either it be the importance of cleanliness, regular practice of *yoga* or utilization of natural medicine of *Ayurveda*. We have to realize the importance of our traditions and customs by visualizing it from the scientific lens. We never thought that we are following physical distancing while bowing for a *Namaskar* and that the classification of society is probably to prevent disease spread. The pandemic is here to change our behaviour, social structure and also the thought process. The nature has shown us that we were on the right path decades back. Our traditional *gamcha,* local food and traditional rituals including even the last rites were all coherent with the scientific rationale. There is definite need of more profound research to study evidence for the hidden scientific underpinnings in favor of our traditional practices so that it be well accepted by the scientific community.

REFERENCES

1. Bhaktivedanta Vedabase. *Bg. 17.8.* Retrieved on 28th December, 2020 from https://vedabase.io/en/library/bg/17/8/.
2. BBC News. (2019, June 19). What is India's Caste System? *BBC News.* Retrieved on 26th December, 2020 from https://www.bbc.com/news/world-asia-india- 35650616.
3. Bihar Yoga, https://www.biharyoga.net/
4. CDC Atlanta. Social Distancing. *CDC Atlanta.* Retrieved on 24th December, 2020 from https://www.cdc.gov/coronavirus/2019-ncov/prevent-getting-sick/social-distancing.html
5. CDC Atlanta. Use Masks to Slow the Spread of COVID-19. Coronavirus Disease 2019 (COVID-19). *CDC Atlanta.* Retrieved on 28th December, 2020 from https://www.cdc.gov/coronavirus/2019-ncov/prevent-getting-sick/diy-cloth-face-coverings.html accessed on 28/12/20
6. Centers for Disease Control and Prevention (CDC) Atlanta. How to Protect Yourself and Others. *Centers for Disease Control and Prevention.* Retrieved on 13th December, 2020 from https://www.cdc.gov/coronavirus/2019-ncov/prevent-getting-sick/prevention.html
7. Chandwani, Nikhil. (2018, October 25). *Sanatan Dharma*- The Way of Living: India's Gift to the World. *Thriveglobal.* Retrieved on 29th December 2020 from https://thriveglobal.com/stories/sanatan-dharma-the-way-of-living/
8. Government of India. (2020, April 3) *Advisory on use of Homemade Protective Cover for Face & Mouth.* Issued by the Office of the Principal Scientific Advisor to the Government of India.
9. Ilie, Petre Cristian; Stefanescu, Simina and Smith, Lee. *The Role of Vitamin D in the Prevention of Coronavirus Disease 2019 Infection and Mortality.* Retrieved on 29th December, 2020 from DOI:10.21203/rs.3.rs-21211/v1 https://www.researchsquare.com/article/rs-21211/v1
10. Lad, Vasant. Ayurveda: A Brief Introduction and Guide. *Ayurveda.* Retrieved on 22nd December, 2020 from https://www.ayurveda.com/resources/articles/ayurveda-a-brief-introduction-and-guide.

11. Live History India. (2018 November 30). What Indians Ate in the 12th Century. *LHI Team*. Retrieved on 28th December, 2020 from https://www.livehistoryindia.com/snapshort-histories/2018/11/30/what-indians-ate-in-the-12th-century
12. *Manusmriti the Laws of Manu*– Introduction. *Hinduwebsite*. Retrieved on 21st December, 2020 from https://www.hinduwebsite.com/sacredscripts/hinduism/dharma/ manusmriti.asp accessed on 21/12/20
13. Ministry of Culture, Government of India. Accessed on 23rd December, 2020 https://www.indiaculture.nic.in
14. Ministry of Health and Family Welfare. *MoHFW*. Retrieved on 2nd December, 2020 from www.mohfw.gov.in/.
15. Morris, Amanda. (2020 May 7). *Vitamin D Levels Appear to Play Role in COVID-19 Mortality Rates*. Retrieved on 29th December, 2020 from https://www.mccormick.northwestern.edu/news/articles/2020/05/vitamin-d-levels-appear-to-play-role-in-covid-19-mortality-rates.html accessed on 29/12/20
16. Nair, R. and Maseeh, A. (2012, April) Vitamin D: The "Sunshine" Vitamin. J Pharmacol Pharmacother. 3(2), 118 126. doi:10.4103/0976-500X.95506
17. *Patanjali Yogasutra*. Retrieved on 16th December, 2020 from https://patanjaliyogasutra.in/article/patanjali-yog-sutra/ accessed on 16/12/20
18. Sadguru. (2018, December 21). *The True Nature of Patanjali's Yoga Sutra. Isha Foundation*. Retrieved on 17th December, 2020 from https://isha.sadhguru.org/in/en/wisdom/article/patanjali-yoga-sutras-true-nature.
19. Sridhar, Nithin. (2020 August 10). The Concept of *Shaucha* or Cleanliness in Hindu Dharma. *Centre for Indic Studies*. Retrieved on 18th December, 2020 from https://www.cisindus.org/2020/03/23/the-concept-of-shaucha-or-cleanliness-in-hindu-dharma/
20. U.S. National Library of Medicine. Yoga for Health. *Medlineplus*. Retrieved on 22nd December, 2020 from https://medlineplus.gov/ency/patientinstructions/000876.htm
21. US History. (2021). The Caste System. *Ancient Civilizations Online Textbook*. Retrieved on 26th December, 2020 from https://www.ushistory.org/civ/8b.asp.
22. *What is the Caste System in India?* Accessed online from https://www.worldatlas.com/articles/the-caste-system-of-india.html
23. World Health Organization. (2020). *COVID-19 Public Health Emergency of International Concern (PHEIC)*. Global Research and Innovation Forum: Towards a Research Roadmap. Retrieved from https://www.who.int/blueprint/priority-diseases/key-action/Global_Research_ Forum_

FINAL_VERSION_for_web_14_feb_2020.pdf

24. World Health Organization. (2020, 29 March). Modes of Transmission of Virus Causing COVID-19: Implications for IPC Precaution Recommendations. World Health Organization. Retrieved on 12th December, 2020 from www.who.int/news-room/commentaries/detail/modes-of-transmission-of-virus-causing-covid-19-implications-for-ipc-precaution-recommendations.
25. Yatharth Sandesh. (2017 August 12), Sanatan Sanskriti Prithvi par Sarvasrestha kyun hai? *Yatharth Sandesh, Ancient Bhartiya Culture*. Retrieved on 13th December, 2020 from https://www. yatharthsandesh. com/blog/detailsnw/361

8

Epidemics and Pandemics: A Case Study of the Indian Experience of Spanish Flu in 1918

Rajkishor

ABSTRACT

If we see throughout the Indian History, it has encountered several epidemics and pandemics. This article discusses about such outbreaks known to have occurred in the twentieth century—Spanish Flu in 1918. The necessity to write this article is because the information is scattered and to source them and compile them into a single article could help the medical practitioners and healthcare workers to understand what this country has been through in the past and what reforms have to be made by them, the community and the government in preventing such outbreaks in the future. In the present Covid-19 scenario, this article has its own importance. Spanish flu, caused by a virus, claimed twelve million lives in India over a period of just three months in 1918. In this case, the British government tried to intervene, advocate social isolation and senitize the population. However, when the enemy is invisible, rapidly advancing and hard to explain, no amount of public or scientific advice, however reassuring it may be, is enough to dispel rumors and fear-mongering. History shows an unchanging pattern in people's reactions— they tend to point the finger of blame at an unknown entity, be it foreigners, another religion, the health system, those who eat meat or drink alcohol, but the British did little endeavours in this direction. There was no known cure, no vaccine, and no certainty how the flu could be contained. Many epidemiologists were looking to 1918-19 pandemic as a likely precedent for another pandemic of flu, and one that would hit countries like India particularly hard, but it did not happened in that expected way. Transport was the key carrier in the pandemics of our past. Spanish flu entered India through Bombay, most likely troops returning from the First World War in Europe, and then spread wavelike across the country from the west and south to the east and north. Covid-19 has reached India through international travel as well.

Keywords: COVID-19, Epidemics, History, Influenza, Spanish Flu, Vaccine.

Life in the submerged and mobile world that we have been looking at was miserable enough in normal times. But the time were often far from normal, for the history of British-ruled India is interspersed by repeated and devastating epidemics and pandemics in which rural landless labourers, migrant workers and artisans were invariably the worst affected. In 2020, after the spread of Corona virus and after completing about a century since 1918–19 Spanish Influenza, scholars are returning to its study to design appropriate pandemic control strategies (Morens and Fauci, 2007). By establishing a baseline picture of how the worst epidemiologic disaster of the modern era unfolded at its global focal point, it is hoped that this study will prompt future research that delves into the complex factors that created and shaped it spatially and temporally (Mills, Robins and Lipsitch, 2004). The lengthening and weakening of the pandemic wave as it swept across India also has broad implications for pandemic control strategies. The duration and intensity of pandemic control measures will need to be judiciously calibrated to the variable nature of any future pandemic wave. In scenarios resembling the 1918 pandemic as it unfolded in India, locations close to an entry point will have extremely short windows of time to deal with a virulent pathogen, placing emphasis on the emergency management of a short and severe wave of illness. While locations that are distant from the entry point will have longer windows of time to prepare for and deal with less lethal variants of the disease, their task will be prolonged by the more gradual build-up and subsidence of the epidemic wave.

Recent Corona virus outbreaks around the world have generated renewed interest in the study of the spread and properties of pandemic diseases with a view to mitigate their impacts (Glass *et. al.*, 2006; Bonabeau, *et. al.*, 1998). The so-called Spanish Influenza of 1918 was the most devastating pandemic in history, with a global death toll of between twenty to fifty million. Caused by a member of the H1N1 family of influenza viruses, the first wave of the disease emerged in the early months of 1918. In the autumn of 1918, a second and severe wave of the disease swept across the globe, leaving no major inhabited region untouched (Johnson and Mueller, 2002). The focal point of the epidemic in terms of mortality was India, with an estimated death toll range of 10–20 million, and an estimate of population loss of 13.8 million for the British-controlled provinces. Surprisingly, no modern study exists that comprehensively characterizes the spatial dynamics of the 1918 influenza in India even though Mills (1986) highlighted its importance through his description of its effects on India. The aim of this study is to use a comprehensive dataset to identify important features of the 1918-19 influenza pandemic in India that are of interest for the understanding of influenza epidemics. Striking findings include a reduction in peak-week mortality, a deceleration in velocity, a prolonging of the epidemic wave, and an overall reduction in virulence of the Spanish Influenza as it spread across India.

In India, it was observed that the phenomenon of two distinct epidemic waves, a mild one in the spring or summer of 1918, and a second and much more lethal one in the autumn or winter (Johnson and Mueller, 2002). Some countries experienced a third wave in 1919 or 1920. In an early attempt to characterize the spread of the pandemic, Pyle (1986) presented diffusion patterns of the disease alongside those of other influenza epidemics of the twentieth century. For England, Mexico and Peru, Chowell, *et. al.* (2010) identified the spread patterns, estimating mortality and transmissibility rates and distinguishing between rural and urban areas. Across Europe, several researchers including Ansart, *et. al.*, (2009) and Erkoreka (2010) estimated the mortality burden of the 1918 pandemic. In addition, early in the second wave, long distance infections were the predominant mode of transmission, with local infections becoming more frequent as the epidemic became widespread.

The Indian experience of the deadly Spanish flu of 1918 shows how pandemics interact with social divide across communities. A ship carrying Indian troops, reached the shores of Bombay on the 29th day of May in 1918. It remained anchored to the city's docks for about forty-eight hours. The world was on its last leg of the First World War, so the Bombay ports were usually busy with the movement of troops and goods back and forth from England. The ship, thus, remained an inconspicuous visitor on its waters among the humdrum of activity around it. However, the city was not prepared for some unusual cargo that had come unknown to anyone on the ship: lethal strains of the H1N1 influenza virus right from the trenches on the Western front. On 10th June, seven police sepoys, one of whom was posted at the dock, were hospitalised with what appeared to be influenza. They were India's first cases of the highly infectious Spanish flu that was rapidly sweeping across the world at the time. Bombay was soon crippled by the virus and railway lines carried it to different corners of the country. By the end of 1920, the pandemic claimed somewhere between fifty to hundred million lives globally – possibly more than both the World Wars combined. India was the country that bore the greatest burden suffering an estimated eighteen million casualties, which accounted for about 6 per cent of the country's population at the time (Singh, 2004).

Such flu pandemics have a peculiar characteristicss of engulfing the world in waves. The first wave is usually mild and resembles the seasonal flu. In the Spanish flu pandemic this wave lasted till July. Then, a second more lethal wave takes over, which began in September and lasted until the end of the year in 1918. The subsequent waves vary in virulence. A final wave of the Spanish flu was witnessed in the early months of 1919 and disease finally vanished by March 1920 (Shaman and Kohn, 2009). From the hilltops of Shimla to the isolated villages of Bihar, no part of the country remained unaffected. The speed and extent of the fatalities were overwhelming. In Bombay, 768 people died in a single day on 6th October in 1918. The Hindi poet, Suryakant Tripathi, popularly known as Nirala, wrote in his memoirs that "Ganga was swollen with dead bodies." He lost his wife and many members of his family to the flu, but could not find enough wood to perform their last rites (Pathak, 2007, 15-16). A report released by the Sanitary Commissioner in 1918 later documented that it was not just *Ganga* that was clogged up with bodies, but all rivers across India (India Sanitary Commissioners Report, 1916–20).

Even Gandhi, who was gaining recognition among intellectual circles as a future leader, came down with the flu in its second wave. "All interest in living had ceased," he later wrote in his autobiography. For a variety of reasons, the second wave proved particularly fatal for India. While the mortality rate for the epidemic stood at 4.7 per 1,000 people in Britain, India's mortality rate climbed to 20.6 per 1,000 people. The country's poor healthcare infrastructure had a key role to play in creating the disparity. But the arrival of the flu also coincided with a drought in 1918, which led to a famine in large parts of the country. Since, hunger weakens the immune system of the body, it made large segments of the population vulnerable to the virus. The colonial regime made matters worse. Despite the famine and the epidemic, Indian-grown food was continued to supply to the war efforts on the British front lines. Doctors were also away for the war (Sanitary Commissioner Annual Report, 1920).

There were other anomalies in the Indian experience with the Spanish flu as well. India was the only country where mortality of women was higher than men across all age groups. It is hard to explain why that was the case? The trend might have been due to the fact that women usually ate less well than men in the average Indian household as the latter gender was prioritised in case there was limitation of food. So, the women were more likely to be malnourished. Moreover, women were more likely to treat the sick as caregivers and, hence, more prone to the disease (Mills, 1986). Apart from gender, the divisions in mortality rates from the Spanish flu also ran across community lines. The mortality numbers from the second wave show the stark impact that birth and affluence can have on surviving an epidemic. Over 61 lower caste Hindus died per 1,000 in the community while merely 18.9 caste Hindus (sic) per 1,000 from the community lost their lives. The same figure for Europeans living in India at the time stood at 8.3. Since the lower caste Hindus were mostly engaged as sweepers and scavengers, it made them highly vulnerable to the spread of the virus. Also, they were usually housed in crowded, unhygienic conditions, and had less access to medical facilities (Chandra, *et. al.*, 2012).

While exposing the deep vulnerabilities that existed across

colonial India, the flu left some long-lasting effects as well. The British found them incapable of handling a crisis at this scale. So, a lot of local and caste organisations collectively mobilised themselves to assist relief efforts. Such grassroots organisations had existed across India for a while, but the flu united them across the country for a single cause. As a result, it was after this crisis that leaders like Gandhi managed to garner support of the grassroots organisations for the national movement as well. Thus, the Spanish flu in its sinister aftermath had a key role to play in paving the way for the freedom movement. India has progressed a lot since the ship carrying the deadly virus docked on the shores of Bombay a century ago. But as another virus – this time from the East – wreak havoc across the globe in 2020, India should look back to let history not repeat itself. The gender and class divide still run deep across Indian society. It is not hard to argue that social distancing and lockdowns come relatively easily for the well-off and they would also be the ones with easier access to healthcare facilities. While this reality has only marginally changed over the last century, the nature of the administration has drastically transformed from the colonial government to a democratically elected one. Only time will tell if the latter has any impact on the eventual outcome.

REFERENCES

1. Ansart, S. (2009). Mortality Burden of the 1918–1919 Influenza Pandemic in Europe. *Influenza Other Respir Viruses*, 3, 99-106
2. Bonabeau, E., Toubiana, L., Flahault, A. (1998). The Geographical Spread of Influenza. *Proc Royal Soc London Ser B: Biol Sci.*, 265, 2421-2425.
3. Chandra, S., Kuljanin, G., Wray, J. (2012). Mortality from the Influenza Pandemic of 1918–1919: The Case of India. *Demography*, 49, 857-865
4. Chowell, G., Viboud, C., Simonsen, L., Miller, M.A. and Acuna-Soto, R. (2010). Mortality Patterns Associated with the 1918 Influenza Pandemic in Mexico: Evidence for a Spring Herald Wave and Lack of Preexisting Immunity in Older Populations. *J Infect Dis.*, 202, 567-575.
5. Erkoreka, A. (2010). The Spanish Influenza Pandemic in Occidental Europe (1918–1920) and Victim age. *Influenza Other Respir Viruses*, 4, 81-89

6. Glass, R.J., Glass, L.M., Beyeler, W.E. and Min, H.J. (2006). Targeted Social Distancing Design for Pandemic Influenza. *Emerg Infect Dis.*, 12: 1671-1681
7. Annual Reports of the Sanitary Commissioners of Assam, Bihar and Orissa, Bengal, Bombay, Central Provinces, Madras, North West Frontier Provinces, Punjab and United Provinces of Agra and Oudh Government Press. 1916–20. Provincial Government Presses: Sanitary Commissions.
8. Johnson, NPAS, Mueller, J. (2002). Updating the Accounts: Global Mortality of the 1918-1920 "Spanish" influenza pandemic. *Bull Hist Med.* 76, 105-115.
9. Mills, C.E., Robins, J.M., Lipsitch. M. (2004). Transmissibility of 1918 Pandemic Influenza. *Nature*, 432, 904-906
10. Mills, I.D. (1986). The 1918–1919 Influenza Pandemic – The Indian Experience. *Indian Econ Soc History Rev.*, 23 (1), 1-40
11. Morens, D.M. and Fauci, A.S. (2007). The 1918 Influenza Pandemic: Insights for the 21st Century. *J Infect Dis.*, 195, 1018-1028
12. Pathak, Vachspati. (2007). *Prasad, Nirala, Pant evam Mahadevi ki Shreshth Rachnaein*. Allahabad: Lokbharti Publication.
13. Sanitary Commissioner. (1920). Annual Report of the Sanitary Commissioner with the Government of India. Calcutta: Superintendent of Government Printing.
14. Shaman, J. and Kohn, M. (2009). Absolute Humidity Modulates Influenza Survival, Transmission, and Seasonality. *Proc Nat Acad Sci USA*, 206 (9), 3243-3248
15. Singh, R.P: (2004). *India Administrative Atlas 1872–2001. A Historical Perspective of Evolution of Districts and States in India*. Delhi: Government of India

9
Women and Pandemic Times: The Biopsychosocial Model

Aparna Pathak

ABSTRACT

The status of women in society has always been changing since ancient times. Their position has been deteriorated and had gone through advanced phases also. The effect of pandemic on women had been huge in the whole world. In India, since females perform many responsibilities, therefore, the effect is a little on the higher side. In the nineteenth century, people witnessed cholera pandemic and flu pandemic. Later in twentieth century, other situations like Asian Flu, SARS, MERS and recently, the Ebola dangers were witnessed. There are various biological, psychological and social factors that changed the life of women during the pandemic times. It has been observed that in earlier times also the females were educated and were involved in extracurricular activities also. Covid-19 is not first pandemic experience that humans faced and it might not be the last one too, but what to be noticed is the difference of its impact on gender basis. While studying the history of epidemics, if biological factors are considered, many studies reveal that females have stronger immune system as compared to men, but their mental health shows high percentage of depression, anxiety and stress.

The pandemic increases emotional distress of women if they already had any mental or physical illness. As far as social factors are concerned, women share more responsibilities in holding the society together by their job, home, school, caring for elderly and other filial duties. Still they are dominated by the males in their jobs and at home as well. The Bio-Psycho-Social model deeply elaborates various aspects of women's condition during pandemic. The most universal role of women that is caregiving, surrounded by people who need care (children, elderly, family), and also their occupation as a health worker bring them to maximum exposure, although their work remains unnoticed.

Keywords: Biological, Psychological, Social Model

Women have a high place in families in India. They have always been the responsibility holders, caregivers and nurturers in their families. It has been observed that in earlier times also the females were educated and were engaged in various other activities. History shows queens like Rani Lakshmibai, Jodhabai, Rani Durgawati etc. Women were getting respect not only in modern era, but since ancient times, still gender seems to play a vital role in Indian society. Although women get respect in their families and society, yet they were not privileged as far as social stratification is considered. They were always disadvantaged and never stood in front when gender equality was considered. Although people had changed their views and now women are empowered. The present century is more concerned towards women. Legislative reforms are introduced to empower women and various government policies are adopted for female education. Still when a birth takes place the point of concern is gender.

At present we all are witnessing difficult periods, physically, mentally and financially. Prior to Covid-19, pandemics occurred many times. In nineteenth century, people witnessed cholera and flu pandemic. Later in twentieth century, other diseases like Asian flu, SARS, MERS and recently Ebola dangers were experienced, but in context to Covid-19, it is observed that it is on dissimilar measure. Its spread was very fast across the world with a disastrous effect in every arena of human civilization. Although the disease has nothing to do with gender, yet all over the world women's freedom is the soundless prey of the pandemic. When the question arises that what is the need of a pandemic patient? The answer is care. Older people who are more vulnerable to infectious diseases had to self-isolate themselves at home. So, what they need? Again – care. All the schools are closed. Children are bound to attend online classes and play indoor games. Who has to look after that? All this care-giving falls on the shoulders of women. This is so because of the present structure of the society. Despite the women entering the workforce, they are considered to be inferior. In comparison to men, there is a big chunk of women population who are doing part time jobs, and the time saved isn't used for leisure activities, but for household activities and looking after their children and other family members. Due to pandemic situations earlier too, there has been employee scarcity which opened access to the job market or labor market for women. The results were that the doors were opened for more jobs outside the home. Working women number increased after First World War. In 1918, influenza pandemic swallowed many people and took away employment of many men and women, who were left devastated. After this, increase in the percentage of women in workforce was witnessed. Now they were in every field like academics, marketing, business, law, medico, engineering and even politics. It was silver lining for them, but as it is said that every coin has two sides. Although they emerged prominently in the workforce of every field, but in commensuration to it their responsibilities too increased. Along with outdoor work they have to deal with the responsibility of homemaker too. Pandemics, then and now, effected women adversely. They have to face many physical, psychological and social problems. Covid-19 is not the first pandemic in history and it might not be the last one too, but the major issue here, is there any gender difference in its effects? The history of pandemics is like a book that has words which elaborates all the conditions. Let's take a brief glance at it.

First Pandemic Outbreak in Athens (430 BC)

In the history of pandemics, the earliest recorded pandemic was the great plague of Athens. This occurred after the Peloponnesian war and resulted in approximately 1,00,000 deaths. It was highly contagious with symptoms, such as rashes, high fever and diarrhea in different ages, gender and nationality. As far as physical health is considered, women were inferior in the male dominant society. Men used to bring diseases with them when they come back to home after travel. Women, who stayed at home, inevitably got infected. When we talk about the treatment, the money was spent on the treatment of males, while females had to take care of themselves. So, without getting treatment and care they use to end up in death. During that time, women had very few rights and no freedom. They would either be a priestess or have certain social responsibilities like, household works and taking care of children and elderly. Most of them were never mentioned by names. They were so much suppressed that, if not by disease, they die due to shame, guilt and psychological outburst of not taking care of their family members properly resulting their death.

Second Pandemic in Rome: Plague of Antonine (165 AD)

Millions of people died due to this strange disease. History records its origin from Huns, further spread to Germans and then Romans. In Rome, its spread was like a forest fire, further dispersing it to other parts. Its symptoms include diarrhea, fever, sour throat and puss filled sores. This disease continued until 180 AD. The physical health of women working at Catholic Church like deaconesses and widow, were affected. It was their duty to care and comfort the infected during epidemic. This was considered as the part of their job as a nurse and little credit was given to them. They became infected very easily and use to die because of no care. Thus, the mortality rate of women was more. Men were said to have positive energy and were protectors and the females had negative energy and were the destroyers. This plague went hand in hand with the first artistic depiction of South Asia's first Goddess, *Hariti*. She was said to be a *yakshi* and the *Mother of the Demons*. It was believed that *Hariti* and her demonic offspring use to steal and kill newborn children. The psychological health of women, then, was bound to be poor because of the emotional torture, blaming them for everything wrong. There are no historical recordings that mentions anything about their feeling or emotions, but a person who is physically and socially discarded could not stand up emotionally.

Third Pandemic Outbreak in Rome: Plague of Cyprian (249-262 AD)

This is called Plague of Cyprian because of the writings of Bishop Cyprian. The symptoms were vomiting, diarrhea, extreme eye burn, throat ulcers and decaying hands and feet. This plague resulted in severe manpower scarcities for food production and Roman army got severely affected. City inhabitants escaped to the country, but instead spread the infection. The status of women during this time also was the same as earlier. The women were inside the doors and were caregivers. Their physical health again suffered due to caring duties. They were nuns in the church who were bound to sacrifice their lives for taking care of others. Their social status didn't change for the good. Neither they could take any decisions nor were they allowed to stand in front and speak. It was an era, where infection was taken as a divine punishment for sins. In case of men, it was believed that they were punished due to alcohol consumption; while for women infection was linked to their character assassination believing that divine acted for their lustful dressing and poor morals. This led to a lot of emotional anguish to women.

Fourth Pandemic Outbreak in Egypt: Plague of Justinian (541 AD)

This plague originated in Egypt and is dubbed after Emperor Justinian, the ruler of Roman Empire. There was a great pandemic situation because during the second half of the sixth century BC, this disease knocked out Europe in at least three waves. Scientists had found that the cause of this plague was pathogen called *Yersinia pestis*. This pathogen disables the immune system. For the first time it was clear that these pathogens survived on small mammals like rats, mice etc. Scientists say that men were more vulnerable than women, but since men carried the disease to their home, where women were caregivers, they also got infected. Women had to stay indoors so they were maximum exposed to the pathogen carriers like rats and fleas and got infected. Studies reveal that the reproductive system of women got affected. It was seen that if women were pregnant, they use to face miscarriage and in future, if they survived, they were not able to conceive. Spending money on their treatment was thought as wastage It was the same society, giving no rights to women but accepting all the care and nurture from them. The psychological health of the women then, must be poor since the plague was affecting their immune and reproductive system.

Fifth Pandemic Outbreak in Europe: Leprosy (Eleventh Century)

Leprosy was present since ages, but it turned into a pandemic in eleventh century and was part of life till 1050. In its dangerous form it caused loss of fingers and toes, decay, blindness, weakness of bones. Some people thought, it was punishment of their sins but others use to view as sufferings, which Christ also went through. They thought that lepers would definitely go to heaven after so much suffering. The impact of leprosy was seen later, and is seen till now in the form of Leprosy hospitals and Leper houses.

Physically, both men and women were equally affected by the diseases, but psychologically and socially women condition was more pathetic when juxtaposed with men suffering from same diseases. They were deprived of any treatment and care, forcing them to beg for food and shelter. Women in early ages got infected because they were caregivers. A study shows that women had complex percentage of distortions in comparison to men. The main problem was that signs and symptoms used to appear late and they continued with their social and filial responsibilities. Thus, they were engaged in cooking, cleaning etc. so, they often repeat ulceration and other chronic deformities. Their mental health was again pitiable because they faced denunciation, isolation and were left to beg. It caused mental trauma because there was a fear of passing the disease to the next generation.

Sixth Pandemic Outbreak in Asia: The Bubonic Plague (1350)

This plague started in Asia and moved towards west. It was called "Black Death". It arrived in Europe when 12 ships with soldiers from the Black Sea stopped at the Sicilian port of Messina. Most of the soldiers were dead and those left were having black boils that oozed black blood and puss. These symptoms further led to other symptoms like vomiting, cold, diarrhea, body ache and then death. The reason was rats and fleas. The whole Europe was highly infected including England and France. Someone has to take care of millions of people falling sick and dying. That duty fell on the shoulders of women. It was decided that women will be kept to nurse those who fell ill or died. These women were elderly or widows. The death ratio during this plague was approximately 10 females for every 9 males. It was said that women use to acquire this disease earlier. Reasons for this difference are vague. Researcher studied the skeleton or remains of the females at that time and found that after recovering the female stature shrinked. A reason suggested for this is post-recovery males might have gained the nutritional food, but women were deprived of that. The social life of females was confined to their home boundaries. Since they were appointed as caregivers without their will, the mental pressure drained them. Researchers found that caregivers often turned into robbers, stole things and caused death to the patients.

Seventh Pandemic Outbreak in India: Third Cholera Pandemic (1852-1860)

Like the first and second Cholera pandemic, the third one also originated in India. It spread through the *Ganges* river delta, passed through Asia, Europe, North America and Africa. Millions of people died in this pandemic. Researchers studied and inferred that contaminated water was the reason behind the disease. The disease spread to Great Britain too where almost 23,000 people died. The symptoms included severe diarrhea, severe vomiting and leg cramps, which caused dehydration, septic shock and even death. It is said it took the life of person within eight hours of appearance of symptoms. The fatality rate was so high that locals struggled to bury all the dead. Studies reveal that adult women and school-age girls suffered more. They were more vulnerable to disease and diarrhea compared to males. It was also observed that if the woman was pregnant, the hormonal changes weaken the immune system and thus, the symptoms worsened. The social epidemiology showed that since women were deprived of resources and were not given the right of decision making, therefore, the spread of cholera in women was higher and the death rate was higher too. The psychological impact of caregiving duties was high. When the girls and women looked after the sick and ill people in the house, they experienced sleepless nights, fatigue and due to this they remained emotionally disturbed.

Eighth Pandemic in Europe: The Spanish Flu (1918)

This flu is considered as the deadliest one in the history. It started in Europe and United States and then swiftly spread its wings across the world. There was no vaccine and medicine and all were bound to stay at home. The flu was known as 'Influenza'. It attacked the respiratory system and was highly contagious. The infected person's cough or sneeze could infect persons near him by inhaling the germs in the air. A simple touch could also led to infection. Young children, elderly people, pregnant women and people previously having some medical conditions were more vulnerable. The symptoms were chills, fever and fatigue. Spain was knocked tough by the flu. Most of the European nations newspapers did not cover the pandemic news due to World War I; while being neutral, Spain media covered the flu news at a high rate, so it was dubbed as Spanish flu. As far as physical health is concerned, there was no difference in men and women mortality rate. Since economy underwent a big drop, the labor market was opened to women due to shortage of workers. Women began to work out along with the household works. This increased the percentage of women employment to almost 21 percent.

It had not been possible without the attack of Spanish flu. Subsequently, the social status of women too changed. They were working in every field—machine, textile, law and everywhere. They started demanding equal salary to men. As their place in society improved, they demanded more rights, especially right to vote. Now their focus was gender equality. This pandemic was overwhelming, but it brought a silver lining to the trodden. It embarked a new phase where women now can think and demand of freedom, employment and decision-making power. This improved their self-confidence and mental health.

Ninth Pandemic in China: Asian Flu (1956-1958)

This was a pandemic attack of Influenza A of H2N2 subtype that originated in China and then spread in the rest part of the world. Approximately two million people died during this pandemic. The symptoms of this flu were unsteady legs, kneeling, high fever, body pain, cough and cold. Pneumonia and bronchitis accounted for 50 per cent of the symptoms and the rest were cerebral and cardiovascular diseases with the after-effect of the disease. Infection rate was highest in young adults, children and pregnant women. There was no gender difference in the infection. Both males and females participated equally in the caregiving process. Male and female nurses and doctors went hand in hand for treatment and caregiving. What drew the attention was the effect on pregnant women. Number of miscarriages increased, hereditary defects, premature births, stillbirths, neonatal morbidity increased. This confirmed the serological effects of the influenza. Besides, now women enjoyed equal status in the society. The psychological problem, if any, was dissimilar to those of males.

Tenth Pandemic in China: Corona Virus (2019)

This is an ongoing pandemic that first originated in Wuhan,

China and spread all over the world. This was declared a public health emergency in January 2020 and a pandemic in March 2020 by World Health Organisation. This is the deadliest of all the pandemics that history had witnessed till now. The death toll is still rising. The public health emergency of international alarm had called the etiology agent as SARS-CoV-2, the serious acute respiratory syndrome-2. It attacked people from all socio-economic status. This disease seems to have three patterns. *First,* moderate adversity involving upper respiratory tract; *second,* non-life-threatening pneumonia; and *third,* severe pneumonia with acute respiratory distress from mild to severe. The studies had shown that Covid-19 infection in spreading regardless of age. Whatever one thinks it is the women who bears most of the responsibilities, be it household work, job market, labor market, children's education, health care and many more. Despite of this fact they are paid less in systems where salary is not prescribed. Research had shown that domestic, sexual and gender-based harassment had increased during the current pandemic times. During quarantine time the dominant or violent males are considered as great physical and psychological danger.

It had been observed that 70% of the health care providers in the frontline are women. Since they had to stay in hospitals or Covid-care cells (specially made for the present pandemic times) they are in direct contact with the infected people. This cause them physical hazard and a fear of getting infected. Also, they are not allowed to go home or outside the hospital since they have to remain isolated because they are in contact with the patient. This resulted in mental agony of being separated from their families and not being able to fulfill their responsibility as a mother, daughter or wife.

Not all the pandemics are discussed, but all had severe economic effect on women. The most universal role of women is caregiving, surrounded by people who need care (children, elderly, family), and also their occupation as a health worker bring them to maximum exposure, although their work remained unnoticed. As per history, nursing job is considered the domain of women with 85 per cent women and 15 per cent men. During Zika virus outbreak there was power difference between men and women thereby meaning that women had no power or independence of their sexual and reproductive lives which was compounded by their medical or financial resources. As far as decision-making is considered the history of pandemics shows that women have insufficient or no rights of decision-making throughout.

For the first time in history of pandemics, it is Covid pandemic during which gender difference had become apparent to the world. Most of the studies on pandemics are either gender specific or gender blind. There is need to understand the effects of pandemic on men and women differently so that difference in coping strategies and psychological effects can be observed. There is another thing which is breaking people, and that is poverty. Education is the best source to eradicate poverty by getting a job. During pandemic girls had to stay at home and due to lack of money, education was made unavailable to them. This leads to emotional torture and feeling of sadness and depression. UN Women, the United States unit had launched the Shadow Pandemic public service campaigns, focusing on the global increase in domestic violence. WHO released a short film *Violence against Women: Strengthening the Health System Response*. It shows domestic violence in pandemic situation. Further, it is required to understand the needs, physical health and mental health of women along with men to maintain peace, harmony and gender equality. Government necessarily should take steps to increase the social safety net and identify the worth of imperceptible and voluntary care work.

REFERENCES

1. Almond, D. (2006). Is the 1918 Influenza Pandemic Over? Long-term Effects of In Utero Influenza Exposure in the Post-1940 U.S. Population. *Journal Political Economy*, 114(4): 672–712. doi: 10.1086/507154.
2. Benedictow, O. J. (2005). The Black Death: The Greatest Catastrophe Ever. *History Today*, 55(3): 42–49.1
3. Cleaning and Disinfecting Your Facility. *Centers for Disease Control and Prevention*. Retrieved from https://www.cdc.gov/coronavirus/2019ncov/community/organizations/cleaning-disinfection.html
4. Sequence for Putting on Personal Protection Equipment. Ministry of Health and Family Welfare. Retrieved from https://www.cdc.gov/niosh/npptl/pdfs/PPE-Sequence-508.pdf
5. DeWitte, S. N. (2014). Mortality Risk and Survival in the Aftermath of the Medieval Black Death." *PLOS One*, 9(5): e96513. doi: 10.1371/journal.pone.0096513.
6. Environmental Protection Agency, USA. (2020). List N: Disinfectants for Coronavirus (COVID-19). Retrieved from www.epa.gov/pesticide-registration/list-n-disinfectants-coronavirus-covid-19.
7. Gottfried, R. S. (1983). *The Black Death: Natural and Human Disaster in Medieval Europe*. NEW York and London: The Free Press of Macmillan
8. History.com Editors. (2020). Pandemics That Changed History. *History.com*, A& E Television Networks. Retrieved from www.history.com/topics/middle-ages/pandemics-timeline.
9. MoHFW, National Centre for Disease Control. (2020). "National Guidelines for Infection Prevention and Control in Health Care Facility." Retrieved from https://www.mohfw.gov.in/pdf/National%20 Guidelines % 20 for%20IPC%20in%20HCF%20- %20final%281%29.pdf.
10. MoHFW. (2020). Novel Coronavirus Disease 2019 (COVID 19): Guidelines on Rational Use of Personal Protective Equipment. Retrieved from https://www.mohfw.gov.in/pdf Guideline sonrationaluseof Personal Protective Equipment.pdf
11. Pittet, D. (2009). Hand Hygiene in Health Care First Global Patient Safety Challenge Clean Care is Safer Care. *World Health*. 30(1): 270.
12. Thucydides. (2017). *History of the Peloponnesian War*. (Crawley R., Trans.) Digireads.com Publishing.
13. WHO. (2007) Addressing sex and gender in epidemic-prone infectious diseases Unpublished manuscript, Geneva.
14. WHO. (2009). "WHO Guidelines on Hand Hygiene in Health Care. Retrieved from http://whqlibdoc.who.int/publications/2009/9789241597906_eng.pdf
15. WHO. Infection Prevention and Control Guidance for Long-Term Care

Facilities in the Context of Covid 19. Retrieved from https://apps.who.int/iris/bitstream/handle/10665/331508/WHO-2019-nCoV-IPC_long_term_care2020.1-eng.pdf

16. World Health Organization. Water, Sanitation, Hygiene and Waste Management for the COVID-19 Virus. 2020; (March):1–9. Retrieved from https://www.who.int/publications-detail/water-sanitationhygiene- and-waste-management-for-covid-19

10
Pandemics and Epidemics: God's Hand? A Biblical View

Chandana John

ABSTRACT

Epidemics and pandemics have been a part of human history and a brief chronology of the various plagues which have affected mankind since recorded historical times, give us a glimpse of the suffering that assailed mankind from time to time. As overwhelmed as we are, dealing with the Covid-19 today, the historical records does point to the resilience of the human race as a whole. The Bible records many plagues and pestilences which affected people who had been disobedient and rebelled against God Almighty, the creator of whole universe. The God of the Bible is a just God who does not pardon sin but is ready to forgive them if the people repent and acknowledge their wrong doings. The uncompromising God who insists righteous living causes Him to warn people again and again through calamities and natural disasters just like a father trying to correct a child headed the wrong way. The Bible does not record any medical facilities. The priests and prophets convey God's displeasure to the people often at the risk of their own lives. This unwillingness to listen to the voice of God and the stubborn reliance on one's own self characterizes mankind throughout the generations and to the end of age. The present pandemic may be another clarion call for humanity to accept God's sovereignty. Interestingly, most people agree that the end times are here, where all the values are upside down and wickedness and evil reigns. The prophecies of Jesus as well as the book of revelation, the last book in the Bible, written by Apostle John speaks about epidemics occurring on earth in the end times. A study of the Bible leads a believer to conclude that pandemics and epidemics are signs of God's anger and point to a final reckoning of good and evil. This chapter is an attempt to delve into the Biblical view of epidemics occurrences.

Keywords: Bible, Epidemic, God, Pandemic, Pestilence, Priests and Prophets.

An epidemic is a disease that affects a large number of people while a pandemic can be defined simply as an infectious disease which spread throughout the world. The words plague and pestilence extensively used in the Bible, has a similar meaning and has been used as synonyms in this paper. Pandemics have been recorded in history from the ancient times. One of the very first pandemic occurred in 430 B.C. during the Peloponnesian war which is said to have decimated two-thirds of the population. Another pandemic called the Antonine plague started with the Huns in 165 A.D and spread through wars and battles to the entire Roman Empire, raging for a span of about fifteen years. 250 A.D. witnessed the Cyprian plague in Carthage and its outbreak continued in intervals for the next three centuries and finally reached Britain in 444 A.D. The Justinian plague erupted in Egypt in 541 A.D. affecting Palestine, the Byzantine Emperor and the Mediterranean. Recurrences over the next two centuries eventually killed about fifty million people which was 26 per cent of the world population.

In the eleventh century, leprosy emerged as a pandemic in Europe. 1350 was the year of Black Death, Bubonic plague, which spread rapidly, decimating one third of the world's population and even forcing truce between two warring countries—France and England. Colonization efforts by the Europeans brought about a recurrence of different diseases in the native populations of the colonies. In the year 1665, London was hit by the bubonic plague which took life of 20 per cent of its population and took almost a year to subside. The second decade of the nineteenth century witnessed the first outbreak of cholera in 1817, beginning in Russia, then spread by the British troops to India and also to Spain, Africa, Indonesia, China, Japan, Italy, Germany and America.

The third outbreak of the bubonic plague began in 1855 in China and spread to India and Hong Kong claiming fifteen million lives. Twenty years later, Fiji measles killed one-third of the island's population, around forty thousand people. The pandemic called Russian flu started in Siberia and Kazakhstan, travelled to Moscow, and made its way to Finland and then Poland, from where it moved into the rest of Europe. By the following year, it had crossed the ocean to North America and Africa. By the end of 1890, three hundred and sixty thousand people had lost their lives. The Spanish flu of 1918 spread throughout the world rapidly. The Asian flu of 1957 is documented as:

> Starting in Hong Kong and spreading throughout China and then into the United States, the Asian flu became widespread in England where, over six months, 14,000 people died. A second wave followed in early 1958, causing an estimated total of about 1.1 million deaths globally, with 116,000 deaths in the United States alone. A vaccine was developed, effectively containing the pandemic.

AIDS was first identified in 1981 claiming thirty-five million lives around the world and a cure is yet to be developed. SARS or severe acute respiratory syndrome was identified in

2003, beginning in China, it spread to twenty-six other countries, infecting eight thousand and ninety six people, with nearly eight hundred deaths. The pandemic that we are still battling in the year 2020 began last year in China and has spread rapidly to more than one hundred and sixty-three countries around the world. On 11th March 2020, the World Health Organization announced that the COVID-19 virus was officially a pandemic after spreading through one hundred and fourteen countries in three months and infecting over one hundred and eighteen thousand people by that time. As it continues to ravage the world, people are trying to come to terms with this situation and adjust to a new way of life. While the medical community is trying hard to find a cure for this virus, God fearing people are interpreting the pandemic as a call to restore spiritual health, a direct intervention of God to bring home to humanity their limitations in spite of the tremendous surge in science and technology throughout the years. Along with natural disasters like floods, tornadoes, droughts, earthquakes, wildfires and the like, pandemics cause widespread devastation and misery and mankind seems so puny and small in their faces. The helplessness of the very situation makes us yearn for a saviour God and the Bible is quite clear in its view that a godless world is headed towards suffering.

The God of the Old Testament chooses the Israelites as his own and is ready to bless them even after they have disobeyed His commands if they turn to Him and cry out for His mercy. The Bible records their suffering as slaves in Egypt under Pharaoh. God empowered his Prophet Moses to lead them out, but it was not easy. Pharaoh was not willing to let go of his bonded labour and so God intervened with ten plagues or disasters which affected only the Egyptians but not the Israelites, making Pharaoh understand that he is dealing with the God Almighty and has no choice in the matter as mentioned below:

> 'Thus says the Lord, the God of the Hebrews, "Let My people go, that they may serve Me." For if you refuse to let them go and continue to hold them, behold, the hand of the Lord will come with a very severe pestilence.' (*Exodus* 9: 1-3, NASB).

We did not come across doctors or medically trained personnel trying to combat an epidemic like the present times, but the priests and the prophets respond to a situation of crisis and they explain why it had happened and the way to healing. For instance, prophet Jeremiah warned King Zedekiah that all the inhabitants of Jerusalem would die by the sword, famine and pestilence due to the Israelites' transgressions. Whereas prophets delivered godly messages, and helped to uncover the reason of illness, priests communicated with God through rituals. If the cause of illness was God's anger, only God could provide way for recovery from it. Therefore, one had to appease His anger. For example, priests advised the Philistines to return the ark of covenant together with a guilt offering in the book of first Samuel, chapter six. Guilt offering was a sacrifice which the priests carried out especially in a situation of an unintentional offence on behalf of the transgressor. Thus, we see that widespread infectious disease which we now term as pandemic may be one of the ways God calls humans to follow His ways rather than the world's at large for it is universally true that mankind tries to make sense of what is happening around him and in this quest can well be led to a higher spiritual wisdom in a time of uncertainty and fear. In the Book of Numbers, we read that God allowed a plague to execute judgment against unrepentant Israelites, and to shake the rest of the nation of Israel in an attempt to draw them closer to Him.

> [T]he Lord spoke to Moses, saying, 'Get away from among this congregation, that I may consume them instantly.' Moses said to Aaron Make atonement for them, for wrath

> has gone forth from the Lord, the plague has begun.' Then Aaron took it as Moses had spoken, and ran into the midst of the assembly, for behold, the plague had begun among the people. So, he put on the incense and made atonement for the people. He took his stand between the dead and the living, so that the plague was checked. But those who died from the plague were 14,700." Numbers 16:41-50 (NASB).

Numbers, 25:1-9 records another instance of plague occurring as a sign of God's displeasure.

> ...Those who died by the plague were twenty and four thousand. And the Lord spake unto Moses saying, Phine has...hath turned my wrath away from the children of Israel...(10,11)

These two instances not only show God's anger, but also how His servants attempt to contain the plague by appeasing God. The first book of Samuel, chapter five, shows, how the God sent a plague against the Philistines living in and around Gaza because of their chronic and unrepentant sin. Now the hand of the Lord was heavy on the Ashdodites, and He made them feel devastated and struck them with tumours, both Ashdod and its territories (*25 : 6*) because they had taken the ark of the God of Israel away.

> ...the hand of the Lord was against the city, creating a very great panic; and He struck the people of the city, from the young to the old, so that tumour broke out on them. (*25 : 9*)

The second book of Samuel, chapter twenty four records another plague which God uses to punish David, the King of Israel for his sin.

> So the Lord sent a plague upon Israel from the morning until the appointed time, and seventy thousand of the

> people from Dan to Beersheba died.. . Then David spoke to the Lord..and said, 'Behold, it is I who have sinned, and it is I who have done wrong'...David built there an altar to the Lord and offered burnt offerings and peace offerings. And the Lord responded to prayer for the land, and the plague was withdrawn from Israel. (*25 : 24*)

In the Book of Jeremiah, the ancient Hebrew prophet speaks a word of great warning to a gathering of apostate leaders.

> [H]ear now this word which I am about to speak in your hearing and in the hearing of all the people. The prophets who were before me and before you from ancient times prophesied against many lands and against great kingdoms, of war and of calamity and of pestilence. (*Jeremiah* 28: 7-8, NASB)

In the Book of Ezekiel, the Lord God warned that the nation of Judah would be struck with terrible diseases as a part of its judgment at the time when the Babylonians would come to conquer the land and destroy Jerusalem. This prophecy came to pass in the period leading up to and during 586 B.C. The prophet Ezekiel says:

> Thus says the Lord God, 'This is Jerusalem; I have set her at the center of the nations, with lands around her. But she has rebelled against My ordinances more wickedly than the nations and against My statutes more than the lands which surround her; for they have rejected My ordinances and have not walked in My statutes.' Therefore, thus says the Lord God, 'Because you have more turmoil than the nations which surround you and have not walked in My statutes, nor observed My ordinances, nor observed the ordinances of the nations which surround you,' therefore, thus says the Lord God, 'Behold, I, even I, am against you, and I will execute judgments among you in the sight of the nations. One

> third of you will die by plague or be consumed by famine among you, one third will fall by the sword around you, and one-third I will scatter to every wind, and I will unsheathe a sword behind them... . So, it will be a reproach, a reviling, a warning and an object of horror to the nations who surround you when I execute judgments against you in anger, wrath and raging rebukes. I, the Lord, have spoken. Moreover, I will send on you famine and wild beasts, and they will bereave you of children; plague and bloodshed also will pass through you, and I will bring the sword on you. I, the Lord have spoken.' (*Ezekiel 5:5-12, NASB*)

The Hebrew prophet Ezekiel continued to warn the nation of Judah over and over again that judgments of plagues and pestilences were coming. In the Book of Ezekiel, the Lord God warned that the city of Sidon (located in the country we now call Lebanon) would be struck with terrible diseases as a divine judgment for unrepentant sin.

> And the word of the Lord came to me saying, 'Son of man, set your face toward Sidon, prophesy against her and say, Thus says the Lord God, 'Behold, I am against you, O Sidon, and I will be glorified in your midst. Then they will know that I am the Lord when I execute judgments in her, and I will manifest. My holiness in her. For I will send pestilence to her and blood to her streets...' (*Ezekiel* 28: 20-24, NASB)

In the Book of Amos too, the Lord God warned the nation of Israel that they would be struck with terrible diseases as a divine judgment for unrepentant sin.

> Hear the word which the Lord has spoken against you, sons of Israel...'Surely, the Lord God does nothing unless He reveals His secret counsel to His servants the prophets. I sent a plague among you after the manner of Egypt; I

> slew your young men by the sword along with your captured horses, and I made the stench of your camp rise up in your nostrils; yet you have not returned to Me,' declares the Lord. 'Seek the Lord that you may live, or He will break forth like a fire, O house of Joseph, and it will consume with none to quench it...' (*Amos*, 3: 1, 7, 4:10, 5:6, NASB)

In the Book of Habakkuk, we again see the Lord God speaking through an ancient Hebrew prophet, warning the nation of Israel that He uses plagues and pestilences to bring judgment to His unrepentant people. "Before *Him goes pestilence, and plague comes after Him...*" (*Habakkuk* 3:5). So it is established that pestilences and pandemics have been used again and again by the almighty God of the Old Testament as a warning to humans to reconsider their ways. The Covid pandemic has certainly resonated a similar call, a new norm with most people rethinking their lifestyles. The lockdown has created a new awareness of conventional values of family, friends and entertainment. Social distancing has helped us to grow closer to our souls and not only the nature rejuvenating during this break, but our souls as well. Surely, the introspection and meditation of our hearts are Godward as we realize the very foolishness of aspiring for things which may be gone with our next breath. Indeed, the necessity to look up for healing and safety is reflected in the Old Testament story of the bronze serpent, put up on a pole by Moses which healed the Israelites of snake bite if they had the faith and wits to look up at it. (*Numbers*, 21)

The uncertainty generated by the nose dive in economy has generated fear, dissatisfaction and disappointment with the very fabric of life and those who have honestly thought about the rat race, most of us are caught up in life are ready to conclude that they are no rats and are getting out of the trap. The Bible holds that the fear of the Lord is the beginning of wisdom and as we wrestle with today's situation, it is gratifying for a believer to turn towards a just but merciful God, especially of the New Testament.

Jesus, in his lifetime as also His disciples, prophesied many terrible things happening as the world comes to an end. The prophecies in the Bible have come to pass throughout history so it is no surprise that Bible scholars are trying to connect the ongoing pandemic with the end time prophecies in the Bible. Jesus prophesied that the last days would see helpless and scared men.

> ...men fainting from fear and the expectation of the things which are coming upon the world; for the powers of the heavens will be shaken. (*Luke:* 21:26, NASB)

Yet Jesus also told us how to respond in such dark times. *Now when these things begin to happen, look up and lift up your heads, because your redemption draws near.* (*Luke:* 21:28)

A Bible scholar states:

> No fewer than 12 times in the Book of Revelation, the Lord God warns that terrible pestilence and plagues will come to the nations of the earth as part of His judgment of sin, prior to the Second Coming of Jesus Christ. This period is known by Bible scholars as the "Great Tribulation" (*Revelation,* 7:14), and it will involve the most devastating period of divine judgment for unrepentant sin in all of human history.

> The book of Revelation talks about a pale horse:

> I looked, and behold, an ashen horse; and he who sat on it had the name Death; and Hades was following with him. Authority was given to them over a fourth of the earth, to kill with sword and with famine and with pestilence and by the wild beasts of the earth. (6:8, NASB)

The ninth chapter of the same book also declares:

> But the rest of mankind, who were not killed by these plagues, did not repent of the works of their hands, that they should not worship demons, and idols of gold, silver, brass, stone, and wood, which can neither see nor hear nor walk. (9:20, KJV)

The eleventh chapter of the book of Revelation talks about the two witnesses of God who would have the:

> power to shut heaven, so that no rain falls in the days of their prophecy; and they have power over waters to turn them to blood, and to strike the earth with all plagues, as often as they desire. (*Revelation* 11:6, KJV)

That God's warning will not be taken heed and is also prophesied:

> And men were scorched with great heat, and they blasphemed the name of God who has power over these plagues; and they did not repent and give Him glory. (*Revelation*, 16:9)

When all these fail to turn mankind to repentance, the God, who is a just God, would have to take account of the Good and the Bad on the great Day of Judgment. Yet, the Almighty God repeatedly promises that He will heal and remove any calamity if humans humbly accept His sovereignty in their lives which of course means to obey His precepts and commands. Chronicles 7:12-14 says:

> Then the Lord appeared to Solomon at night and said to him, 'I have heard your prayer and have chosen this place for Myself as a house of sacrifice. If I shut up the heavens so that there is no rain, or if I command the locust to devour the land, or if I send pestilence among My people, and My people who are called by My name humble themselves and pray and seek My face and turn from their wicked ways, then I will hear from heaven, will

> forgive their sin and heal their land." (*NASB)*

Jeremiah, 18: 7-8 reiterates the same promise of God:

> At one moment I might speak concerning a nation or concerning a kingdom to uproot, to pull down, or to destroy it. If that nation against which I have spoken, turns from its evil, I will relent concerning the calamity I planned to bring on it. (*NASB*)

Pandemics and epidemics are certainly God's doing to a believer but harsh as it may seem, it comes from the hand of a merciful God who wants mankind's attention and obedience as a father, for in that, mankind would be blessed with peace and prosperity. The Bible depicts pandemics as a punitive measure, physical misery leading to a correction in the spiritual relationship with Him. Atheists and agnostics may well scoff at the very idea of seeing God's hand in a pandemic and call it foolish but even scientists and doctors at the cutting edge of technology can be baffled at times with a dimension which is beyond the capacity of the human intellect to grasp. So when a believer in the God of the Bible thinks of Him as his heavenly father and clings to the promise in psalm ninety one : *I will say to the Lord, My refuge and my fortress, my God in whom I trust! For it is He who rescues you from the net of the trapper and from the deadly plague.* (Psalm 91 : 2), His hope and faith is surely a better direction to take than wallowing in despair.

REFERENCES

1. https://theconversation.com/how-the-ancient-israelites-dealt-with-epidemics-the-bible-tells-of-prophecy-and-rituals-135803
2. https://www.history.com/topics/middle-ages/pandemics-timeline
3. https://www.joshuafund.com/downloads/FACTSHEET-BibleAndPandemics
4. The bible verses are quoted from the New American Standard version.

11
Representation of Epidemics and Pandemics in the Art of Europe

Paromita Das

ABSTRACT

As the entire world today is in the grip of a pandemic, resulting in large scale decimation of the human species, many believe that this is an unprecedented event in the history of the world. Yet a century earlier after the First World War the Spanish Flu had created havoc on a similar scale. Moreover, if we look back in history we find that even two thousand years ago pandemics and epidemics had periodically wiped out sizeable numbers of people around the world and these episodes are graphically depicted in art objects and paintings. Without recourse to antibiotics the people who were affected, turned for deliverance to divine intervention. They often turned to the holy men or Saints to intercede with God on their behalf and death, destruction, prayer and saints that are represented in the art of Europe down the ages.

Keywords: Pandemic, Pestilence, Prayer, Plague Saints.

Since the month of December 2019, the Covid-19 pandemic has been wrecking havoc in all corners of the globe with the exception perhaps of the Polar Regions. As of 24th December,

2020 more than seventy-nine million have been affected and nearly eight million have lost their lives*. Today, quarantine and "lockdown" have entered everyday parlance and people have utilized social media to reach out to one another. In an attempt to cope with the present existential crisis, where the future of humanity itself appears to be at stake, many have expressed themselves through cartoons and memes. Many believe that this present global crisis is unprecedented in its sheer dimension and that their experiences are indeed unique. Yet, when we look back in time, we find that humanity had faced similar situations and on a similar global scale throughout the pages of history. Not only do we encounter graphic details of epidemics and pandemics in literature, but also in the field of art.

Art holds up a mirror to society. Each and every artistic object/artefact represents the belief system of the society that produced it. In present times, with the advancement of science and modern medicine, human beings have a much better understanding of the causes and remedies for diseases that afflict mankind. But in the remote past, in ancient and medieval times, very often, the causes of diseases were attributed to the wrath of the Divine. Hence, succour too was sought in the form of Divine intervention. Therefore prayers were one of the chief means to combat disease, besides the use of conventional medicines and the service of doctors. To intercede on one's behalf in front of the Divine, besides priests, the saints were also invoked. And in art we find numerous saints whom the people believed, would protect them from the devastating effects of the plague. Other artworks are graphic representations of death and despair due to the pandemic. It is proposed to examine the representation of plague and pestilence in the art of Europe.

One of the earliest references to an epidemic is found in the writings of the Greek historian Thucydides. In 430 BCE

Worldometers, 24 Dec, 2020

when the Athenians were engaged in the Peloponnesian War, the city state of Athens was ravaged by a pestilence that reportedly killed nearly a quarter of its citizens. Thucydides describes the Athenian Plague in his *History of the Peloponnesian War* which had such devastating effects thus

> *On the outside the body was not hot to the touch, nor was there pallor; the skin was rather red, livid, and broke out into small blisters and ulcers (helkoi)...those suffering from this pestilence did not recognise 'themselves or their friends' (In the Athenian Plague, he claimed) , physicians were useless, ignorant of how to treat the disease, and particularly vulnerable as a result, but no other human art was any more help, nor were appeals to the divine; all were eventually abandoned by the afflicted populace, despair dominated. (Thucydides 2.47.4., cited in Fleming, 2019)*

He claimed that social morals deteriorated as...*the catastrophe was so overwhelming that men, not knowing what would happen next to them, became indifferent to every rule of religion or law* (Thucydides, 2.52 cited in Flemming, 2019).

The painting "Plague in an Ancient City" by the Flemish artist Michiel Sweerts (c. 1618-1664) is believed to represent the Athenian Plague described by Thucydides. **Fig. 11.1** vividly depicts the dying population of the beautiful city of Athens juxtaposed against its classic architecture. Measuring 118.7 cm (height) × 170.8 cm (width) executed in oil on canvas, it is at present on display at the Ahmanson Building in the Los Angeles County Museum of Art. Many people are shown with their hands raised towards the heavens beseeching for succour. In the foreground we find the corpses lying about on the public street. A tragic site is that of an infant suckling at the breast of its dead mother. In the lower left hand corner are two figures with despair writ large upon their faces. Others are holding their hands covering their nostrils to protect against the stench of dead and decaying bodies that

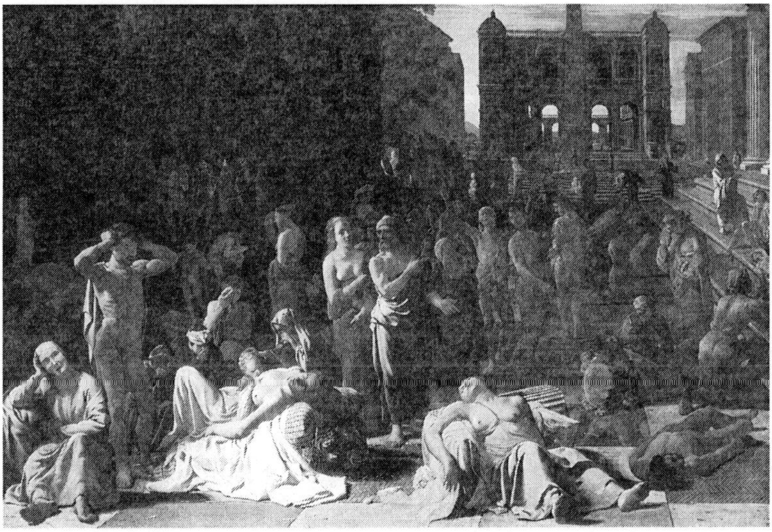

Fig.11.1: Painting Depicts the dying population of the city of Athems. *SOURCE:* http://collections.lacma.org/sites/default/files/remote_images/piction/ma-31770455-O3.jpgGallery:http://collections.lacma.org/node/183358 archive copy, Public Domain, https://commons.wikimedia.org/w/index.php?curid=27201183

are too many to merit a decent burial probably also due to the fear of contagion. In the background towards the left we find a cross-section of different strata of a devastated city.

Another early reference to plague is found in the treatise *Methodus Medendi* by the Greek physician Galen, who was a contemporary of the Roman Emperor Marcus Aurelius Antoninus Augustus, who flourished in the second century CE. Hence, it is referred to in history as the "Antonine Plague" or the Plague of Galen, as the latter first identified the symptoms of this pestilence as "great" and of long duration, and mentioned fever, diarrhoea, and pharyngitis as well as a skin eruption, sometimes dry and sometimes pustular, that appeared on the ninth day of the illness. He states :

> Those easily restored to health from the plague seem to me to have been previously dried and purged in respect to the whole body, for vomiting occurred in some of them and the stomach was disturbed in all. And, in the same way, in those already purged who were going to be saved, dark pustules (*exanthemata*) appear clearly over the whole body, in most ulcerous, in all dry. And it was obvious to the observer that, what was left of the blood which had been putrefied during these fevers, had, like a kind of ash, been forced through the skin by nature, just like many other superfluities (Flemming, 2019, 229).

This unknown disease was brought back to Rome by soldiers returning from a campaign against the Parthians. They spread the disease that resulted in the loss of over five million people and decimated the Roman army. Galen claimed that there was no medicine to combat the disease, which was in all probability smallpox. He writes :

> On my arrival in Aquileia the plague attacked more destructively than ever before, so the emperors fled immediately to Rome with a small force of men. For the rest of us, survival became very difficult for a long time. Most, indeed, died, the effects of the plague being exacerbated by the fact that all this was occurring in the middle of winter. (Flemming, 2019, 224)

To placate the Gods many a time votive objects would be offered. These would often be in the form or representation of the injured or diseased part of the body and would be left at the temple of a God. A terracotta votive offering measuring 32 cm x 21 cm depicts a male torso (Fig 11.2). The sculpture is clearly dissected to show the infected viscera. It was reputedly recovered from the Isola Farnese, Italy and belongs to the period 200 BCE to 200 CE.

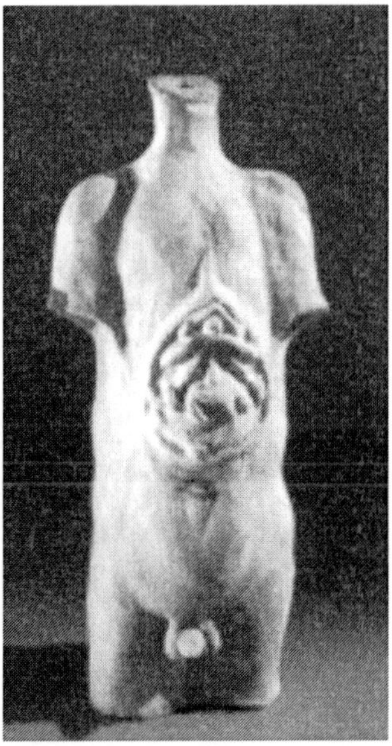

Fig. 11.2: Sculpture dissected, showing the infected viscera. Source: https://www.ssplprints.com/image/86234/votive-male-torso-roman-200bc-200ad

An engraving measuring 33.2 x 44.9 cm by Levasseur is based upon a painting, oil on canvas, by Jules-Elie Delaunay(1828-1891) (Fig.11.3) at the Musee d'Orsay in Paris. Measuring 131 cm × 177 cm it depicts the Angel of Death striking at a door during the plague. In the background is Marcus Aurelius upon a horse. On the right hand side we see a fair angel directing the Angel of Death to strike at the house indicated, a harbinger of pestilence and death. On the extreme right can be seen the lower part of a statue of Aesculapius, a Graeco-Roman deity associated with healing. He is usually depicted as a standing figure in a long cloak, bare chest and holding a staff with a snake coiled around it. Below him are afflicted devotees praying for succour. In the upper left hand corner we see a procession of white robed figures, probably

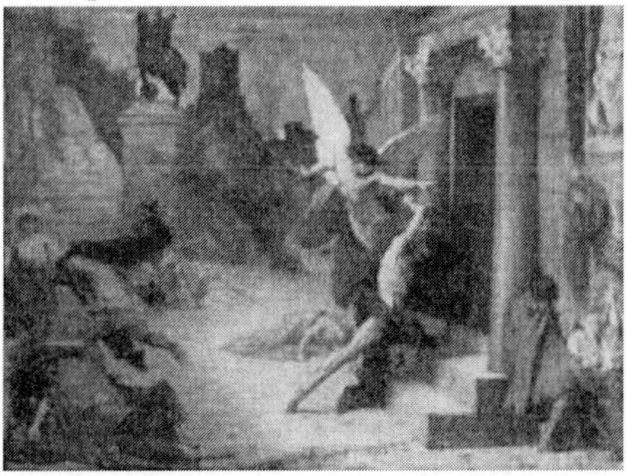

Fig.11.3: Painting despites the Angel of Death striking at a door.
Source: Wikimedia/commons, public domain

priests, carrying a cross.

The imagery of an angel of death (Fig. 11.4) has survived till contemporary times.

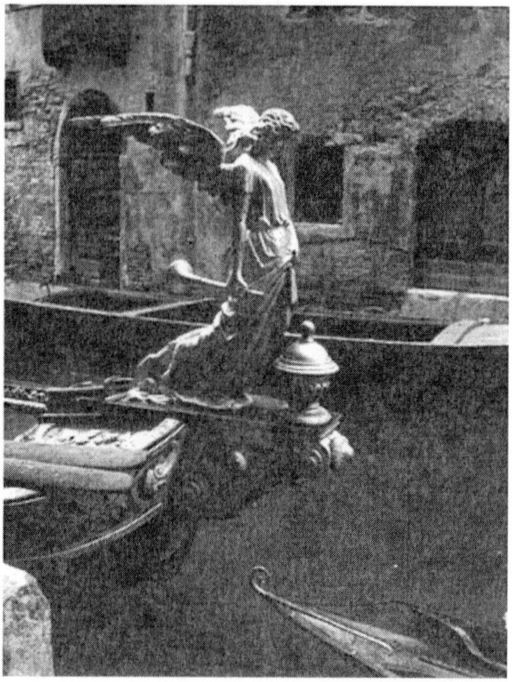

Fig.11.4: The Angel of Death, sculpture as found in a funeral Gondola in Venice.

Source: https:/commons. wikimedia.org/w/index.php?curid=48059400

Another painting by an unknown artist vividly depicts the destruction cause by the Antonine Plague (Fig.11.5). This painting is similar in theme to the one depicting the plague at Athens (Fig.11.1). Dead bodies litter the street and citizens are covering their faces with their hands to avoid the stench of rotting bodies. To invoke a sense of pathos, here too we find a child at the breast of its dead mother whose body has a sickly greenish gray pallor, while another child lies dead near her. In the background men are shown carrying corpses into the crypts for burial.

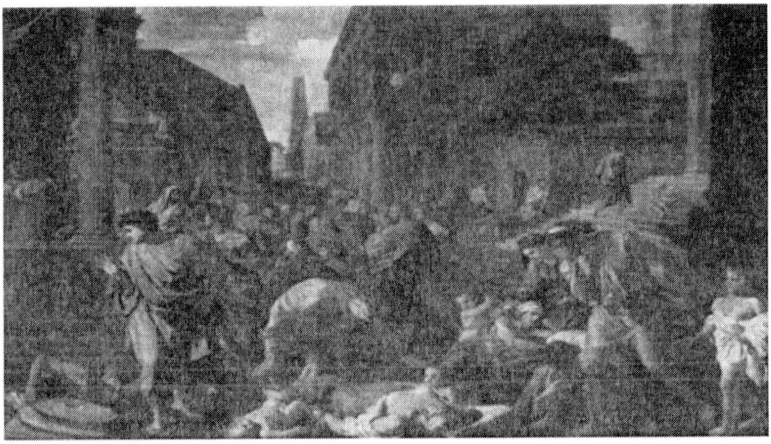

Fig. 11.5: Painting depicts the destruction caused by the Antonine Plague
Source: Wikimedia/commons: public domain

Fig.11.6 depicts Galen in consultation with a group of physicians in an image from the *Vienna Dioscurides* an early sixth century Byzantine Greek illuminated manuscript of *De Materia Medica.* The original five-volume work was written between 50 and 70 CE by Pedanius Dioscurides, a Greek physician in the Roman army.

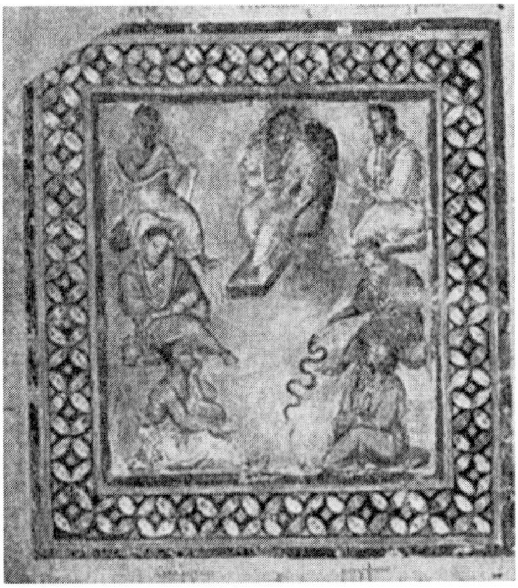

Fig.11.6: Glam in consultation with a group of physicians
Source: Wikimedia commons/ public domain

In 541 CE the Eastern Roman Empire was visited by another pandemic. There was an outbreak of bubonic plague during the reign of Justinian I (527- 565 CE). This Justinian Plague lasted for }nearly a year and was documented by the emperor's court historian Procopius

(500-565 CE) in his *History of the Wars*, Book II. The latter traced its origin to Egypt from whence it spread to Constantinople (modern Istanbul), the capital of the Byzantine Empire. However, new scientific evidence traces it probable origins to China in Asia, and not Africa. Generally regarded as the first recorded incident of the Bubonic Plague, it decimated up to a quarter of the population of the Eastern Mediterranean and nearly forty per cent of the population of Constantinople. This Black Death or Justinian Plague is vividly depicted in many paintings of medieval Europe. Fig. 11.7 vividly depicts victims with the typical manifestation of the disease on their faces seeking blessings of a priest.

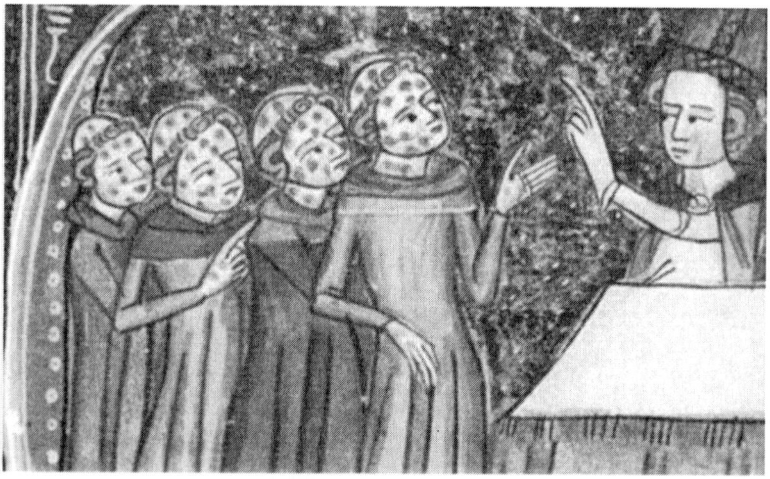

Fig.11.7: Victims seeking blessings of a priest
Source: Wikimedia commons/ public domain

In 1346 there was an outbreak of the Bubonic Plague in Europe that lasted for nearly seven years. It is popularly known as the Black Death due to blackening and death of tissue (gangrene) in the extremities, most commonly fingers, toes and nose and the presence of black buboes as shown in Fig. 11.7. The Black Death is believed to have originated in Asia and spread via the fleas living on the rats that lived aboard merchant ships. Ports were major urban centres at that time and were very crowded. From the crowded sea ports that were the perfect breeding ground for the rats and fleas this plague decimated the population of Europe, Africa, and Asia. *The Triumph of Death* (Fig. 11.8) in the Museo del Prado in Madrid is an oil panel painting measuring 117 cm × 162 cm, by Pieter Bruegel the Elder painted in c. 1562. It reflects the social upheaval and terror caused by the Black Death which devastated medieval Europe. In a desolate landscape, Death is personified as skeletal ghostly figures attacking the hapless people. In the centre of the painting we find the dead and dying lying upon one another in a heap while in the foreground a dog is eating a corpse. In the centre left are people in shrouds with a cross representing the helplessness of the Church to save the dying populace. In the upper left hand corner two skeletons ring a bell signifying the knell of death, i.e. tolling of bells to signify death is approaching. In other paintings on a similar theme, as for instance Jan Brueghel's 1597 version death is similar shown as skeletons with scythe riding a skeletal horse. Some artists also depict the four horsemen of the apocalypse or end of the world.

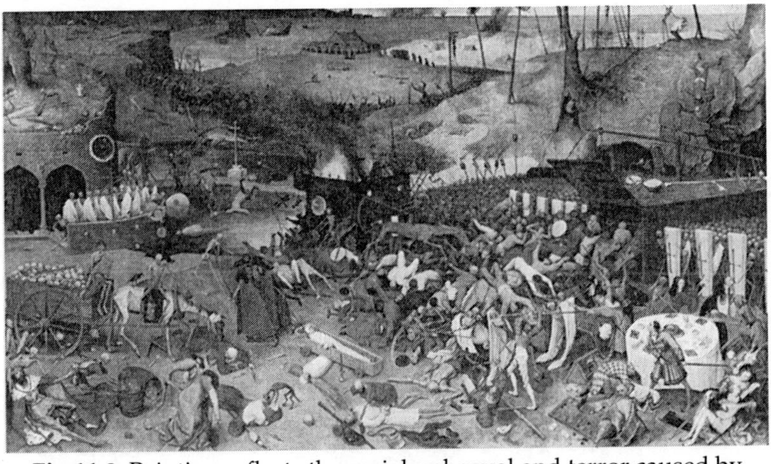

Fig.11.8: Painting reflects the social upheaval and terror caused by Black Death

Source: Wikimedia commons/public domain

The *Antiquitates Flandriae*, a manuscript dated 1349 contains illustrations of the Black Death. A miniature painting (Fig.11.9) depicts the burial of the dead. The great number of coffins carried in a fashion similar to Christ carrying the cross indicated the heavy burden the people had to bear. Steeped in medieval superstitions the people of Europe sought scapegoats, people to blame for the plague and deaths.

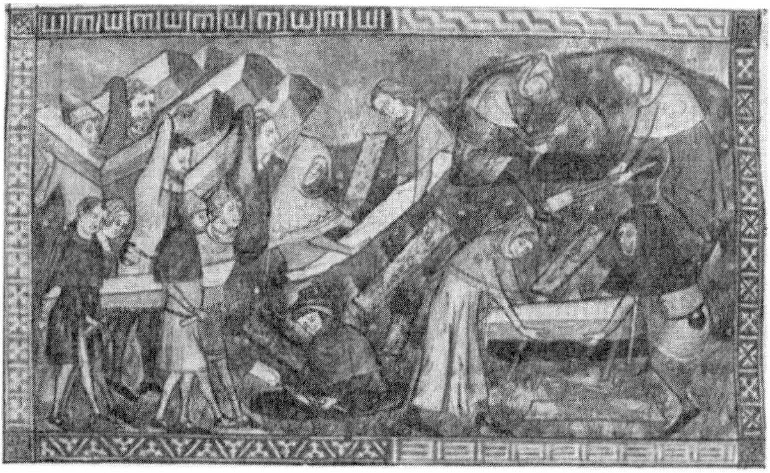

Fig. 9: A miniature painting depicts the burial of dead
Source: Wikimedia commons/ public domain

Another miniature in this fourteenth century manuscript (Fig. 11.10) is a graphic depiction of Jews being burnt alive by Christian fanatics.

Unable to deal with death on a large scale many people turned to the Church and the Christian faith to relieve their sufferings. This resulted in a renewal of religious fervour and fanaticism and some Europeans blamed the merchant class such as the Jews and other wandering groups like the friars, foreigners, beggars and pilgrims, as well as lepers and the Romany people (i.e. Gypsies). Many Jews and lepers, and others with skin diseases such as acne or psoriasis, were killed throughout Europe. One of the worst massacres of Jews during the Black Death occurred in February 1349 in Strasbourg, when 2,000 Jewish were burned alive. In the spring, 3,000 Jews defend themselves in Mainz against Christians but were overcome and slaughtered (Seven: 2020).

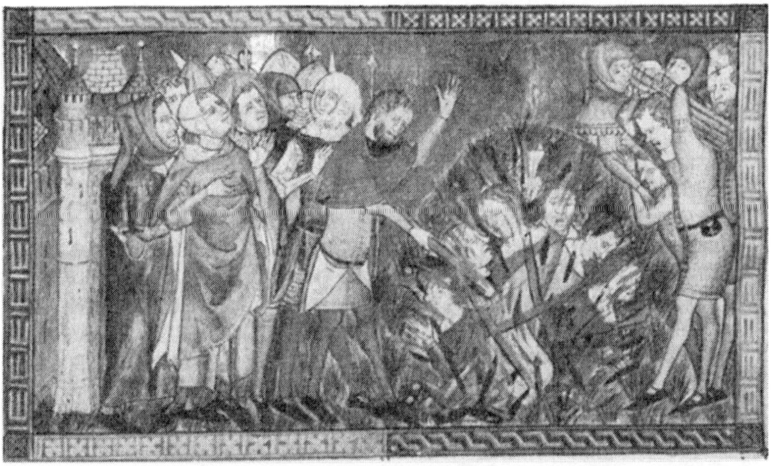

Fig. 10: Depiction showing Jews being burnt alive by Christian fanatics
Source: Wikimedia commons/ public domain

Another feature of the art of medieval Europe following the bubonic plague was the depiction of saints and the mythology associated with them. The idea of praying to saints to intercede with the Gods was not uncommon in Greco-Roman history. We also find this phenomenon in Christianity. Many pagan healers, both mythical and historical were also invoked by Christians and we find images of popular saints depicted in the art of medieval Europe. A painting by Josse Lieferinxe, (c.1497–1499) of Southern Netherlands of the earlier Justinian plague (Fig.11.11) shows St. Sebastian pleading with Jesus for the life of a gravedigger afflicted by the disease. His bare body is pierced with arrows. According to legends, St. Sebastian flourished in the 3rd-4th century and secretly practiced Christianity. When his secret was discovered by the Roman Emperor he was given the death penalty and the royal archers supposedly shot him dead, but he recovered and was later clubbed to death. During the Black Death his martyrdom was viewed symbolically as the ability to "draw away the arrows of plague" from others to himself and he was one of the earliest saints to be associated with plague.

The imagery of the arrows is an ancient one. *"The arrow is not merely a weapon, but traditionally a carrier of disease, especially the plague."* (Hall cited in Ortega, 2012). The arrow as a symbol of the plague has its origins in the legend of Apollo and his sister, Diana, shooting and killing the fourteen children of Niobe who had tried to persuade the women of Thebes not to offer prayers to Leto, the mother of the siblings. The "Christianization" of the symbol of the arrow was a continuation of the Greco-Roman tradition. The symbolism of the plague-arrow also appears in ancient Hebrew literature and God's anger or wrath is manifested in plague laden arrows that reign down pestilence upon the world (Ortega, 2012).

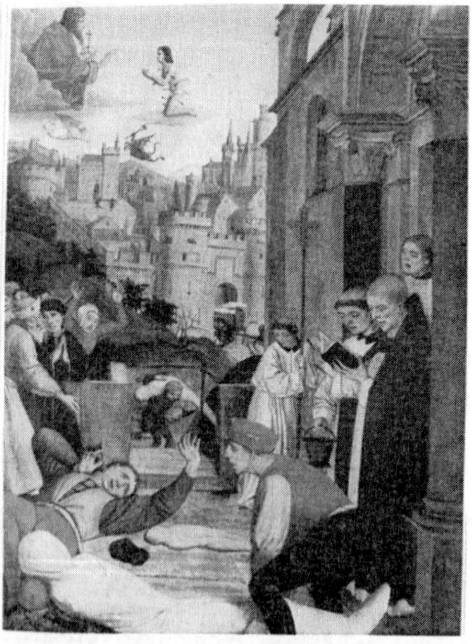

Fig. 11 .11: St. Sebastian pleading with Jesus for the life of a gravedigger
Source : Wikimedia commons/ public domain

In the upper section of the painting the saint's body riddled with arrows is seen beseeching Christ to spare the people whose eyes are turned heavenward, praying to the saint for deliverance from the plague. Below them in the sky a battle rages between the fair good angel and the dark angel of death. Below can be seen dead bodies that await burial as the gravedigger too is afflicted with the disease. Fig.11.12 is a statue of the saint, his body pierced with arrows in the Museum of Archeology at Herne. In both the depictions St. Sebastian has a peaceful look upon his face, of someone who has surrendered to the Divine and accepted his fate. In Fig. 11.13 the saint who is tied to a tree to be used as target practice for the Roman soldiers is offered a crown by an angel.

In many altar panels we find St. Sebastian along with other

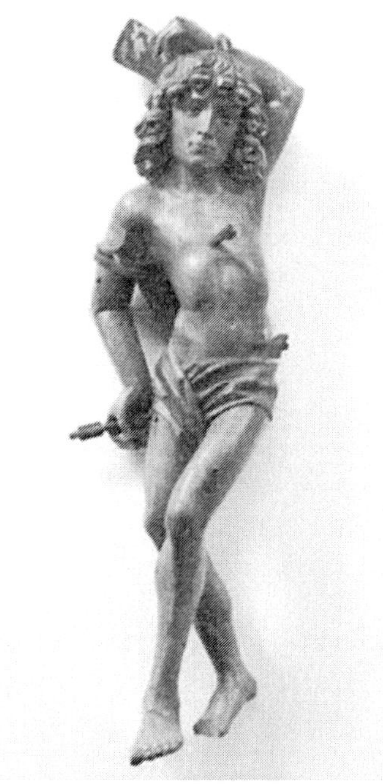

Fig. 11 .12: Statue of saint, his body pierced with arrows.

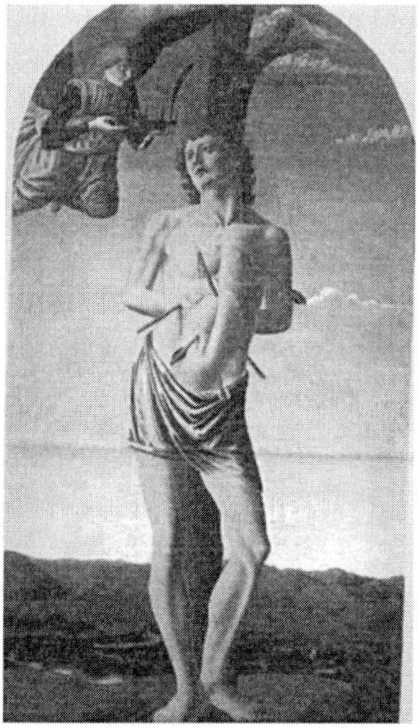

Fig. 11 .13: Saint tied to a tree is offered a crown by an angel.

Source : Wikimedia commons/ public domain

saints who were also called upon to save the people from the wrath of the Divine. In Benozzo Gozzoli's *Saints Nicholas of Tolentino, Roch, Sebastian, and Bernardino of Siena, with Kneeling Donors* (Fig. 11.14) the plague saints are in a *sacra conversazione* or "holy conversation". Sebastian can be "identified by his name inscribed in his halo and the iconic arrow he holds in his hand. Behind the saints, angels are flying in the sky, directing plague-arrows down to the city below. The donors, kneeling in the foreground, clearly commissioned this work to invoke the saints because the artwork included angels afflicting the town with disease in the background." (Ortega, 2012).

Another popular saint was St. Roch who lived in the fourteenth century and was regarded as the patron saint of invalids, many of whom he was said to have miraculously cured by invoking Christ and the cross and prayer (Sauerlander, 2014). According to popular legends he himself was contacted by the dreaded bubonic plague and forced by people to live in a forest. He miraculously recovered, continued to minister to

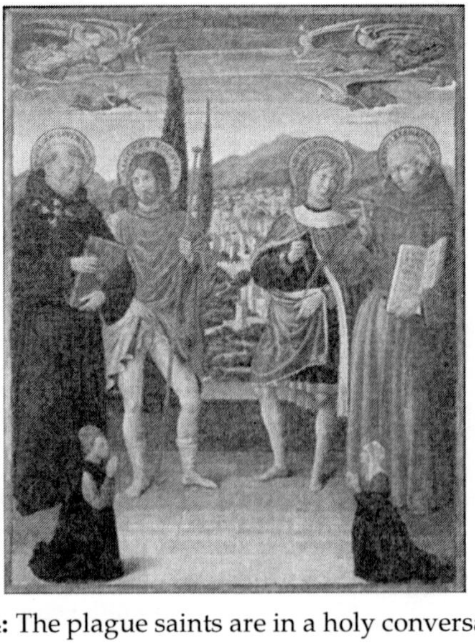

Fig. 11 .14: The plague saints are in a holy conversation.

Source : Wikimedia commons/ public domain

the sick. In art he is generally "*portrayed as a pilgrim with a hat and staff, and a bubo* on his thigh (a relic of his illness). He is often accompanied by a dog, representing the dog that brought bread to him and licked his wounds when he was ill" (Marshall, 1994). In an altarpiece (412 cm × 258 cm) by Sir Peter Paul Rubens, painted between 1623-1626 CE in the Church of St. Martin in Aalst, Belgium, titled *Christ Appointing Saint Roch as Patron Saint of Plague Victims* (Fig.11.15) two groups of figures are depicted. In the upper half we find St. Roch praying to Christ who appears along with a messenger and points at an inscription that reads "*Eris in peste patronus*" (Thou shall be the patron in the plague). The lower group who is afflicted by the plague, look upwards at this miracle with hope on their faces (Sauerlander, 2014). St. Roch can be identified by the prominent bubo on his thigh, his staff and the dog.

In *Saint Roch Interceding with the Virgin for the Plague-*

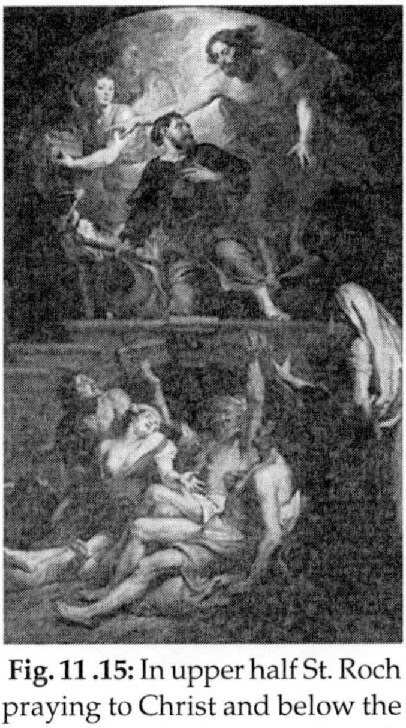

Fig. 11 .15: In upper half St. Roch praying to Christ and below the lower group look upwards with hope on their faces.

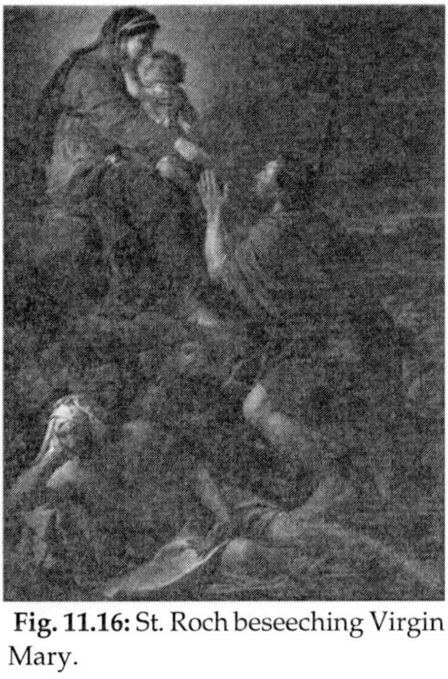

Fig. 11.16: St. Roch beseeching Virgin Mary.

Source of photos: Wikimedia/commons

Stricken, a 1780 painting by French artist Jacques-Louis David, the afflicted people appear desolate and forsaken. Although Roch is seen beseeching Virgin Mary on behalf of the afflicted, her attention is focused upon the child Jesus and she appears deaf to his prayers and appeal (Fig.11.16). The Virgin Mary is clad in bright blue and red in contrast to the dull brown and grey clothes of the plague victim who have lost all hope (Sauerlander, 2014).

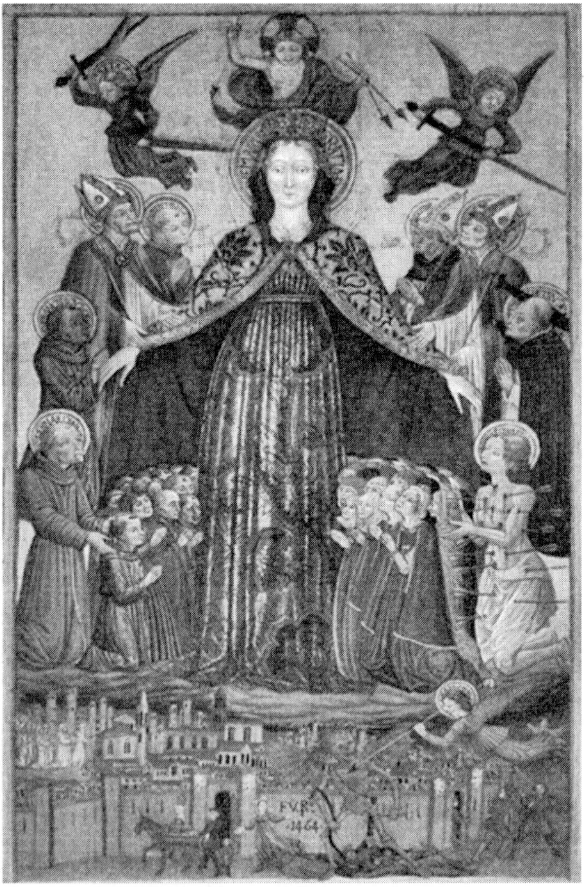

Fig. 11. 17: Virgin Mary shielding Citizens from plague-arrow with her cloak.

Source: Public Domain)

But, very often Virgin Mary, mother of Jesus, is also found protecting people from the plague in medieval art (Hall: 2008). Benedetto Bonfigli's *Madonna della Misericordia* (Fig.11.17) shows the Virgin shielding citizens from plague-arrows with her cloak. The angels are shown wielding swords while Christ has arrows. There are a multitude of saints surrounding the Virgin, assisting her to protect the people. In the foreground, below the Virgin and saints, an angel torments citizens of a walled city and bodies are strewn across the earth.

We also find female saints in art. Thecla, a companion and disciple of the apostle Paul, is the patron saint of the north Italian city of Este. Surrounded by plague victims, she beseeches God to deliver the city from disaster. Thecla's prayer is answered: angels chase away the Plague, a satanic creature with a pointed crown. St. Thecla Liberating the City of Este from the Plague depicts her face uplifted toward heaven, as all around her, people are picking up their dead and small children cling to decayed greenish corpses of their parents (Fig.11. 18). This 18th-century painting is by Giovanni Battista Tiepolo, also

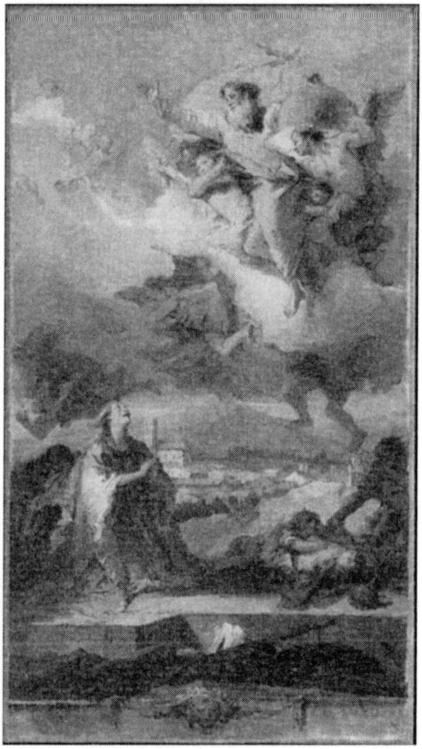

Fig. 11. 18: Thecla beseches God to save city from plague.
Source: https://images. metmuseum. org/CRDImages/ep/original/ DT11803.jpg)

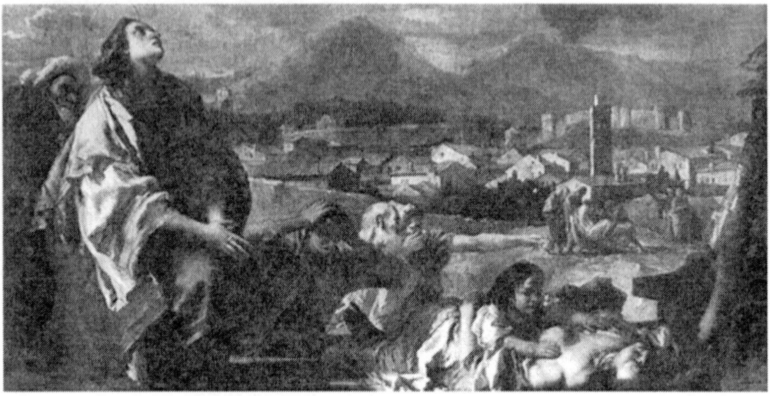

Fig. 11.19: (Source: Public Domain)

known as Giambattista (or Gianbattista) Tiepolo, an Italian painter and printmaker from the Republic of Venice. Another painting by the same artist measuring 81.3 x 44.8 cm, titled *Saint Thecla Praying for the Plague-Stricken* (Fig.11.19) is found at the cathedral at Este, near Padua. Commissioned in 1758 and installed on Christmas Day, 1759, the picture commemorated the devastating plague of 1630 with the citizens of Este praying for the intercession of Saint Thecla. The first-century saint is shown among the victims while the town is depicted in the background.

Besides the depiction of plague scenes in paintings and sculptures, we also find wood engravings depicting a grim humour like the "Dance of Death", composed of grinning skeletons (Fig. 11.20) that can be termed as "grave humour". This artwork engraved by German artist Michael Wolgemut of Nuremberg is a printed leaf measuring 46 cm × 31.7 cm from the Nuremberg Chronicle dated 1493 CE and is presently housed in the Metropolitan Museum in New York, USA. In the foreground is a skeleton, partially covered by a shroud and apparently buried under the ground. Above the ground, three skeletons dancing on this grave are while a fourth, personifying Death itself, is playing upon the pipes, leading the marked victims to their ultimate destination. Another woodcut depicts a Jew poisoning a well (Fig.11. 21), a reflection of the prejudiced attitude of Christian Europeans. Above the well is the figure of the Devil and a Christians is shown impaled upon a crucifix. As mentioned earlier, Jews and other non-Christian communities were persecuted and often burned alive as they were held responsible for the plague or Black Death and suspected of being in association with the Devil.

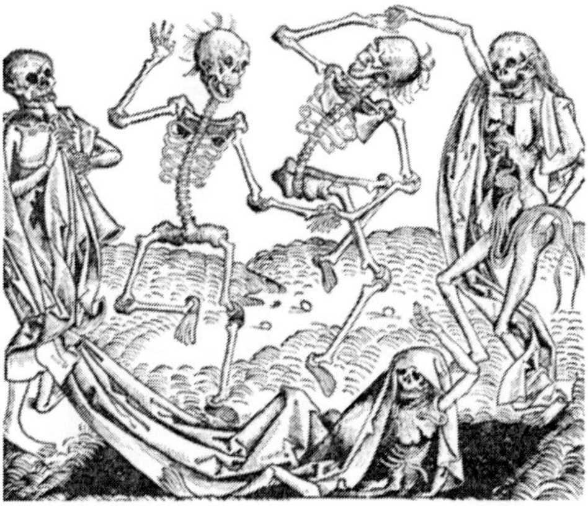

Fig. 11.20: Wood engraving depicting a grim humour like the Dance of Death.

Source: Wikimedia commons/public domain

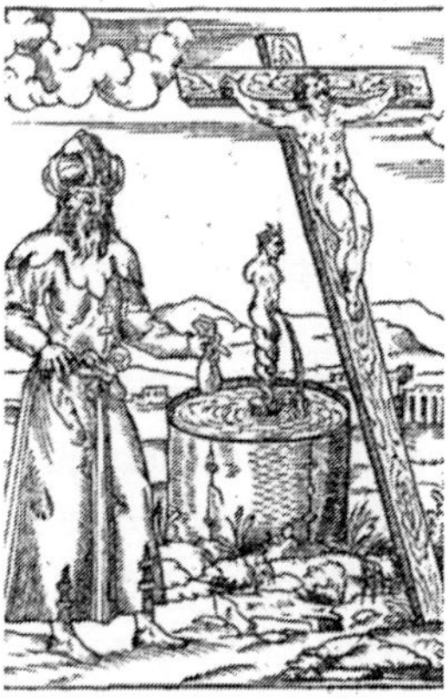

Fig. 11.21: Woodcut depicts a Jew poisoning a wall.

Another figure closely associated with the Black Death was the doctor. His arrival at a home was of regarded as a portent of death. To avoid contamination and inevitable death in case of falling victim to the plague, in view of the absence of treatment, (expect the present system of isolation of the afflicted) the plague doctor is generally depicted in paintings as a grim figure, clad in a long robe of black or other dark colours, wearing gloves and a penguin like mask (Fig. 11.22) quite similar to the modern personal protection equipment.

From the foregoing discussion we can conclude that epidemics and pandemics were vividly depicted in art, mainly in paintings that were often used as objects of veneration in churches and shrines. Sculptural depictions were also not uncommon. These artworks reflect the contemporary social scenario as a result of the plague and pestilence. The motif of death and desolation were the main features of the paintings. Being overwhelmed by large-scale death, people turned to the divine, to their faith and to saints, to intercede with the divine to protect them. Hence a large number of paintings portray these themes. Other paintings also indicate social prejudices like the suspicion of Jews causing the plague and the terrible repercussions, the burning alive of the "hated Jews". Painting of "plague doctors" in protective clothes and other equipment, and of associating the ancient physician Galen with an epidemic also provide interesting facets of how Europeans viewed the plague, especially in medieval times.

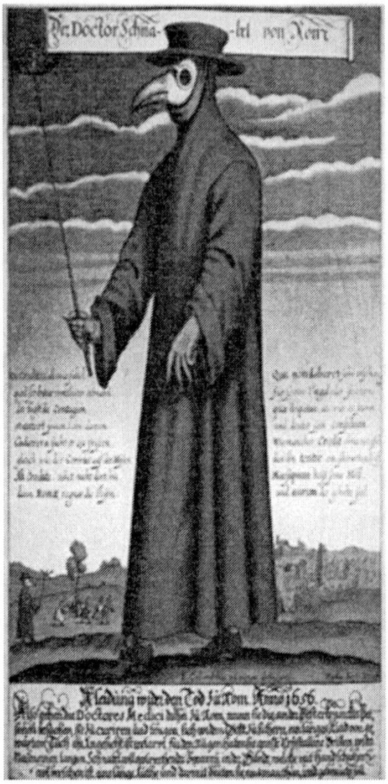

Fig. 11.22: A depiction of the plague doctor.
Source: Wikimedia/commons

REFERENCES

1. Coronavirus Cases: *Worldometer.* Retrieved on 24th December, 2020 https://worldometers.info/coronavirus.
2. Flemming, Rebecca. (2019) Galen and the Plague. In Caroline Petit (Ed). *Galen's Treatise (De indolentia) in Context (A Tale of Resilience).* Brill Publications. Retrieve on 23rd December 2020. https://www.jstor.org/stable/10.1163/j.ctvrxk2wj.12.
3. Kosloski, Philip (2017). *5 Colors and their Symbolism in Sacred Art.* Retrieved from https://aleteia.org/2017/09/25/5-colors-and-their-symbolism-in-art/

4. Lawler, Andrew, *et. al.* (2016). How Europe Exported the Black Death. *Science.* Retrieved on 22nd December 2020 https://www.sciencemag.org/news/2016/04/how-europe-exported-black-death
5. Marshall, Louise (1994). Manipulating the Sacred: Image and Plague in Renaissance Italy. *Renaissance Quarterly*, 47 *(3), 505.* Retrieved on 20th December, 2020 doi:10.2307/2863019. JSTOR 2863019 PMID 11639337
6. Marshall, Louise (2012). A Plague Saint for Venice: Tintoretto at the Chiesa di San Rocco. *Artibus et Historiae,* 33 (66), 153-187. Retrieved on 23rd December, 2020 https://www.jstor.org/stable/23509749.
7. Ortega, Jessica. (2012). *Pestilence and Prayer Saints and the Art of the Plague in Italy from 1370 -1600.* University of Central Florida. Retrieved on 23rd December, 2020 https://stars.library.ucf.edu/honorstheses1990-2015/1367
8. Sauerlander, Willibald. (2014). *The Catholic Rubens: Saints and Martyrs.* Getty Publications. 136–141.
9. Seven, John. (2020). The Black Death: A Timeline of the Gruesome Pandemic. *History.com,* A&E Television Networks, Retrieved from https://www.history.com/news/black-death-timeline
10. Sussman, George D. (2015). Scientists Doing History: Central Africa and the Origins of the First Plague Pandemic, *Journal of World History,* June, 26(2), 325-354, University of Hawai'i Press on behalf of World History Association. Retrieved on 23rd December, 2020 https://www.jstor.org/stable/43901755
11. Theilmann, John and Cate, Frances. (2007). A Plague of Plagues: The Problem of Plague Diagnosis in Medieval England. *The Journal of Interdisciplinary History.* 37 (3), 371-393. The MIT Press. Retrieved on 23rd December, 2020 https://www.jstor.org/stable/4139605
12. Yeomans, Sarah K. (2020). Pandemics in Perspectiv, *Biblical Archaeology Review,* 26 August. Accessed on 23.12.2020.

12

Virus Versus Women

Historical Introduction to Gender Dimension of Migration at the time of Disease

P.K. Yadav

ABSTRACT

Paul Farmer, the well-known author of "Pathologies of Power", once said that the epidemics and pandemics are "biological expressions of social inequality". And history says that crisis tests humanity in its worst form. But during the time of a disease and epidemics, women as a social group are most badly tried, tested and terminated from their rights, roots and aspirations. Their vulnerability and marginalization is also strikingly visible like never before when they are forced to face the denial of identity, dignity and opportunity. This aspect of women in a society can be studied by looking at the gender dimension of migration in the time a disease.

Keywords: Development, Epidemics, Marginalisation, Migration, Opportunity, Women

"Women around the world face with tough choices. They are the disproportionate group that observes stress and impact. Some nights women sleep with tears to wake up with smile to a new day. Many don't have shoulders to cry on, many don't have safe places to go, many don't have means to support themselves or their children."

—Amanda Neikam, University of Maryland

Amidst the Covid-19 Pandemic and nationwide lethal lockdown, one of the images that came out of India was of a girl child of about six years of age, walking with her worldly possessions, tied in a small piece of cloth on her head. Parents trekked with infants, even the elderly. This was an unexpectedly heartbreaking image enough to inspire an effortless conscious thought processes. Last few months have also witnessed the fight of magnanimous man and woman against the microscopic microbe called Covid-19. This global existential crisis of unparalleled magnitude has unearthed and brought to the surface several unnoticed issues that are otherwise lost in the class hatred, caste divide and communal consideration. This can be located in the axis and praxis of man, microbe and migration which traces the human and historical question about how and why India migrate. This specifically refers and responds to a class of people who are most underappreciated, overworked and underpaid. They are not a part of our collective imagination: they are the migrants from the length and breadth of India. Therefore, it is pertinent to see and make a sense of the question of migration in a proper historical perspective with reference to gender question.

Movement of people is not new in human history. Migration has been a particularly peculiar feature of human existence for centuries. Humans have often migrated in groups as well as individuals. Migration has been one of the most positive means of greater global interaction and integration. This rich trajectory of population movement on account of seasonal or circular migration for hunting, agriculture or pastoralism, migration in search of greater security and subsistence, to escape natural disasters and warfare, for trade and pilgrimage have tremendously shaped and changed the course of human experience, its exigencies and the patterns of human to human cross border cultural contacts and collaborations. Women have been a closely related part of the global migration history. However, women dimension of migration has not received its due share in historical scholarship, analysis and explanation. Gender specific migration trends and their analysis deserve adequate historical light, insight and specifically targeted grounded research, besides some of the recent works that are being done on account of women diaspora studies with regard to South Asia.

This chapter is an attempt to examine and explain the gender dimension of migration in the time of a disease in a historical introductory outline. Looking through a historical lens, this foregrounds some of the perturbing social and psychological issues related with the gender dimension of population movement. The article considers the relationship between migration and gender roles and relations (Premi, 1980). Census of India 2011 revealed that women form almost 70 per cent of the internal migrant community and gender influences reasons for migrating, who migrates and to where, how people migrate and the networks they use, opportunities and resources available at destinations, and relations with the place of origin. Risks, vulnerabilities and needs are also shaped in large part by one's gender, and often vary drastically for different groups. The roles, expectations, relationships and power dynamics associated with being a man, woman, boy or girl, and whether one identifies as lesbian, gay, bisexual, transgender and/or intersex (LGBTI), significantly affect all aspects of the migration process, and can also be affected in new ways by migration (International Organisation for Migration, 2020).

It is therefore important to understand how gender interacts with migration and to respond accordingly. Taking into consideration gender-specific migration patterns can mean the difference between implementing a project that successfully addresses the specific needs and capacities of all, and one that fails to do so and perpetuates inequality (Banerjee and Raju, 2009). Given the gender-specific nature of migration, it is pertinent to think, and act on advocating for equal rights under the law in employment and mobility; combatting discriminatory migration practices; understanding how gender affects the types of migration undertaken; responding to how gender influences access to social services, economic growth, capacities, risks and vulnerabilities; ensuring diversity and inclusiveness in consultations and participation in activities; and addressing how migration influences gender roles and relations (International Organisation for Migration, 2020). The issue of migration, intra and interstate, can also be located from the point of economic exigencies, inefficient and insensitive institutional policy positions, and willfully ignoring political perspective which is associated with the fate of 395 million interstate migrants in India, of which 62 million and 31 million are Dalits and Adivasis respectively. They moved to cities precisely on account of caste violence, atrocities, poverty or loss of ownership over forests and land. Migration is also linked with the humanly quest for upward socio-economic mobility. However, disadvantaged sections are disproportionately tried, tested and failed by the systematic urban spatiality (Yengde, 2020).

Peruse Dirk Hoerder's *Cultures in Contact* (2002), a prize-winning historical overview of global migrations during the last millennium, where one will find throughout close attention to gender dynamics. Not only migration systems characterized as predominantly male or female, but the author suggests how the interplay of individual circumstances, familial relationships, larger economic cycles, and existing circuits of knowledge and transportation are gendered and how that interplay encourages or discourages certain types of migration at particular point of time, in particular places, and even at times for particular individuals. As an example of global history, *Cultures in Contact* a far cry from Arnold Toynbee's *A Study of History* (1948), a 12-volume chronicle of "civilizations" in which women, let alone gender analyses, do not appear, or even from Immanuel Wallerstein's *The Modern World-System* (1974, 3 volumes), to which Hoerder pays intellectual homage. In some ways, *Cultures in Contact* most calls to mind the early work of geographer E. G. Ravenstein (1885) with his laws of migration, written in the 1880s – both for its striving toward an inclusive definition of migration and for the attention it pays to men and women in migration circuits, though Ravenstein viewed women as primarily involved in short-distance migration compared to longer-range migration for men, a point that Hoerder disputes. Yet Hoerder also echoes Ravenstein in seeking patterns and in building theory – hallmarks of social science methodology shared across the century and across disciplines (Sinke, 2006).

The gender dimension of migration is crucial as women have notably different migration intensions, motivations, patterns, options, and obstacles from men. Men and women tend to experience migration differently; the challenges of re-negotiating work and care in a new setting often led to a 'feminization' of women's roles, as women find themselves taking up more traditional gender roles as wives and mothers. In many cases, men make autonomous decisions while women migrate as part of family strategies where they are not in full control. The most common cause for female migration in India is considered to be marriage and largely explained by the twin factors of marriage and dependency on the principal bread-winner. Internal migration in India is highly differentiated, and women's involvement in geographic mobility is also highly variable, their tendencies to migrate and forms of migration depending on their social and economic positions at origin; cultural differences and prescriptions for female behavior; demands for female labor;

and other social and economic factors (Singh, 2015).

Women currently make up around half of the world's migrant population, and this is without taking into consideration short-term and seasonal movements, many of which are unrecorded. Globally, the number of female migrants has been large and increasing, both in terms of sheer number of women involved and in terms of their share of world's migrant stock. There is a remarkable diversity of migration patterns among women, and such diversity has increased along with recent economic and social changes in both sending and receiving locations. Women migrate for long and short periods, over short and long distances. They move for many reasons, of which marriage is only one and among which work is becoming increasingly significant. Young women dominate in migration, but older women migrate as well. They move with or without their families. Both single and married women migrate. Indeed, there is growing evidence of women who have borne children moving for work, leaving the care of their children with family members who remain at home (Ghosh, 2012).

As a discipline, history had its own rigidities and these became particularly visible as discussions of globalization and transnationalism emerged in the 1990s. For historians of migration – a phenomenon that typically crossed national boundaries – the organization of the discipline around national fields (notably in the modern era) has been problematic. A student who does not follow chronological and regional criteria risks never getting into a graduate program (for lack of an advisor) and more importantly risks the chance of not getting a tenure-track job, for until the late 1990s practically no positions existed outside national paradigms. Even today the vast majority of positions in history are both region- and time-specific, although positions requiring expertise in world history or in several world regions continue to increase in number. The flowering of theoretical interest in global, international, and transnational approaches to migration in the 1990s was a welcome development to those interested in women and in gender, but it was also one that challenged them to examine gender in a wide range of locations. No longer would historians examine gender mainly or exclusively through study of immigration to North American nations, or through analyses of gendered adaptation to single national states. Instead, analysis of gender is pursued at a variety of regional, global, and transnational levels (Sinke, 2006).

According to UN, the proportion of women migrants has increased over the years. In 2005, nearly half of the world's migrants were women: there were more female than male migrants in Europe, Latin America and the Caribbean, North America, Oceania and in the former USSR. Whereas, women traditionally migrated to join their partners or families or migrated together with their family in the earlier periods, an increasing number of women are migrating independently. These women are labour migrants, often the primary earners for their families. However, there is a difference of global and local historical perspectives when it comes to women migration.Until the late 1970s, most writings on international migration either focused explicitly only on male migrants (usually conceived of as workers) or seemed to assume implicitly that most migrants were male. That assumption was particularly prevalent when attention was focused on the economic aspects of international migration, because it was widely believed that the participation of women in international labor migration was negligible. Of course, such beliefs were rarely based on statistical evidence since, both then and now, data on international migrants often were not classified by sex. Consequently, when scholars began to call attention to the participation of women in international migration, one of their tasks was to refute those beliefs (Zlotnikthe, 2003).

Historically, women were thought to migrate primarily for marriage or family reunification, both internationally and nationally. Marriage migration is particularly sought when the ratio of women to men is low, such as in rural northern India, where women from eastern India and Nepal are sought for marriage. According to International Organization for Migration (IOM), China's one child policy resulted in a dramatic gender imbalance, leading to foreign wives being sought from Vietnam, as well as Lao P.D.R. and Myanmar (Fleury, 2016). As a matter of fact, for more than 40 years, female migrants have been almost as numerous as male migrants. In 1960, there were 35 million female migrants and 40 million male migrants; by 2000, although the total number of migrants had more than doubled, the gap between female and male remained about the same, 85 million female migrants versus 90 million male migrants (Zlotnikthe, 2003). .

The globalization of the care economy – and the international division of household work is a good example to understand the nature of work, role and place that are occupied by women in the historical migration story. Domestic service is one of the most common occupations of women migrants from developing countries to developed ones. This is particularly true in some European countries like France, Italy, Spain and Greece, as well high and middle-income countries in Asia and the Gulf states. In the 1990s, this was also encouraged by official policies: a significant proportion of the migrants who entered Italy, Greece and Spain through the quota system, were women domestic workers, and they also dominated among those migrants who were subsequently regularised. For some developing countries, this is now the major component of migration in the Philippines and Sri Lanka (Ghosh, 2012). Many such women perform domestic tasks – the labour involved in social reproduction – that is still seen as the responsibility of women in the more developed industrial societies in Europe or North America, or the more dynamic and rapidly growing developing parts of Asia such as Hong Kong, Singapore and South Korea, or the oil-exporting countries of West Asia and the Gulf. They thereby potentially free such female labour for more active participation in the paid labour market, and contribute to the economic growth of the receiving country. At the same time, the migrant women's own household responsibilities back home must be fulfilled by other women, since the gender division of labour at both ends of the migratory spectrum still leaves women primarily responsible for doing the domestic work (Parrenas, 2001, 37). This housework back home is often performed by women relatives, such as mothers, sisters and daughters. But the very large wage differentials across sending and receiving countries can allow such migrant workers in turn to relegate their own domestic work by hiring poorer local women to care for their own children and perform necessary household tasks. In turn, such women may even be migrants from rural areas who have come into cities and towns in search of income (Ghosh, 2012).

Men account for over 80% of all internal migration for work in India. But between 2001 and 2011, female migration more than doubled from around 4.1 million to 8.5 million, Mazumdar and Neetha (2020) wrote in a paper published in *The Economic and Political Weekly* in May. In 2001, 47 per cent of women migrating for work, were headed to urban areas. By 2011, it was 58%. "Notwithstanding the visibility of women among these migrants, the gender dimensions of the migrant question and the special conditions of women's labour migration remained largely ignored or sidelined in the public policy debates and interventions that were pushed to centre stage by the Covid-19 pandemic". The failure of "official macro data to delineate the scope, scale and patterns of female labour migration" and thus incorporate gender in development approaches to internal migration, was also highlighted in an IWWAGE report in May 2019 (Bhandare, 2020).

These failures could prove costly. "Emerging trends underline how the convergence of poverty, gender and marginalisation has played out during the pandemic, to render women, and specific categories amongst them, especially vulnerable," write Indu Agnihotri of Centre for Women's Development Studies and Asha Hans, founding director, School of Women's Studies, Utkal University, Bhubaneswar, in a forthcoming book on Covid-19 and migration. Women pay the highest price during any major economic shock, said Mahesh Vyas, managing director and CEO of the Centre for Monitoring Indian Economy, whose Consumer Pyramids Household Survey has collected weekly data at a national level since January 2016 from close to 175,000 households. Of the 6.7 million women displaced from the labour force during this period, 2.3 million were rural women while 4.4 million were urban women. In fact, urban women saw the deepest loss with a labour force contraction of 27.2%. For urban men, the contraction was 2.8% (Bhandare, 2020).

According to recent paper by Indrani and Neetha, it should be axiomatic that the spectrum of labour laws that govern wages, employment relations, and social security apply to both migrant and non-migrant workers; so also do the unique provisions for the countervailing force of collective action by workers against the inequalities of power in employment relations, as argued by Otto Kahn-Freund (1972).

> The relation between an employer and an isolated employee or worker is typically a relation between a bearer of power and one who is not a bearer of power. In its inception it is an act of submission, in its operation it is a condition of subordination, however much the submission and the subordination may be concealed by that indispensable figment of the legal mind known as the "contract of employment". The main object of labour law has always been, and we venture to say will always

> be, to be a countervailing force to counteract the inequality of bargaining (Mazumdar and Neetha, 2020).

While the Constituent Assembly was in session, the Factories Act, 1948 set the benchmark for the regulations regarding conditions of work, the Minimum Wages Act, 1948 (MWA) for the statutory minimum wage for all workers, including the outworkers and employments outside factories. The Employees' State Insurance Act (ESI), 1948 provided a framework for health benefits (including maternity), and the provident fund for coal workers in 1948 followed by the Employees' Provident Fund Act (EPF), 1952 made provision for post-employment/retirement. These social rights were however, not independent of the conflicts between labour and capital, given the cognizance by the Industrial Disputes Act, 1947. Male migrants are more often employed in construction and are paid more than female migrants, who work mostly in trade and services. However, men and women show almost no difference in complying with migration laws, vulnerability in interactions with the state, relations with employers and apartment owners as well as transnational practices (Rocheva and Evgeni, 2018). Further, a narrow outreach of labour laws has long undermined and limited its democratising force by denying a majority of workers' access to key entitlements, such as women workers. Despite the constitutional direction to the state to ensure "equal pay for equal work for both men and women" (Article 39), the Equal Remuneration Act (ERA), 1976 was enacted only after the recommendation of the Committee on the Status of Women in India (CSWI) in the 1970s. Even today, the ERA remains insubstantial in implementation. Feminised paid domestic work (mostly migrant) and female intensive home-based manufacturing remain bereft of the regulations for providing the minimum rights granted in the labour laws (Mazumdar and Neetha, 2020).

Even as a strong male bias in labour migration persists, with men accounting for more than 80% of migrant labour in India, the rising numbers and proportions of women migrating for work are no less striking. Census figures showed a spurt in female migration for employment and business (from around 41 lakh in 2001 to 85 lakh in 2011), and an increased female share of such migrants from 12% to 16%. Census data also showed a shift in the pattern of female labour migration from predominantly rural destinations to a distinctive tilt towards urban destinations. Forty-seven per cent of all women migrating for work/business were in urban areas in 2001. By 2011, migration to urban destinations had jumped to 58%. Such a trend is likely to have been further enhanced since 2011, with the Periodic Labour Force Survey (PLFS) data for 2017–18, showing a further dramatic fall in work participation rates (WPR) among rural women by 7 percentage points from 24.8% to 17.5%, reflecting an absolute drop by close to 25 million women workers in rural India after 2011–12 and by just short of 47 million, if 2004–05 is taken as the benchmark year. Although the decline is notable across all social groups, it is most for women from Scheduled Caste (SC) and Scheduled Tribe (ST) categories, with the WPR of ST and SC women dropping by about 10 percentage points during 2011–12 to 2017-18 (Bhagat, 2010). Such a large-scale, and historically unprecedented eviction of women from the rural workforce, especially of the most oppressed castes/communities, highlights the negative impact of neo-liberalism's growth paradigm—ramping up of agrarian distress, and an employment crisis that is highly gendered. Stagnation in urban India, where female WPR are even lower, hovering between 15 per cent and 14 per cent across the decade of 2007–08, with just a small increase in absolute numbers, can hardly compensate. Nevertheless, the shift towards the urban in women's migration is obviously a key phenomenon of the times (Muzumdar and Neetha, 2013).

Ipsita Sapra from TISS says that the migration of single women for work has been on the rise with the middle-class-isation of the Indian cities. This middle-class-isation, an outcome of the growth of the service sector, has spurred a series of consequences. It has created jobs for both men and women. Large numbers of nuclear families with both spouses working in professional spaces have created a set of service demands in the family. Single women work as live-in domestic help in the metropolis of Delhi, Mumbai, and Chennai. Women in the service economy work in salons and beauty parlours. Women work in restaurants as waitresses and usherettes. Women work as assistants in large stores. The cooks, the cleaners, and the co-workers in construction sites or family units working in brick-kilns. The piece-rate worker at the lowest rung of a global supply chain. The silently accompanying 'other' in an overwhelmingly male phenomenon of mobility. These are women who are still captured in the camera lens as walking with their husbands and children. However, the single women migrants while being a ubiquitous part of our daily existence are completely invisible from the media gaze. What brought single women to the cities? This chapter is an attempt to steer the gaze to the women question in migration in the wake of the COVID-19 situation (Sapra, 2020).

However, the macro-data sets fail in helping us understand the nature of women's employment, especially in urban areas. Of the three broad categories of regular, self-employed and casual workers, the share of regular employment among women workers in urban areas is the category that shows consistent increase for more than three decades. It rose from 28.4 per cent in 1993–94 to 42.8 per cent in 2011–12, and then to 52.1 per cent by 2017–18. Prima facie, it is assumed that this denotes better forms and conditions of work for women workers. However, regular work is defined only in terms of duration of employment, irrespective of wages and other conditions of work. Thus, paid domestic work and other service sector employees, who may be working continuously during the year without minimum wages and on completely insecure terms, are counted as regular workers. The actual growth of temporary and casual employment is thus not adequately captured by the macro data, especially in the case of female employment. The occupational profile of women's employment in the PLFS 2017–18, however, gives us a useful insight into the contemporary pattern of urban women's employment. Manufacturing constituted the single largest occupation for the female workforce in urban areas (45 lakh), of which 20 lakh were textile and garment workers, and another 16.5 lakh were in food processing, tobacco products (beedi workers) and leather goods. Teachers constituted another big chunk, with those in pre-primary to secondary education numbering around 21 lakh, and another 6.5 lakh in higher education. Domestic workers were around 20 lakh, with *ayahs* and childcare workers constittute 4 lakh, while 11.3 lakh were shops and salespersons, another 11 lakh were in housekeeping and restaurant services, and 10.5 lakh were clerical workers. Around 10 lakh were construction workers. A little over 5 lakh were health professionals, of which more than half were nurses. Close to 4 lakh were garbage collectors and another 4 lakh were beauticians. Some 4.5 lakh were occupied in finance, business, administrative, police, social work, etc, and a surprising 16.6 lakh were directors and chief executives. Together, these workers constituted around 79 per cent of the 2.19 crore urban female workforce. Further, some 20 per cent of urban women workers were home-based (Mazumdar and Neetha, 2020).

Historical scholars across time and space unanimously agree that migration is the hallmark of modern times along with its intrinsic aspects for development. In recent times, women have been the pioneers in migration not only through marriage to different towns and cities but also in search of better livelihood for themselves and their families. However, women's migration brings issues of restricted movement, vigilance and control. These restrictions, vigilance and control act as obstacles on women's migration especially in Indian society. The present study aims to enhance the understanding of migratory process with special focus on gender dimension between two migration related rounds (55th and 64th) of the NSS. Starting with an illustration of changes in migration at macro level reveals that migration men are less than that of women. There has been increase in women's migration with increasing age. The difference, however, between the levels of migration during the period of 1999-2000 to 2007-2008 is not so high. Migration from rural to urban is more dominating than urban to urban streams, which is also the main reason of urbanization. One significant finding that emerges from this study is that, factors such as low income and low literacy are the common determinants of migration for both sexes, but low level of social status is found to be associated significantly only for men's migration. On the contrary, marriage is not the only most critical factor for women migration but high income, high literacy and higher social status are also some major pull factors associated with women's migration in urban India (Singh, 2015). Here, it is very touchy to mention that migration can improve the autonomy, human capital, and self esteem of women, as well as women's authority and worth in their families and communities. Migration has the potential to advance more equitable social norms and improve women's rights and access to resources. Although migration is largely beneficial, there are many constraints that limit its gains, such as restrictive social norms or laws, gender and racial discrimination, and gender specific vulnerabilities.

The depiction of women's migration today is complex, representing the apparent advantages to women of higher incomes and acknowledgment of work as well as the dangers and difficulties linked with migrating to new and unknown situations with the potential for various kinds of exploitation. The desperation that drives most such economic migration, and the exploitative conditions that it can result in, deserve desired historical examination, understanding and explanation. But it is also true that the categorical knowledge of conditions and possibilities elsewhere can have a liberating impact upon women, which creates a momentum for positive social change and gender empowerment. Even if we are not convinced by Good Economics for Hard Times: Better Answers to Our Biggest Problems where the authors dispute the alarmist narratives and argue that, far from being a major threat, migration should be welcomed if not encouraged, we need to recognize and realize if not respond to the migrant workers' crisis in the time of Corona. Migration is also an important way of transformation with its compellingly contrasting incidences and phases. The most appealing among them is: the migration will never stop. But the quality of migration will improve every generation.

REFERENCES

1. Anna Rocheva and Evgeni Varshaver. (2018) Gender Dimension of Migration from Central Asia to the Russian Federation. *Asia-Pacific Population Journal*, Volume 32, Issue 2, Nov 2018, p. 87-135. https://doi.org/10.18356/e617261d-en
2. Banerjee, A. and Raju, S. (2009). Gendered Mobility: Women Migrants and Work in Urban India', *Economic and Political Weekly*, 54(28): 115-123. Retrieved December 29, 2020 from https://www.epw.in/journal/2009/28/special-articles/gendered-mobility-women-migrants-and-work-urban-india.html
3. Bhandare, N. (Dec. 16, 2020). Although men too lost jobs, the pandemic affected Indian women in the workforce harder. Retrieved from https://scroll.in/article/981291/although-men-too-lost-jobs-the-pandemic-affected-indian-women-in-the-workforce-harder
4. Fleury, Anjali (February 2016) Understanding Women and Migration: A Literature Review (KNOMAD Working Paper 8), KNOWMAD. p. 3
5. Ghosh, J. (2012) The Gender Dimension Of Migration and Global Crisis. Retrieved from https://www.ingenere.it/en/articles/gender-dimension-migration-and-global-crisis

6. Hania, Zlotnikthe. (2003). *Global Dimensions Of Female Migration.* Migration Policy Institute. Washington, DC: Retrieved from https://www.migrationpolicy.org/article/global-dimensions-female-migration
7. International Organisation for Migration. (2020). Gender and Migration. Retrieved on December 29, 2020 from www.iom.int/gender-and-migration.
8. Mazumdar, I., Neetha N. (2020) Crossroads and Boundaries: Labour Migration, Trafficking and Gender. *Economic and Political Weekly*, 55 (20), Retrieved December 29, 2020 from https://www.epw.in/journal/2020/20/review-womens-studies/crossroads-and-boundaries.html
9. Mazumdar, I., Neetha, N. and Agnihotri, I. (2013) Migration and Gender in India, *Economic and Political Weekly*, 48(10): 54-64.Retrieved December 29, 2020 fromhttps://www.epw.in/journal/2013/10/special-articles/migration-and-gender-india.html
10. Parreas R. (2001) *Servants of Globalization: Women, Migration and Domestic Work,* Stanford, CA: Stanford University Press, p.37
11. Premi, M. (1980). Aspects of Female Migration in India. *Economic and Political Weekly, 15*(15), 714-720. Retrieved December 30, 2020, from http://www.jstor.org/stable/4368564
12. Sapra, I (April 25, 2020) Why don't we see women? The untold story of covid-19 migration." *The Indian Express.*
13. Singh, N., Keshri, K., & Bhagat R.B. (2015). Gender Dimension Of Migration In Urban India. In S. Irudaya Rajan (Ed), *India Migration Report 2015: Gender and Migration* (ed.) Rutledge, New Delhi, pp. 176-190
14. Sinke, S. (2006). "Gender and Migration: Historical Perspectives. *The International Migration Review,* 40(1), 82-103. Retrieved December 29, 2020, from http://www.jstor.org/stable/27645580
15. Yengde, S. (2020 April 5). Dalitality: The Caste Factor in Social Distancing. *The Indian Express.*

13

Women and Pandemic

History behind the Humanly and Heroic Contribution of Women

Anuradha Thakur

ABSTRACT

Women have been playing significant role during any pandemic all over the globe. Countries like Finland, Germany, Denmark, and New Zealand have done far better to handle Coronavirus pandemic. The female leadership has been fighting more efficiently than their male counterparts in other countries. The number of deaths due to virus is far less than the male-dominated states. If we turn the pages of history, we will find that women have been contributing in epidemic, such as plague since time immemorial. Catherine the Great, Empress of Russia, was the first to be inoculated against the smallpox vaccination during Russian plague in 1768. She had also established first Russian College of Medicine and hospitals for the civilians. This chapter deals with the prominence of the unending continuity of contribution of women from past to present in twenty-first century. It highlight women and their role of leadership combatting epidemics since decades of history. Women have remarkable association in the healthcare services worldwide. The able management, collaboration and preparedness define the effective administration of women in such tragic times. Such things with regard to gender participation and women contribution have historical antecedents and precedents that reach to this day.

Keywords: Catherine, Jacinda, Pandemic, Savitribai, Women Warriors

The narratives of unsung heroes, *Women* find no mention in history books. However, they have travelled time and history and still are contributing to the frontline healthcare warriors. The fourteenth century's plague, probably the most deadly disaster in human history, set free many serfs in Europe, forced the wages for labourers to rise, and caused a fundamental shift in the economy along with an increased standard of living for survivors (Blackburn and Parker, 2018). The history of epidemics and pandemic portray the forgotten past of the women warriors. Highly exposed to the risks of infection, they steps out in a gender-biased landscape to save lives. They are the living contemporary figures of humanity tracing lives to recreation and rejuvenation. Today, we face the global outbreak of a disease that has the potential to catalyse what the historian Eva Schlotheuber terms a *pandemic of the mind* (Miller, 2020). The creation of such sort of pandemic arose due to the strict nationwide lockdowns. Humans find it difficult to be under the safe walls of their houses. Many were trapped in different nations, held the desire to reach to their real homes. Unfortunately, the fabric of mankind is at the stake. The history has repeated itself nearly after a century of occurrence of the Spanish Flu pandemic. The different aspects of the socio-political, economical, and cultural life seemed to be devastated.

Diseases have been part of humans and their histories ever since they have been on the earth and history has infinite number of examples with Women Warriors in medical wars of world. The frontline healthcare staffs are women nurses in majority, according to the statistics. Women, the Creator of Civilization, have not been only nurturing the lives, but risking their own amidst this Corona virus pandemic. Giovanni Boccaccio, the author of *The Decameron* illustrates the narratives of seven women who fled plague driven Florence in his book. This chapter is an attempt to locate the historical legacy, agency, and exigencies of womanly quest for a better, sustainable and healthy world that has an unbroken history and hence, it deserves our sincere historical investigation and application of research insight. This paper also tries to apply scholarly inquiry techniques that can bring into light the roles, responsibilities and conviction that the women have showed in times of crisis, emergency and distress from the pages of the past to the canvas of the present.

'Her' Story during Epidemic Times

Women warriors have shown tremendous efforts in lifting mankind in pandemic. One such name is Catherine, the Great, who finds great historical relevance. She established standard professional healthcare in Russia. Empress Catherine II established 'a medical commission' and personally introduced 'vaccination' (Alexander, 1981). She hailed great scientific temperament and rationality in professional medical care. Her interest in the public health was derived from the problem of high infantile mortality rate. She opened hospitals with multi-beds out of her personal interest. The first permanent public hospital in the empire was Paul's Hospital (Alexander, 1981). The lack of sufficient skilled surgeons had caused unnecessary suffering and loss of life during the Seven Years' War, the Empress lamented; she recommended increasing surgical cadres and improving their status (Alexander, 1981). The Bubonic Plague by the end of eighteenth century took death toll in severe conditions. Empress was more convinced in the public medical healthcare infrastructure after the plague. She opened medical institutions and increased recruitment of medical staffs.

Catherine didn't stop at Moscow Plague. She actively conducted meetings with medical council to understand the nature of disease. After studying medical records, she proposed her own "method", ice baths or wrappers (Proskurina, 2011). Her method proved to be effective in some cases and even came into some medical reviews under her name as *Remedium Antipestilentialae Catharinae Secundae* (Mikhail, 2008). In one incident, Empress even risked her life. On October 12, 1768, the British physician Thomas Dimsdale inoculated Catherine with tissue taken from a recovered boy by the name of Alexander Markov (Proskurina, 2011). She emerged as the warrior and saviour of Russia by setting an example for the entire European nations. The successful inoculation placed her reign dynamic forever in the pages of history. She defeated 'hydra' and saved Russia twice in the battle against plague. She was awakening at the plague riot. However, considerable efforts were taken in concern. Catherine, the Great is remarkably a pioneer in the resolution of public health and Black Death.

Woman Position and Movement Advanced along with 1918 Flu

The 1918 influenza pandemic, commonly known as the Spanish Flu, is estimated to have infected 500 million people, or one-third of the world's population (*Women: The Unsung Heroes of the 1918 Flu Pandemic*, 2020). However, it was seen as the phase of opportunities for women. The era also witnessed First World War at the same time. As the nurses, women became the primary caregivers of the pandemic. Taking charge of the day-to-day care, they risked infection while ventilating rooms, administering remedies the doctor had recommended, and ensuring patients were warm, nourished, and hydrated (Sachan, 2017). We have not mentioned such crucial participation of women in our history books nor have we documented her story. This won't largely affect women contribution in medicine. Not only did their role in this pandemic help shape the future for women in medicine, it proved female nurses of the time with a sense of professional fulfilment (*Women: The Unsung Heroes of the 1918 Flu Pandemic,* 2020). The soldiers were infected with the flu virus in parallel with war. This created a gap and shortage of labour was the immediate consequence. This gap enabled women to play a new and indispensable role in the workforce during the crucial period (Blackburn and Parker, 2018). When the influenza pandemic hit, many doctors were serving in the First World War so nurses and volunteers stepped in, including these women at the Red Cross Emergency Ambulance Station in Washington, D.C (Dubois, 2020).

Women Nurses in the Spanish Flu in America

Women were enrolled as nurses to help during the influenza pandemic (Dubois, 2020). Mable Chilson was one of these professional nurses. As the epidemic raged in the Midwest, Mabel Chilson was one of many student nurses at Fort Des Moines, who decided to help the needy. In *The Spanish Influenza Pandemic of 1918-1919: New Perspectives,* Nancy Bristow shares some passages Chilson wrote for her school yearbook: "*We wondered, 'were we helpless or could we fight?' With eager determination we entered the ranks*" (Baldwin, & Taylor, 2020). In Bristow's book *American Pandemic: The Lost Worlds of the 1918 Influenza Epidemic,* we learn of more of these nurses, including Miss Condell, a nursing student in Boston, who said

> "All of us who had any part in helping in the epidemic must look back upon it as one of the most immediately satisfactory experiences of our lives, and this is true even though we were borne down with the knowledge that,

do all we might, the pressing, tragic need for nursing was much greater than could possibly be met. (Nanthini, & Nair, 2020).

Women, thus, led this pandemic phase by administering care and emerged as the major workforce in those times.

Woman Serving in Epidemic: Crossing the Caste Barriers in India

Savitribai Phule is a great social reformer of India. Her life is a testimony to the social cause and upliftment of women. The Black Death or Bubonic Death hit the Indian sub-continent severely in the nineteenth century. The historic pandemic has caused irresistible damages. An anecdote mentions, how Savitribai carried a 10 year old boy from Mahar settlement in Mundhwa to her son's clinic in Pune's outskirts. Although the little boy survived, Savitribai caught the infection and succumbed to it on 10th March 1987 at the age of 66 (Kandukuri, 2019). When doctors were not ready to treat patients due to the caste prejudice prevalent in India. Savitribai took a step ahead to treat *Shudra* and *Dalit* patients. She urged her son, Yashwantrao Phule to start a clinic in Pune. While treating patients, he was also caught by plague and eventually lost his life on 13 October 1905. Her work is really commendable in spite of caste dynamics.

From the Past to the Present

The women warriors have arrived here from history. Even today, after hundred years, a new virus has taken death toll in millions and women have been so effective in tackling the scenario. Here, an attempt has been made to establish the connection between the *forgotten histories to facing here, via her efforts* (Walsh, 2017). Women leaders have shown remarkable genius in controlling spread of Corona virus infection in their respective countries. The study carried out by Supriya

Garikipati, University of Liverpool, and Uma Kambhampati, University of Reading, revealed that policy measures in the initial three month of the pandemic in female-led countries saved nearly two times more lives than those run by male leaders despite having similar number of cases. This study is published in the economic Policy Research and the World Economic Forum analysing 194 countries hit by Covid-19 (De, 2020). The study also highlighted that women leaders and saved more lives imposed lockdown immediately. However, their male counterparts risked lives of their people for economy.

Youngest Woman Leader Tackling Covid-19

Jacinda Ardern became the Prime Minister of New Zealand at the age of 40. She has been the youngest women leader in 2017. New Zealand, with 1,514 confirmed cases of Covid-19 and just 25 deaths in a population of 5 million, has been hailed along with South Korea and Taiwan for its success in combating the novel Corona virus partly due to shift lockdown measures (New Zealand PM Jacinda Ardern touts success in tackling Covid-19 pandemic in poll push, 2020). With the sheer determination, Jacinda made it possible to handle Corona virus. Her government took immediate action of imposing lockdown as early as 15th March. Moreover, the country ramped up its testing capacity to 8,000 tests per day, one of the highest testing rates per capita in the world at that time (De, 2020). This also made her to win election and re-elected as Prime Minister for one more term. Women around the globe have made the impossible as possible. However, society is critical in addressing her major contribution in severe life-threatening times of the pandemic.

Herself a Scientist: Woman Leader in Germany

As we see cases take a surge, Germany with a better healthcare system also collapsed. Although, Angela Merkel,

Chancellor of Germany took succeeding steps to tackle Covid-19 death rates in Germany. A lady of composure made sure that the country must get all the necessary medical aid and information. She kept track of misinformation and rumours from creating havoc among the people in the state (Krishnadas & Taha, 2020). Trusted by her people to navigate the murky waters of outbreak, without inciting or succumbing to a pandemic of the mind, one politician is less commander in chief and more a scientist in chief: Angela Merkel (Miller, 2020). Her political persona coupled with scientific background was very cautious in handling the entire healthcare infrastructure coping up with corona death rates. Moreover, high mortality rate cannot be debated against her charismatic personality. The pandemic has brought the entire mankind on toes. It's only where we can really appreciate the association of women leaders putting in so many efforts to handle Covid-19 with effective results.

Quick Response of Taiwan

Tsai Ing-Wen holds the command in Taiwan with such a quick response that resulted relatively less death in the state. They mechanised the healthcare system with digitalisation of citizens' records (Marindo, 2017). In January 2020, Taiwan established a response team for the disease and activated the Central Epidemic Command Centre. To cater to the demand for masks, the government introduced maps with real-time updates about mask inventory nearby (De, 2020). Here again, the woman leader started the implementation of healthcare infrastructure from quarantine to masks inventory immediately at the outbreak of Covid-19. This shows the far-sightedness and presence of mind of women warriors in the pandemic.

Women Workforce in Covid-19

The pandemic that has shocked the global leaders and left

economy to agonize, couldn't defeat women in the frontline. Women comprise 70 per cent of the global healthcare workforce, and yet they only hold 25 per cent of the senior roles in the healthcare profession (Miyamoto, 2020). Healthcare workers are at a greater risk of transmission of virus as they are attending the patients. A higher proportion of healthcare workers diagnosed with Covid-19 were women, reflecting workforce demographics. In Spain 72 per cent (5,265) of infected healthcare workers were women and in Italy 66 per cent (10,657) of infected healthcare workers were women (Miyamoto, 2020). Similarly, in the United States, the Centres for Disease Control and Prevention found that 73 per cent (6,603) of infected healthcare workers were women (Miyamoto, 2020). Policymakers must come up with gender inclusion programmes to tackle the existing scenario. We are losing a bunch of professional and trained, skilled workforce in the pandemic.

Humanly Contribution of Half of the Population

On the other side of the coin is *Shadow Pandemic* for women as described by United Nation. Ironically, major workforce is also the section of the society which is facing increased number of violence. Emerging data shows an increase in calls to domestic violence helplines in many countries since the outbreak of Covid-19 (Guidorzi, 2020). So far, we have seen how women from different parts of the world has contributed in epidemics and pandemics. Women find no especial mention in the history. However, unnamed fighters have a footmark in the survival of mankind amidst pandemic Archibong & Annan, 2017). Catherine, the Great to Savitribai Phule, to modern Jacinda and many more women leaders have done marvellous jobs in the healthcare system. The Spanish Flu Nurses have toded the path instead of World War to serve the needy. From the *pages of past to the present book,* pandemics have always witnessed women warriors, contribution in frontline health care workers (Rahmaty, & Jaghab, 2020).

Epidemics are "not random events that afflict societies capriciously and without warning," says historian Frank Snowden in his book *Epidemics and Society: From the Black Death to the Present*. "On the contrary, every society produces its own specific vulnerabilities" (Baruah, 2020). All of that remind us that disease is still shaping and changing human history and has the potential to be the most powerful and provocative force in human history. When cholera started to make its way out of India in the 1820s, "It," as the historian Mark Harrison wrote, "defined the contours of a new world economy, revealing its connections and also, more starkly, its divisions."

The same will be true of the Corona virus. Historians of disease are unlikely to spend much time on epistemology, and given the richness of our sources for historical exploration, analysis and understanding, the nature of our concerns, and our unstable disciplinary diversity, this should not surprise anyone. Most of us are not inclined to question the biological presence of disease and death, but we need to stand and speak for the courage, patience and persistent sacrifice that women had showed for this planet and its sustainability, especially in the times of crisis. Historical scholars also needs to be louder and plane in terms of women intellectual articulation and also for its circulation because Chinua Achebe, the prominent Nigerian novelist and author of *Things Fall Apart*, once said in an interview in 1994 with the *Paris Review* that, "until the lions have their own historians, the history of the hunt will always glorify the hunter". Therefore, the cultural and social responses to these undeniable conditions of existence have provided us with a wealth of thought provoking ideas for historical analysis and scholarship about women across historical time and space and Covid-19 is one such pertinent recent burning scene on the unending records of thinking, research and womanly quest for a better equal world. Thucydides, the well-known Greek Historian, declared human nature as a constant victim as well as a constant actor. It is natural human nature which carries out atrocities and which suffers them. In this realization lay its particular value to the historian as a constant in the historical process.

REFERENCES

1. Alexander, J. (1981). Catherine the Great and Public Health. *Journal of the History of Medicine and Allied Sciences,* 36 (2), pp. 185-204. Retrieved on December 26, 2020 from https://www.jstor.com/stable/24631585
2. Archibong, B., & Annan, F. (2017). Disease and Gender Gaps in Human Capital Investment: Evidence from Niger's 1986 Meningitis Epidemic. *The American Economic Review,* 107(5), 530-535. Retrieved on January 31, 2021 from http://iproxy.inflibnet.ac.in:2060/stable/44250455
3. Baldwin, G. and Taylor, S. (2020). Uniformed Women in Peace Operations: Challenging Assumptions and Transforming Approaches. *International Peace Institute.*doi:10.2307/resrep25267. Retrieved January 31, 2021, from www.jstor.org/stable/resrep25267
4. Baruah, S. (2020, May 28). The Fortune of Others. *Indian Express,* Retrieved on January 30, 2021 from https://indianexpress.com
5. Blackburn, C and Parker, G. (2018, March 1). How the devastating 1918 Flu Pandemic Helped Advance US Women's Rights. *The Conversation.* Retrieved on December 26, 2020.
6. De, A. (2020, August 21). Why Women Leaders Have Fared Better Than Men In Handling Covid-19. *The Indian Express.* Retrieved on December 26, 2020, from https://inidanexpress.com/article/world/women-leaders-jacinda-adern-angela-merkel-fared-better-in-handling-covid-19-6562933
7. Dubois, E. (2020, April 20). A Pandemic nearly derailed the Women's Suffrage Movement. *National Geographic, History.* Retrieved on December 26, 2020, from https://www.google.com/amp/s/api. national geographic.com/distribution/public/amp/history/2020/04/pandemic-nearly-derailed-womens-suffrage-movement
8. Guidorzi, B. (2020). The 'Shadow Pandemic': Addressing Gender-based Violence (GBV) During COVID-19. In Cannon C. (Author) & Carmody P., McCann G., Colleran C., & O'Halloran C. (Eds.), *COVID-19 in the Global South: Impacts and Responses* (pp. 117-126). Bristol: Bristol University Press. doi:10.2307/j.ctv18gfz7c.18
9. Kandukuri, D. (12 January, 2019). *The Life and Times of Savitribai Phule.* Retrieved on December 26, 2020, from https://www.livemint.com/Leisure/DmR1fQSnVD62p4D3eyq9mO/The-life-and-times-of-Savitribai-Phule.html

10. Krishnadas, J. and Taha, S. (2020). Domestic violence through the window of the COVID-19 lockdown: A public crisis embodied/exposed in the private/domestic sphere. *Journal of Global Faultlines,* 7(1), 46-58. doi:10.13169/jglobfaul.7.1.0046
11. Marindo, R. (2017). Gendered Epidemics and Systems of Power in Africa: A Feminist Perspective on Public Health Governance. *Africa Development / AfriqueEtDÈveloppement*, 42(1), 199-219. Retrieved on January 31, 2021, from http://iproxy.inflibnet.ac.in:2060/stable/90013906
12. Mikhail, A. (2008). The Nature of Plague in Late Eighteenth-Century Egypt. *Bulletin of the History of Medicine,* 82(2), 249-275. Retrieved on January 31, 2021 from http://iproxy.inflibnet.ac.in:2060/stable/44448549
13. Miller, S. (2020, April 20). The Secret to Germany's COVID-19 Success: Angela Merkel Is a Scientist. *The Atlantic.* Retrieved on December 26, 2020 from https://www.theatlantic.com/international/archive/2020/04/angela-merkel-germany-coronavirus-pandemic/610225/
14. Miyamoto, I. (2020). *Covid-19 Healthcare Workers: 70% are Women*. Inouye Asia-Pacific Centre for Security Studies. Retrieved from https://www.jstor.org/stable/resrep24863
15. Nanthini, S., & Nair, T. (2020). *COVID-19 and the Impacts on Women*.S. Rajaratnam School of International Studies, 2020,doi:10.2307/resrep26875.Retrieved January 31, 2021, from,www.jstor.org/stable/resrep26875
16. New Zealand PM Jacinda Ardern touts success in tackling Covid-19 pandemic in poll push. (2020, Oct 11). *DH Deccan Herald*. Retrieved on December 26, 2020, from https://www.deccanherald.com
17. Proskurina, V. (2020). *Catherine the Healer*. Academic Study Press. Retrieved December 26, 2020 from https://www.jstor.org/stable/j.ctt1zxsj03.7
18. Rahmaty, M., & Jaghab, J. (2020). *Peace building during a Pandemic: Keeping the Focus on Women's Inclusion*. International Peace Institute. Retrieved on January 31, 2021 from www.jstor.org/stable/resrep26635, doi:10.2307/resrep26635
19. Sachan, D. (2017). Zeda Rosenberg: Determined to Empower Women to Prevent HIV Infection. *BMJ: British Medical Journal*, 359. doi:10.2307/26950625
20. Walsh, J. (2017). Dubliners and the Influenza Epidemic of 1918/19. *Dublin Historical Record*, 70(1), 81-95. Retrieved January 31, 2021, from http://iproxy.inflibnet.ac.in:2060/stable/44985463
21. *Women: The Unsung Heroes of the 1918 Flu Pandemic*. (2020, May 18) *WIMLF*. Retrieved on December 26, 2020 from https://www.wimlf.org?blog/women-the-unsung-heroes-of-the-1918-flu-pandemic

14
Pandemics and Epidemics in Colonial India

Kamlesh Singh and Pranshu Mathur

ABSTRACT

In the domain of irresistible infections, a pandemic is the direct outcome imaginable. At the point when an epidemic spread across a nation's borders, that is the point at which the illness authoritatively turns into a pandemic. Transferable sicknesses existed during mankind's agrarian days; however the move to agrarian life 10,000 years back made networks that made pestilences more conceivable. Malaria, cholera, leprosy, plague and others previously showed up during this period. The more civilized humans became, building cities and forging trade routes to connect with other cities, and waging wars with them, the more likely pandemics became. India has encountered several epidemics and pandemics throughout history. This chapter talks about such outbreaks known to have occurred in the 19th-21st century.

Keywords: Cholera, Colonial India, Leprosy, Malaria, Pandemic, Plague.

During the Age of Discovery (from the beginning of seventeenth century till eighteenth century), India gradually in phasing manner came to be governed under the jurisdiction of European colonial powers. By the first half of the nineteenth century, the subcontinent came to be known as Colonial India. The wealth and prosperity of India (as India was called *Sone* ke Chiriya) attracted the French, Portuguese, Dutch and finally the British who invaded our country and till 1947 when India attained its independence but got divided ruled into two countries, i.e., India and Pakistan. In the second half of eighteenth century, Britain and France struggled for dominance, partly through proxy Indian rulers but also by direct military intervention. The defeat of the formidable Indian ruler Tipu Sultan in 1799 marginalised the French influence. This was followed by a rapid expansion of British power through the greater part of the Indian subcontinent in the early nineteenth century. By the middle of the century the British had already gained direct or indirect control over almost all of India. Colonial India, consisting of the directly-ruled British presidencies and provinces were the most populous and valuable parts of the British Empire and thus became known as "the jewel in the British crown".

Establishment of the Indian Medical Services

The historical backdrop of western medication in India goes back to 1600, when the first medical officials showed up in quite a while alongside the British East India Company's first fleet as the ships'surgeons. In 1757, the East India Company emerged as political power in India, which prompted the improvement of common and military administrations. A clinical office was set up in Bengal as far back as 1764 for delivering medical services to the soldiers and workers of the Company. It comprised of around 4 head surgeons, 8 associate surgeons, and 28 surgeons' mates. In 1775, hospital boards were formed to oversee European clinics involving the Surgeon General and Physician General, who were in the staff of Commander-in-Chief of the Royal Indian Army. In 1785, clinical offices were set up in Bengal, Madras, and Bombay administrations with 234 surgeons. The clinical divisions included both military and civil medical services. In 1796, hospital boards were renamed as medical boards to take care of the undertakings of the civil parts of the medical departments. In 1857, the Indian Rebellion prompted the handing over of the administration of India to the Crown and various departments of civil services were created. It wasn't until 1868 that a separate civil medical department was formed in Bengal. In 1869, a Public Health Commissioner and a Statistical Officer were named to the Government of India. In 1896, with the abrogation of the official framework, the three presidential medical offices was amalgamated to shape the Indian Medical Services (IMS). After the formation of IMS, clinical obligations for the Royal Indian Army were performed by the Army Medical Department, later called the Royal Army Medical Corps (RAMC) (Government of India, 1909, 457-80).

Medical offices were heavily influenced by the imperial government until 1919. The constitutional reforms introduced in 1919 after the Montgomery-Chelmsford Report prompted the exchange of public health, sanitation, and vital statistics. This was the initial phase of decentralization of health administration in India. In 1920-21, Municipality and Local Board Acts were passed containing legitimate arrangements for the advancement of public health in provinces. The Government of India Act 1935 gave further self-sufficiency to provincial government. All the health activities were arranged in three sections: federal, federal-cum-provincial, and provincial. In 1937, the Central Advisory Board of Health was set up with the Public Health Commissioner as secretary to facilitate the public health activities in the nation. In 1939, the Madras Public Health Act was passed, which was the first of its kind in India. In 1946, the Health Survey and Development Committee (Bhore Committee) was appointed by the Government of India to survey the existing health structure in the country and make recommendations for the future developments. The Committee submitted its report in 1946 and the health of the nation was reviewed for public health, medical relief, professional education, medical research, and international health. (Park, 2005, 679-80; Harrison, 1994)

Disease Control and Prevention

At the point when the British Empire came into power in India, they confronted the challenge of new set of infections that were endemic in that region. India is a vast nation with the geography ranging from the world's most noteworthy mountains to green plains, and from tropical forests to infertile deserts. Such a diverse locale had its own impossible-to-miss maladies, which were hard to prevent with the restricted assets of the IMS. Colossal measures of work were accomplished for the counteraction of scourges to spare the lives of individuals in India by and large, and the imperial soldiers and officials specifically. Pestilence sicknesses that had decimating impact during that period were plague, leprosy, cholera, and malaria. The British government took incredible endeavours to forestall infections yet, because of dearth of medical officials and funds, the significant objective was to ease the enduring and render curative services as it was exclusively a state obligation during that period with, for all intents and purposes, no volunteer or private-area associations. Counteraction and natural cleanliness had for quite some time been ignored. It wasn't until the late nineteenth century that the Government understood that numerous deaths could be prevented and public health services were fortified.

Plague

Plague is an infectious disease caused by the *Yersinia pestis* bacteria, usually found in small mammals and their fleas. The disease is transmitted between animals via their fleas and, as it is a zoonotic bacterium, it can also transmit from animals to humans. Humans can be contaminated by the bite of infected fleas, through direct contact with infected materials, or by inhalation. Plague can be a very severe disease in people, particularly in its septicaemic and pneumonic forms, with a case-fatality ratio of 30 per cent—100 per cent if left untreated (WHO, Plague). There are reports of various plague outbreaks in India but authentic information is available for 1812 outbreak in Kutch that spread to Gujarat and Sind, and lasted for approximately 10 years. A disease having all the symptoms of plague was reported in 1828 and 1829 in Hansi in the Hissar district of Punjab. In 1836, it was reported that plague was prevalent in the Marwar state of Rajputana. The first official records dates back to 1896 when an epidemic of bubonic plague broke out in Bombay. Initially, it was reported in the port cities of Bombay, Pune, Calcutta, and Karachi. In the first year, it was confined to Bombay except for minor occurrences in other parts of the country. In the second year, epidemic was reported in Bengal, Madras, United Provinces, Central Provinces, Punjab, Mysore, Hyderabad, and Kashmir. It devastated almost whole of India until about 1899. By the end of 1903, this deadly epidemic took the lives of about 2 million people according to state records but the actual figures might be much more staggering. (Government of India, 1909; Nathan, 1898; National Library of Scotland).

Being on the international trading route, there was huge pressure on the British imperial administration of India to control this crisis. The Plague Commission was established in 1896 under the chairmanship of T.R. Frasor, Professor of Material Medical at the University of Edinburgh. It involved individuals from different departments including J.P. Hewett, Interior Secretary to the legislature of India, A.E. Wright, Professor of Pathology at Army Medical College Netley, and others. The report of the Plague Commission in 1904 reasoned that the malady was exceptionally infectious and considered human transit as a significant source of spreading the illness as they conveyed the germs with them. The commission prescribed fundamental preventive measures to purify and clear contaminated spots, to put a control over mass travel, and to improve sanitary conditions. The commission likewise recommended reinforcing of general well-being administrations and improvement of labs. (Lamb, 1908)

According to the Account of Plague Administration in the Bombay Presidency from September 1896 till May 1897 (General Department Bombay, 1897), the Epidemic Diseases Act was passed in 1897 and the Governor General of India gave uncommon forces to local authorities to execute the vital measures for control of pandemics. There was a vivacious execution of the Act. Provincial force was utilized for intense isolation of infected people, sanitizations, evacuations, and even destruction of contaminated spots was undertaken. Medical and administrative authorities reserved the right to inspect any presumed individual on spot; they may have called for detainment of any people from boats and railways. This alarmed the locals resulting in riots in certain zones yet the administration utilized the military power to guarantee legitimate enforcement of important preventive measures. Intensive research work was carried out (Lamb, 1908; General Department Bombay, 1897; Madras Marine Plague Regulations, 1910; 1902)

The Plague Research Committee was anointed. As demonstrated in reports of Surgeon Maj. Lyons, President of the Plague Research Committee and by Surgeon Capt. Childe, different kinds of researchs were carried out in 1897. The investigations of Hankins inferred that plague bacillus was not spread by saprophytic methods from the rest of the world. Its principle sources were poor sanitation and the resultant spread from discharges of people and animals (Lyons and Childe, 1897). Haffkine's Anti-Plague vaccine was utilized and vaccinations were made at a huge scale that proved to be helpful as detailed by W.B. Bannerman, Superintendent of the Bombay Plague Research Laboratory (1897-1900). Professor Lusting's therapeutic serum was likewise utilized and discovered to be compelling as depicted by the reports of G. Polverine, Officer in–Charge of Parel Municipal Laboratory and Col. J. S. Wilkins, Special Medical Officer for Plague Operations (Bannerman, 1900).

Leprosy

Leprosy was one of the major issue of colonial India. IMS clinical officials did gigantic amounts of research on the scientific treatment for disease. Notwithstanding its impediments and difficulties, leprosy research in India got overall acknowledgment; numerous Indian remedies for leprosy have been consolidated into western medication. In the light of G.A. Hansen's discovery in 1873, leprosy is spread by contact, H.V. Carter of the Bengal Medical Department increased an authority over leprosy control in India. He acquired extraordinary acknowledgment in the central imperial government of India and proposed separating of lepers. He encouraged the foundation of Leper Asylums in India as were formed in Norway then. (Carter, 1887, Memorandum; Observations). After the 1889 Leprosy Bill, the National Leprosy Fund was comprised by the British Empire under chairmanship of the Prince of Wales. A Leprosy Commission was framed to explore the etiology and epidemiology of leprosy. The Leprosy Commission presumed that leprosy is a disease *sui generis* brought about by a bacillus having striking likeness to tuberculosis. It's anything but a genetic sickness, it spread by infectious methods yet the odds of are little. However, its spread is in a roundabout way impacted by poor sanitization and malnourishment. The Commission proposed that isolation probably won't be productive in India. It recommended preclusion on the sale of food articles, prostitution, and different occupations including direct obstruction with individuals like hair stylists or watermen by the infected individuals. It demanded the improvement of sanitary and living environments (Report of Leprosy Commission, 1893). Notwithstanding, the administration of India passed the All-India Leprosy Act in 1898 and Leper Asylums were set up in significant parts of the nation and coercive isolation of lepers was undertaken. Various territories outfitted different overviews and reports. Extreme reconnaissance and research work were done on the distribution of lepers, genetic transmission, and predisposition possibilities, infectiousness, and connection of disease with sterilization and diet and reports were published. It includes *A Collection of Reports from various Provinces on the Distribution and Causation of Leprosy* was published in 1879 by the Department of Revenue and Agriculture, Government of India; *Leprosy and its Control in Bombay Presidency*, published by Government of Bombay in 1914; *Report on Leprosy in North-Western Provinces* a published in 1876. In 1881, there were approximately 120,000 patients with this infection in India that diminished to 102,000 in 1921. These were implausible measurements keeping in view the high birth rate in India.

Cholera

Officials of the British East India Company were inexperienced about cholera. Prior to 1817, cholera was restricted to Bengal but the 1817-1821 cholera epidemic in India bewildered the company. By the 1830s, cholera was known to be a life-threatening ailment in the western world. In India, it became the focal point of medical services because of its serious effect on the soldiers and officials of the company; else, it was an ailment of poor individuals. Because of the absence of viable treatment for cholera at that period, the fundamental spotlight was set to its prevention (Government of India, 1909; National Library of Scotland). The British India government adhered to meteorological speculations about cholera after the

Constantinople International Sanitary Conference of 1868, accepting that barometrical conditions are the essential reason for spreading the infection. After the 1868 cholera epidemic in India, the Cholera Committee was set up under G. O. no. 216 on 27th February 1867, to delve into the reasons for the malady and report upon the arrangements that should be made to give practical effect in the Madras Presidency to the recommendations and suggestions of the International Sanitary Conference. It included the Principal Inspector General of the Indian Medical Department, Sanitary Commissioner for Madras, and Col. A.C. Silver. The cause and generation of cholera, the epidemicity and endemicity of the malady in India, contagiousness and proliferation of cholera, and measures fundamental for its counteraction were examined. The Committee presumed that cholera was frequent particularly at religious festivals and fairs. Epidemics were inferable from the importation of malady by explorers, voyagers, and troops. The Committee recommended

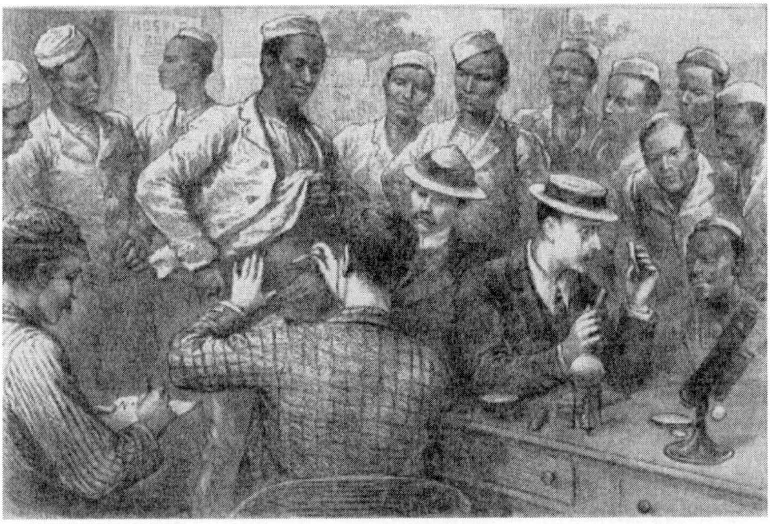

Fig. 14.1 Cholera vaccination of Third Gurkhas in India at the time of the 1893 epidemic.

Source: Wellcom Collection/CC BY-SA 3.0

improving sanitation, guaranteeing appropriate administration of celebrations, and creating sterile conditions in foundations like emergency clinics, prisons, and military cantonments. *Rules regarding the Measures to be adopted on the Outbreak of Cholera or Appearance of Small-pox* were also issued by G.O.C.C. No. 193, dated 3rd August 1870 (Sanitary Commissioner, Madras, 1868; Government of India, 1870). Dr. S.C. Townsend, Sanitary Commissioner for Central Provinces and Berar, additionally detailed his 1868 cholera epidemic investigations (Townsend, 1868).

Several cholera pandemics occurred during the British rule in India and in many other parts of the world starting from early 1800s till 1920s. Since the pandemics were so widespread and occurred at intervals of every six-seven years, they were named First, Second, Third and so on according to their order of occurrence. Deaths in India between 1817 and 1860, in the first three pandemics of the nineteenth century, are estimated to have exceeded 15 million people. Another 23 million died between 1865 and 1917, during the next three pandemics. Cholera deaths in the Russian Empire during a similar duration exceeded 2 million.

First Cholera Pandemic

It was also known as First Asiatic Cholera Pandemic or Asiatic cholera and it occurred during 1817-1824. The word cholera was used in the texts of the previous centuries but there was no true evidence of the cholera in the south asian subcontinent, so the pandemic of this time was named as Asiatic cholera. This pandemic started near Calcutta and spread throughout south and southeast Asia to the Middle East, eastern Africa and the Mediterranean coast. The total deaths in this pandemic remained unknown. Many scholars have estimated death toll. Hundreds of thousands of Indians and ten thousand British troops died during this pandemic. As for India, the initially reported mortality rate was estimated to be 1.25 million per year, placing the death toll at around 8,750,000 (Alexandre, 1831).

Second Cholera Pandemic

The second cholera pandemic (1826–1837), also called the Asiatic Cholera pandemic, was a cholera pandemic that came to India across western Asia to Europe, Great Britain, and the Americas, as well as east to China and Japan. Second Cholera caused more deaths, all the more rapidly, than some other epidemic infections in the nineteenth century. The medical fraternity presently accepts cholera to be only a human disease, spread through numerous methods like travel during the time, and sent through warm fecal-contaminated river waters and contaminated foods. During the second pandemic, scientific researchers fluctuated in its convictions about the reasons for cholera. Although not much is known about the journey of the cholera pandemic in east India, many believe that this pandemic began, like the first, with outbreaks along the Ganges Delta in India. From there, the disease spread along trade routes to cover most of India.

Third Cholera Pandemic

The third cholera pandemic (1846–60) was the third significant flare-up of cholera beginning in India in the nineteenth century that came to a long way past its fringes, which specialists at UCLA accept, may have begun as right on time as 1837 and lasted until 1863 (Frerichs). In Russia, more than 1,000,000 people died of cholera. In 1853–54, the pandemic in London took more than 10,000 lives. This pandemic was considered to have the most noteworthy fatalities of the nineteenth century epidemics. It had high fatalities among populaces in Asia, Europe, Africa and North America. In 1854, which was viewed as the most noticeably terrible year, this disease took the lives of 23,000 individuals in Great Britain.

Fourth Cholera Pandemic

The fourth cholera pandemic (1863-1875) started in the Ganges Delta of the Bengal district and headed out with Muslim explorers to Mecca. In its first year, the pestilence claimed 30,000 of 90,000 Mecca pilgrims' lives. Cholera spread through the Middle East and was conveyed to Russia, Europe, Africa and North America, for each situation spreading from port urban communities and along inland streams.

Fifth Cholera Pandemic

The fifth cholera pandemic (1881–1896) was the fifth major international outbreak of cholera in the 19th century. It spread throughout Asia and Africa, and reached parts of France, Germany, Russia, and South America. It claimed 200,000 lives in Russia between 1893 and 1894; and 90,000 in Japan between 1887 and 1889. During the pandemic, Robert Koch isolated *Vibrio cholerae* and proposed postulates to explain how bacteria caused disease.

John Murray, who was Inspector General of Civil Hospitals in North Western Provinces and Bengal, led detailed studies on cholera. Despite the fact that there was proof of infectiousness, Murray accepted that ecological variables accelerated the attacks of cholera; however he gave important treatment guidelines for cholera in that period. (Murray, 1869). Surgeon W.R. Cornish, Sanitary Commissioner for Madras, tested meteorological hypotheses about the spread of cholera and did point by point reconnaissance and exploration work to build up the infectiousness of the malady, which is obvious from his reports on cholera in southern India in 1871 and his examinations of cholera flare-ups in H M's 18th Hussars in Secunderabad in 1871 that killed 115 individuals in one month including 20 soldiers of the Royal Indian Army (Cornish, 1871).

Malaria

Fever was one of the main sources of fatalities in India. The circumstance declined in the mid-nineteenth century. One of the contributing components was the foundation of the railways and water system network (irrigation) by the British administration of India without keeping in view the effective drainage systems for floods and rainwaters. This made numerous new water reservoirs for the spread of mosquitoes. Because of the weighty loss of life, financial misfortune, and danger to the lives of British officials serving in weak regions like Punjab, a ton of research was accomplished for jungle fever (malaria) control. During the 1840s, consideration was given to appropriate waste management and chemoprophylaxis was begun with Quinine. (Government of India, 1909; National Library of Scotland). In 1900, Christophers, Stephens, and James conducted detailed research on mosquitoes in the military cantonments in Punjab. All-India Malaria Conferences (1900-1909) and Punjab Intestinal sickness Surveys (1909-1911) were conducted under the oversight of Christophers (National Library of Scotland). From 1903 to 1908, Capt. S.P. James led research on the causation and anticipation of malarial fevers. He composed valuable reports for the avoidance and treatment of jungle fever for medical care suppliers (Cornish, 1871; James, 1908). In 1909, the Central Malaria Bureau was formed in Kasauli for intestinal sickness control and examinations (James, 1903).

Conclusion

Epidemiological examinations on the colonial time frame uncover that between 1896 and 1921, more than 30 million individuals fell prey to epidemic illnesses – bubonic plague, cholera, malaria, smallpox and flu. Of these, around 10 million belonged to Punjab, North-Western Provinces and Bombay. The containment of epidemics didn't rely just upon the state activity; it likewise relied upon the public response. Sure enough, the very presence of colonial and 'native' dictatorial structures is firmly connected to the major substantial causes (mass pauperisation, primitive clinical infrastructure, poor disinfection, shortage of clean drinking water, instructive backwardness, and so forth) behind the monstrous detailed fatalities. The colonial generalizing of individuals as 'notoriously filthy', 'insensible' and 'savages' additionally had an impact. Interestingly, the fear of forced isolation and the stigma attached to being a carrier of the disease induced people to smuggle out their symptomatic relatives to 'safer' areas, hide them in attics, inside cupboards, under furniture, or in secret rooms whenever the state's search parties showed up. Some of these tactics still reverberate in our society.

REFERENCES

1. 1881–1896 cholera pandemic. (2020, July 19). https://en.wikipedia.org/wiki/1881%E2%80%931896_cholera_pandemic.
2. Bannerman, W.B. (1900). *Statistics of Inoculations with Haffkine's Anti-plague Vaccine 1897-1900*. Compiled from records in the Plague Department of the Secretariat and the Plague Research Laboratory, Bombay. Bombay: Government Central Press.
3. Carter, H.V. (1887). *Memorandum on the Prevention of Leprosy by Segregation of the Affected.*
4. —— *Observations on the Prevention of Leprosy by Segregation.*
5. Cornish, W.R. (1871). *Cholera in Southern India: A Record of the Progress of Cholera in 1870 and Resume of the Records of Former Epidemic Invasions of the Madras Presidency*. Madras: Government Gazette Press.
6. Department of Revenue and Agriculture, India. (1879). *A Collection of Reports from various Provinces on the Distribution and Causation of Leprosy*. Department of Revenue and Agriculture, India.
7. Frerichs, Ralph R. *Asiatic Cholera Pandemics during the Life of John Snow: Asiatic Cholera Pandemic of 1846-63*. UCLA Department of Epidemiology, Fielding School of Public Health.
8. General Department, Bombay (India: Presidency). (1897). *Supplement to the Account of Plague Administration in the Bombay Presidency from September 1896 till May 1897*. Bombay Government Central Press.
9. Government of Bombay. (1914). *Leprosy and its Control in the Bombay*

Presidency. Bombay: Government of Bombay.

10. Government of India. (1870). *Rules regarding the Measures to be Adopted on the Outbreak of Cholera or Appearance of Small-pox*: Calcutta: Superintendent of Government Printing.
11. —— (1893). *Leprosy in India: Report of the Leprosy Commission in India, 1890-91*. Calcutta: Superintendent of Government Printing India; 1893.
12. Government of India. (1909). *The Imperial Gazetteer of India. Vol. IV Administrative*. Published under the authority of His Majesty's Secretary of State for India in Council. Oxford: Clarendon Press, 457-80.
13. Harrison M. (1994). *Public Health in British India: Anglo-Indian Preventive Medicine 1859-1914*. Cambridge: Cambridge University Press.
14. James, S.P. (1903). *The Causation and Prevention of Malarial Fevers: A Statement of the Results of Researches drawn up for the use of Assistant Surgeons, Hospital Assistants and Students*. Office of Superintendent of Government Printing.
15. —— (1908). *Malarial Fevers: A Statement drawn up for the use of Assistant Surgeons, Hospital Assistants, and Students*. Calcutta: Superintendent Government Printing India.
16. Lamb G. (1908). *The Etiology and Epidemiology of Plague: A Summary of the Work of the Plague Commission* (issued under the authority of the Government of India by the Sanitary Commissioner with the Government of India, Simla). Calcutta: Superintendent Government Printing, India.
17. Lone, S.R. (2020, April 8). *What Epidemics from the Colonial Era Can Teach Us About Society's Response?* The Wire. Retrieved from https://thewire.in/history/colonial-era-epidemics-india.
18. Lyons R.W., Childe L.F. (1897). *I- Report by Surgeon-Major Lyons, I.M.S., President of the Plague Research Committee. II - Report by Surgeon-Captain Childe, I.M.S. III. - Summary of work carried on by Mr. Hankin*.
19. Moreau de Jonnes, Alexandre. (1831). University of Lausanne: Chez les FrËres Reycend et Comp. 75–76.
20. Murray J. (1869). *Report on the Treatment of Epidemic Cholera*: From information collected by the Governments of Bengal, Madras, Bombay, N.W. Provinces, Punjab, Oudh, and Central India. Calcutta: Superintendent of Government Printing.
21. Nathan R. (1898). *The Plague in India, 1896, 1897*. Simla: Government Central Printing Office.
22. National Library of Scotland. *Medical History of British India*. About the Medical History of British India Collection - Retrieved from https://digital.nls.uk/indiapapers/about.html
23. Park K. (2005). *Park's Textbook of Preventive and Social Medicine*. 18th edn., Jabalpur: Banarsidas Bhanot Publishers.
24. Planck, C. (1876). *Report on Leprosy in the North-Western Provinces*.

25. Sanitary Commissioner, Madras. (1868). *Report of Cholera Committee.* Madras: Gantz Bros.
26. *The Madras Marine Plague Regulations.* (1910). Madras: Superintendent Government Press.
27. *The Madras Plague Regulations and Rules for District Municipalities and other Towns and Villages.* (1902). Madras: Superintendent Government Press
28. *The Madras Plague Regulations and Rules for the city of Madras.* (1902) Madras: Superintendent Government Press.
29. Townsend, S.C. (1868). *Report on the Cholera Epidemic of 1868.*
30. World Health Organization *Plague.* World Health Organization. Retrieved from www.who.int/health-topics/plague#tab=tab_1.

15

Colonizing the Indigenous During Epidemic Times

Interventions, Responses and Ramifications

Shreya Pathak

ABSTRACT

Though much has been researched and written about health policy and epidemics in colonial India, but not a deserving space and attention has been given on the ways and methods adopted by the alien rulers and how they availed these times of epidemic urgencies to fasten up the colonizing process by reinforcing the policy of racial discrimination and cultural interventions through western science and medicines. Health policy and western medicines were always projected by the rulers as benevolence of colonial governance. The British wanted to establish their own cultural hegemony to assure that the British Empire sun never sets in this most scintillating gem of the Crown. This chapter is an endeavour to delve into the available study sources and answer few questions: Firstly, how the policies adopted by the rulers in different arenas of administration became the underlining cause for aggravating the spread and severity of the epidemics during the colonial period; secondly, how these epidemic times were availed by them to consolidate their imperial structure of domination; and thirdly, what were the responses of the Indians towards the intervening and coercive policies of the rulers into the daily life of the individuals.

Keywords: Cholera, Colonial India, Epidemics, Imperialism, Health Policy, Plague, Western Medicine.

As the societies were evolving, changes were witnessed in the diseases and its spreading pattern. With the introduction of industrial revolution and increase in territories under political hegemony of the imperialist nations, there was shifting of millions of people to urban centers for employment and to colonies where indentured system was introduced like Fiji in 1879 (Alam, 2016). This movement of people globally also led to disease movement through travel, ships and trade routes (Morens, *et. al.*, 2009). This was witnessed with the first outbreak of cholera pandemic in 1817-24 that started in Calcutta and adjacent areas, which was the major center of British trade in India and it has been more than fifty years since English East India Company had established its ascendancy in Bengal province. This epidemic soon spread throughout southeast Asia, Middle East and eastern Africa. The world soon witnessed outbreak of second cholera pandemic in 1829-37 that crossed from India to Asia, Europe, Britain and America. According to Mumtaz Alam, Fiji faced the outbreak of measles epidemic within a year of British possession over this colony in 1875 that claimed about 40,000 lives as Fiji people have never encountered the disease before and people have not developed the immunity against it. The probability of the outbreak of diseases like cholera and smallpox was on higher side with the introduction of Indian Indentured System in Fiji in 1879 under which indentured Indian labours were being transported to British colonies. All this led the British to plan for a vaccination campaign in Fiji (Alam, 2016). These vaccination campaigns included mainly European medical staff, though local inhabitants were also trained for vaccination, but very less in number and were mainly recruited at the lower rung of the whole structure. The initiative behind the campaign was never for the well-being of the Fiji people, but it was important to keep the Indian indentured system in continuity, who were required as labours for plantations and other works as a substitute of slave labour that ended in 1833. So, the vaccination system in the British colony of Fiji was more a strategy to induct Indian indentured labours and suppress the possible resistance and discontent of the local inhabitants due to spread of disease.

The first cholera epidemic in India occurred in 1817 that continued till 1824 with second wave in 1827. Both originated in the province of Bengal spreading towards central and north India. Due to these outbreaks, India lost population of 25 million during the span of 19th century and first quarter of 20th century. The condition of Indians during Cholera epidemic was much worst where human suffering was added with all-India famine of 1877-78. Recording the pathetic condition of Madras Presidency, one of the sanitation officers reported, *it was not uncommon for district officers in their tours across country to come upon numerous bodies and skeletons in the course of a morning's ride.* (Watts, 1997, 173). On 30th June, 1889, British Government appointed Indian Leprosy Commission with three Commissioner members, one each appointed by Royal College of Physicians, the Royal College of Surgeons and Executive Committee of National Leprosy Fund. They visited Bombay on 17th November, 1890 to study the condition. The report published in 1893 used cholera hit regions as a barometer to test the climate, local healthiness and sanitary state of that particular area. As according to this Commission (Surgeon Major Thomson of Bengal Medical Service, Drs. B. Rake and G. Buckmaster) cholera was occurring more as an epidemic in certain climatic regions and tracts of the country and was considered as an endemic disease in those regions, while in other tracts of the country cholera was not always active and rampant. They reported that the regions where cholera was an endemic disease, general life and habits of the population were unhealthy and one of the dominant reasons of cholera spread. These regions includes Bengal, Assam, Orissa, Konkan, Malabar, Low Burma, North-West Provinces, Oudh and some districts of Punjab and Central Provinces (Rake, 71-73).

The educated Britons were mainly having the imprint of India as it was mentioned in Mill's *History of British India* written in six volumes in 1817, where the author had presented an extremely demeaning picture of the nation by criticizing every institution, every idea and every action of the Indians holding them responsible for all ills and backwardness of the society and the only panacea to all this was through introduction of enlightened despotism. This book was introduced as a textbook in Haileybury School of England, an institution established to educate the young Englishmen coming to India as administrators and civil servants. It could be surmised that with this education, mental conditioning and training, an European officer having a perception of India as the homeland of diseases that threatened the West was nothing strange. For them Indian villagers were filthy, having unhealthy habits, unhygienic living, poor sanitary conditions that led to spread of epidemic. Historians like Mill and Co. endeavoured to deprive Indian land of its glorified past history and culture of being the most ancient civilization of human race, her incredible achievements in the field of architecture and engineering. They recorded every word in the books to portray the dark age, black history, barbarous society and diseased people. The 5000 years old advanced civilization, well-structured administrative system of the dynasties, the widely spread consolidated rule of the Mauryas and Guptas, advanced technology, military strategies, ancient medicines, literary achievements, spiritual epitome, well developed and highly profitable trade, internal and external both, to far away countries all are now well recorded with archeological-literary evidences that are hard for denial and speaks itself of the negationism in British writings of Indian history during colonial period. Hobson in his study of imperialism had revealed the nakedness of the British civilizing presence.

> The idea that we are civilizing India in the sense of assisting them to industrial, political and moral progress along the lines either of our own or of their civilization is a complete delusion, based upon a false estimate of the influence of superficial changes wrought by government and the activity of a minute group of aliens. The delusion is only sustained by the sophistry of Imperialism, which weaves these fallacies to cover its nakedness and the advantages which certain interests suck out of empire. (Hobson, 1902, 303),

The British postulated for politico-administrative superiority, but the reality exposed when the province that was their launching pad as a political power i.e., Bengal, faced famine in 1769-70 within four years of the grant of *diwani* to the East India Company in 1765 by Mughal Emperor. The severity of the famine can be surmised by the fact that it ended almost 10 million people of Bengal. Stavorinus, a Dutch naval commander in Chinsura in 1770, later recorded the pathetic tragedy that he witnessed.

> This famine arose in part from the bad rice harvest of the preceding year; but it must be attributed principally to the monopoly the English had over the last harvest of this commodity, which they kept at such a high price that most of the unfortunate inhabitants- who earned only a sou or a sou-and-a-half a day to sustain their family-found themselves powerless to buy the tenth part of what they needed to live. To this scourge was added smallpox, which spread among persons of all ages and of which they died in great numbers. (Nicholas, 1981, 33)

In 1825, Dr. Annesley one of the English doctors with an experience of 25 years of medical practice in India, communicated to his London friends about the investigations that he conducted on the history of cholera. He surmised that there was no evidence of the prevalence of cholera in India as a wide spreading epidemic before 1817, though few local outbreaks were reported by Europeans traders in ports before 1817, but never as an epidemic. He asserted that cholera was a new phenomenon in most of Asia. An article on his report was published in Medical and Surgical Journal in 1826 that reveals about this investigation report that was obviously suppressed by the imperial ideologues who believed India to be the mother of all diseases and postulated occurrence of cholera epidemic as a common phenomenon in this country. A committee of 18 medical doctors in Britain unanimously expressed in a medical report about the disease that it was a variant of an English fever and not an Indian epidemic. After Bengal, cholera outbreak was witnessed in central India among the army men that was led by Hastings against the Marathas and severity of this disease can be surmised by the details that Hastings had mentioned in his Diary on 15th November, 1817 that 500 men of his army died in one single day. (Watts, 1997, 178, 193)

Thus, other than railways, shipping and trade, British army movement was also one of the major reasons of the spread of disease. British always regarded India as a quagmire of epidemics like plague, malaria, smallpox, cholera, while H. Webb in *Health of European Soldiers in India* published in 1864 clearly stated that overcrowding in Indian barracks was the dominant cause of insalubrities in India. E. Parkes (1866, 294-98) in his *Manual of Practical Hygiene* prepared for the use in army medical service, clearly mentioned that mortality was not mainly due to diseases but poor living facilities of the British troops in most insanitary conditions.

India had witnessed the worst famine in the history during

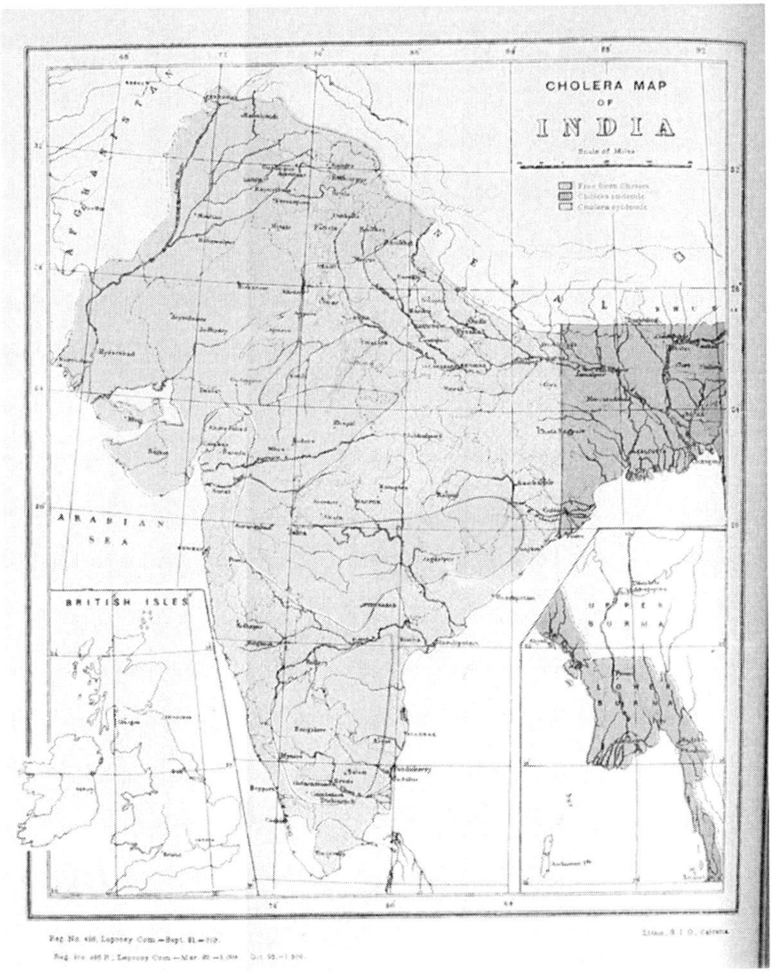

Map. 15.1: Map of Cholera in India with dark grey showing the endemic areas

Source: Leprosy in India: Report of the Leprosy Commission in India, 1890-91

the closing decade of 19th century when there were two all-India famines within a short span of time, first in 1896-97 and second in 1899-1900. During these famines, there were government orders that all starving people should move to

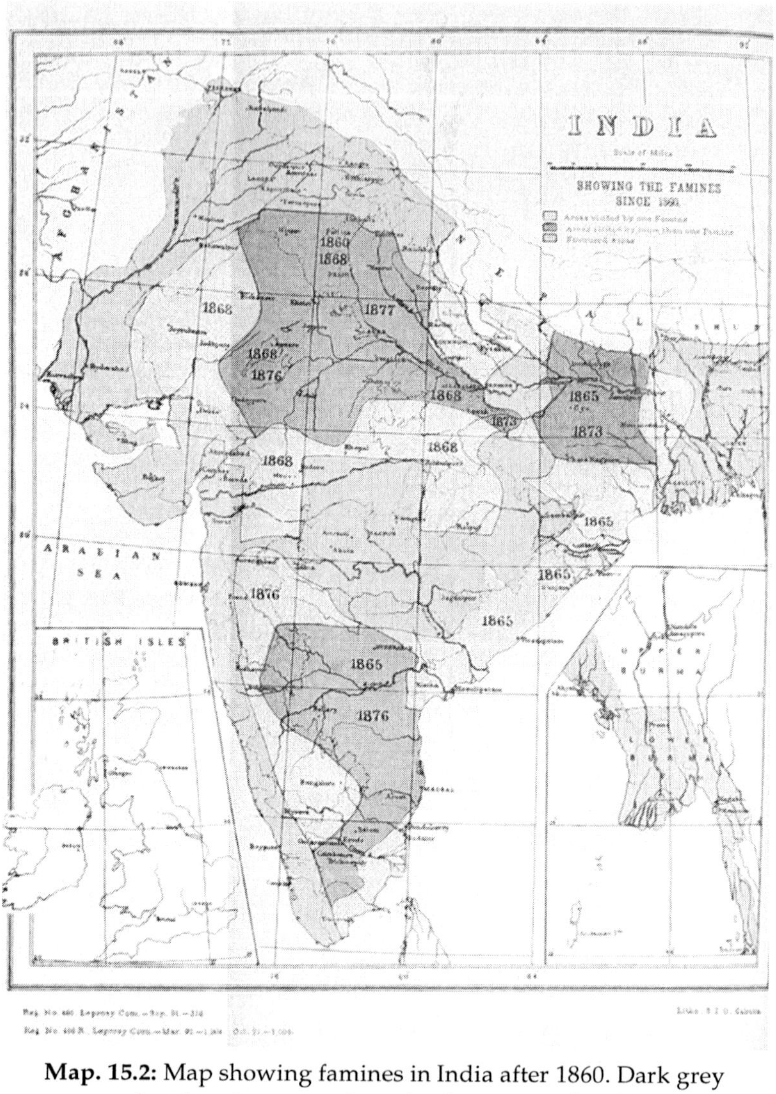

Map. 15.2: Map showing famines in India after 1860. Dark grey showing the areas where famine occurred twice

Source: Leprosy in India: Report of the Leprosy Commission in India, 1890-91.

central camps where they were provided work by Public Works Department in lieu of which they were provided food for living. These orders were given as one of the relief measures recommended by Strachey Famine Commission in 1880. The commission report stated that state should provide work to able-bodied persons and in lieu of labour they should be provided food grains as per requirement. Though it may sound very magnanimous and sensitized policy of the government, but reality speaks something else. The work given included strenuous physical jobs like road construction, irrigation canal works etc. that physically weak, ill and aged people were unable to do. Those who refused to do work or were physically incapable of doing such strenuous jobs, their names were written off from the list of workers and with that also ended their possibility to procure food during famine. Needless to say, the living conditions and facilities provided in these overcrowded camps were insalubrious. (Watts, 1997, 201-202).

Thus, low morale of the local inhabitants due to British administrative exigencies, excess of revenue imposition, coercive methods of revenue collection, malnourishment and suffering due to famine, all provided the conducive environment required for any disease to struck and spread its tentacles to an extremity of epidemic. Sheldon Watts rightly put in his words.

> As a direct result of British policies of compulsory settlement and moneterization, tens of thousands of people became demoralized, hunger-weakened wrecks whose inner organs seemed incapable of generating the acids and alkali needed in time of emergency to fight off the cholera vibrio. (Watts, 1997, 182)

The frequency, severity and spread of famine worsened in India due to British irrigation policy that emphasized much on productive irrigation works that guarantees high dividends on invested capital rather on protective irrigation works. The places where irrigation projects were undertaken, British engineers failed to create a proper parallel drainage system to drain out the surplus water that entered the nearby fields. These water pools became the breed house of malaria mosquitoes and was the major reason for the spread of the disease in nearby areas. Such conditions were also seen where railway lines crosses the water drainage path leading to creation of water pool and then spread of malaria mosquitoes. Malaria had such a killer element that *makes the poor malarious and the malarious poor* (Watts, 1999)

Here it is important to know that the British who boastly talk, write and report about their civilizing presence in India, what and how they were reacting towards their subjects when the first cholera epidemic outbreak was faced by them in the year 1831-32. Knowing about the spread of cholera in other parts of the world, British introduced an Anatomy Bill in the Parliament in 1828, according to which the unclaimed bodies of poor people in workhouses would be legally given to local medical school for study. This bill got Royal assent in 1831. All this created a phobia among the British poor people of becoming a part of an *anatomy soup*. There were innumerable incidents reported of people's resistance and unrest who blamed of legal murders of the poor patients of cholera by medical professionals. One single city of Liverpool experienced about eight major riots with other minor disturbances within a short time span from 29th May to 10th June 1832. The public unrest was mainly because cholera victims were being forcefully hospitalized where they were killed by the doctors to use the bodies for anatomical dissection. There were cases where bodies were digged out at night and sold for dissection to local anatomy schools. In 1826, 33 bodies were found in docks of Liverpool that were being shipped to Scotland for dissection. These riots demonstrate the social responses and discontentment due to cholera epidemic in Britain and the level of social-administrative insensitivity in this boasted civilized society where people were less fearful of cholera than of medical professionals (Burrell and Gill, 2005).

High land revenue, insensitive and intervening administrative system, indifferent famine and irrigation policy of colonial government had played their own part in aggravating the spread of different epidemic in India, but what was most important was the British policy of health and sanitation that was directly responsible for an epidemic status, its spread, severity, mortality and frequency. If we look back since the commencement of British rule, it was in 1785 when East India Company established its medical department in three presidencies with 234 military surgeons. In due course of time, more British doctors were imported for medical aid of British officials and troops that were engaged in battles with regional powers for their territorial expansion. The progress in this field was really very slow with meager number of hospitals that were mainly concentrated either in the presidencies or in towns where there was availability of sufficient funds and a medical officer to be as in-charge. Military and political considerations were always dominant factor in determining the British policy towards health, hospital and medicine. Even Indian Medical Service, started in 1896, was primarily a military service where all medical officers were commissioned officers of the army (Government of India, 1907, 458-64). The rural population was completely untouched and neglected with no medical and sanitation facility. For the first time, government's focus was diverted towards the sanitary reforms only after the investigations of the Royal Commission and publication of its report on sanitary state of army in India in 1863. It was only after the publication of this report that application of sanitary principles became one of the concerns of the Government in its own circle and later, it was further extended to towns and villages (HoC, 1894, 374). Though, the reality of sanitary conditions in the densely populated towns and villages is not a hidden fact. The tables given below shows a picture of the medical institutions during the closing two decades of the 19th century:

Table 15.1: Statistics of Public Hospitals and Dispensaries under Government Control

Years	**1880**	**1890**	**1900**	**1902**
Institutions	1,212	1,736	2,364	2,456
Patients (indoor and outdoor both)	7,409,000	12,977,000	20,905,000	22,412,000
Surgical operations performed	372,219	604,140	831,806	895,226
Income:				
From government fund	19,03,000	20,73,000	27,76,000	29,89,000
From Municipal and Local Funds	12,90,000	22,07,000	31,64,000	37,15,000
From subscriptions, endowments, fees and other sources	5,02,000	5,69,000	13,36,000	14,65,000
Total	**36,95,000**	**48,49,000**	**72,76,000**	**81,69,000**

Source: Imperial Gazetteer of India (1909), Vol.IV, p. 480.

Table 15. 2: Statistics of other Hospitals and Dispensaries in 1902

	Institutions	**Patients**
Private independent institutes	480	3,007,000
Railway, Police, & C, hospitals	506	1,111,000

Source: Imperial Gazetteer of India, Vol.IV, 1909, p.480

Before English medical system, there were well-established two principal medical systems in India that British never promoted—one was the ancient *Ayurveda* practiced by *vaids* and other was *Unani* system that came from Arab after fourteenth century and was practiced by *hakeems*. Two European medical professionals who travelled Francois Bernier and John Fryer India in 1660s and 70s decades, had regarded Indian medical professionals as knowledgeable and skilled as their European counterparts (Watts, 1997, 184). Even the Imperial Gazetteer that was published under the authority of His Majesty's Secretary of State for India in Council could not stop themselves to appreciate the advance medical system of Hindus by stating, *The Hindu medical system, though not devoid of errors and absurdities, shows, at its best, a surprising degree of progress in all branches of the science* (Government of India, 1907, 457).

Government's preference for western medicine and encounter between the indigenous and western medicine became more evident in 1912 with the passing of Registration of Medical Practitioner Act in Bombay presidency. The Act was related to qualification and mandatory registration of legally qualified medical practitioners, but it excluded all indigenous practitioners i.e. *Ayurvedic* and *Unani* practitioners, from their right to get registered. This led to protests by Indian medical practitioners of *Ayurved* and *Unani*. In 1915, Poona Ayurvedic dispensary was closed on the grounds that its medical in-charge, an *Ayurved* graduate, was irregularly qualified. All this incited resentment, where prominent leaders like Tilak also gave their active participation and all native newspapers were inundated with criticism of Government's decision. Due to vociferous protest, government was forced to introduce an amendment in the Act by which previous order was repealed and Poona dispensary was restored by Governor's order stating that Poona municipality was permitted to maintain the dispensary (Ramanna, 2006). All this exposed the British scheme of sheer westernization of the medical system in India by jeopardizing the existing native system that enjoyed the faith of people since centuries by providing successful treatment at cheap rate. Where on one hand, western medical system enjoyed official patronage with high salary and high positions reserved for its practitioners; on the other hand, the indigenous medical practitioners were incessantly struggling with the limitations and demarcations posed by the government itself in spite of enjoying the faith and trust of the people. Anil Kumar in his study on medical policy of colonial India wrote about the ulterior motive of the imperial masters behind their policy of science, technology and medicine.

> ...the coming of British with their renaissance 'science and culture' initiated the process of subjugation and captivation of India's traditional scientific systems. With the colonial power at the apex, the western sciences, without facing any recognizable resistance, gradually dethroned and outdistanced the indigenous scientific systems and stamped the seal of superiority. The British made full use of their sciences both in the creation as well as in the maintenance of empire. (Kumar, 1998, 10)

Here it is pertinent to mention an example of Orissa province in order to understand the degree to which government was heeding to the health policy. Orissa, separated from Bihar in 1936, the health conditions can be envisaged by the fact that the Administration Commission Report proposed to have one officer as in charge of public health and prisons both in spite of the fact that the subjects were not related to each other. The Committee held this decision of composite charge inevitable as the new province with limited resources could not provide sufficient field for individual charges. Their health policy was clearly determined to be more preventive rather than curative. (Nanda, 2015) Dr. Sheldon Watts had rightly expressed in these words.

> Whether openly admitted or not, Development itself was intended solely as a means of providing London with an uninterrupted flow of dividend returns on capital investment. Impacting most heavily on the ability of cholera to slaughter millions were gentlemanly capitalists' very substantial investments in irrigation, in railways and port facilities and, equally decisively, the near absence of investment in public health. (Watts, 1997, 168)

Medical science was used to indisputably legitimize European imperialism in Afro-Asian colonies and to maintain European authority since medicine is always seen as something that is universal and neutral. Ascendancy of western medicine was a progressive tool of empire, while indigenous practices of colonies were regarded as something that was superstitious, lethal, backward and hindrance to European progress (Arnold, 1988, 16-18). Epidemic had played an important part in propagation of western medicine and maintaining strong withhold of colonialism as Roy MacLeod opined in his words:

> When they threatened the status quo, epidemics also created conditions favourable to the consolidation of imperial or government rule... Empires which based their claims of occupation and settlement in part on the moral superiority of European civilization, and saw an obligation to secure the safety of their subjects, found their credibility as purveyors of European culture and rational government intricately tied to their power to control the spread of disease. (MacLeod and Lewis, 1988, 10-11)

Another important epidemic was smallpox that British physicians ranked as the *scourge of India* claiming relatively more victims that what was the result of all diseases combined (David Arnold, 1993, 116). Before British, smallpox was generally treated by variolation, but this was considered lethal by Smallpox Commission 1850. Later, Vaccination Act 1880 was passed to prohibit inoculation and promote vaccination by making it mandatory for children in certain municipalities and cantonment areas. This was certainly resisted by many Indian who considered it colonial medical intervention and cultural encroachment. Anil Kumar aptly stated,

> "It was fairly clear since the beginning of the British rule that the colonial medicine derived authority from the state and not from the consent of the people. Though, chiefly dependent upon the coercive agencies of the army and the police, the British desperately needed the people's consent for the legitimation and longer survival of its newly founded Empire (Kumar, 1998, 220).

Table 15.3: Percentage of each cause of death on total annual deaths in India.

Year	1881-82	1886-87	1891-92
Cholera	3.53	4.16	9.81
Small pox	1.62	1.02	1.67
Fevers	69.70	69.24	64.20
Bowel Complaints	5.72	5.30	4.11
Injuries	1.00	1.75	1.49
Snakes and Wild Beasts	.48	.50	.40
Other causes	17.37	18.08	18.32

Source: Statement Exhibiting the Moral and Material Progress and Condition of India, House of Commons, 24th March, 1894.

Table 15.3 includes data of Bombay, Madras, Bengal, North Western Provinces, Punjab, Central Provinces, Lower Burma,

Assam and Berar.

The last decade of the 19th century had been the most deadly unfateful period in the history of India that not only witnessed couple of all-India famines, but also epidemics. In September 1896, an outbreak of virulent plague epidemic was witnessed in the port city of Bombay where the coercive discriminating ways in which colonial government responded from the very outset of the epidemic led to political and social agitation to a level that was not seen in colonial India since the suppression of 1857 revolt in different parts of India. It was on 10th October, 1896 when British Government got the report confirming that what they were dealing with in Bombay was a bubonic plague (British Medical Journal, 1896). Local conditions like over populated and ill-ventilated dwellings, filthy and squander living conditions, poor sanitation, environmental pollution of water, air and soil were considered as predisposing factors for the origin of plague epidemic. Much was not known about the etiology of the disease initially for which a five member Scientific Committee was appointed in November 1896 to study the Bombay plague with Surgeon-Major Manser as its President (British Medical Journal, 1871). Initially the disease was considered contagious from human to human, but later with the studies and investigations conducted it was found not so much contagious as was assumed, though British still hesitated to totally take it as non-contagious. Thus, in January 1897, local medical practitioners presented a memorandum to Government of Bombay that:

> the bubonic plague now prevailing in the city is under certain conditions only slightly contagious or infectious and "the facts observed in connection with individual cases and those associated with the general progress of the disease warrant us in concluding that its incidence is greatly due to local conditions (Kidambi, 2004).

A Bombay Plague Committee was appointed under the Chairmanship of Sir James Campbell by Government Resolution No. 1204/720P that submitted its 250 pages report covering time span from 1st July, 1897 to 30th April, 1898. The exhaustive report gives a detail of mortality rate in Bombay during two epidemics: First from 11th November, 1896 to 30th April, 1897 and second from 12th December, 1897 to April 1898.

Table 15.4: Death Rates in Bombay during Plague Epidemics in 1896-97 and 1897-98

Month and year	Total Mortality	Death rate per 10,000 per month
December 1896	6,243	84.4
January 1897	7,627	158.9
April 1897	3,578	61.6
December 1897	8,794	48.4
April 1898	5,097	68.5

Source: Report of Bombay Plague Committee on Plague in Bombay, 1898, p.102

The preventive measures that were adopted by the Government includes enforcement of elaborative rules regarding railway inspections, detention in observation camps and disinfections of passengers coming from infected areas, movement restrictions on in-comers and out-goers of Bombay, inspections in coast ports, mandatory hospitalization of suspected victims, intrusive house visitations in search of cases, rigid segregation of contacts with patients, evacuation of infected houses, shifting of family members to other places, disinfecting of houses, demolition of building etc. On 10th February 1897, Municipal Commissioner and local authorities' powers and authorities were immensely increased with greater control under Epidemic Diseases Act, 1897 that was enacted on 4th February, 1897 for better prevention of spread of dangerous epidemic diseases. All these measures created a lot of discontentment among the masses that brought them on the streets for protest against the colonial plague policies (Kidambi, 2004). Increasing restriction in leaving Bombay and difficulty in getting exit pass, too frequent house visits for search and disinfection purpose, continuous presence of troops, segregation of family members and forced hospitalization without family consent, all these aggressive sanitation and containment measures stirred opposition among the people who grew more and more sullen and hopeless with time. They even started opposing death registration for which they had no objections previously. This ever-growing discontentment culminated and exploded in the form of riot on 9th March, 1898 with inspection of corpse as the immediate reason. (Bombay Plague Committee, 1898, 51-52).

The violent and strong resistance of people during epidemic questioned the powers of administrators and medical professionals, who were authorized for every interventions under the cloak of epidemic combating measures. The incidents of protests and riots forced the government to retreat and relax its plague policy. A Circular dated 17th March, 1898 was issued to the District Plague Officers for limited Plague Operations where clear instructions were given that no compulsory search or frisking should be executed in any house unless confirmed that it was a plague infected house; no mandatory hospitalization of suspects and only plague victim confirmed by certified Medical Officer should be shifted to hospitals with the consent of family; in case of any property damage during search and disinfection process, compensation was to be given on the spot to the family. Thus, a reversal of plague policy was witnessed after riots in Bombay and as per circular, this new policy was adopted with instructions to all District Plague Officers on 22nd March, 1898 with detail rules regarding house visit. (Bombay Plague Committee, 1898, 186-87)

Mortality rate in India was 41.3 per thousand in the decade of 1880 that increased to 48.6 per thousand in the decade of 1911-21. Many regards India's increased exposure through brisk trade and transport, to new invading pathogens like plague and influenza as the major cause behind high mortality, while others regarded it as repercussions of incessant deteriorating state of economic-social-environmental conditions due to British profit-oriented policy (Arnold, 1993, 200). The table 15.5 clearly shows that in 1896-97 major percentage of total plague mortality of India was occurring in Bombay city that later reduced. India's plague mortality crossed one million in 1904, but afterwards a decline was seen in Bombay and India both.

Table 15.5: Plague mortality in Bombay city and India for the period 1896-1914

Year	Bombay	India
1896	1,936	2219
1897	11,003	53,816
1898	18,185	116,285
1902	13,820	5,83,937
1904	13,538	1,143,993
1914	2,941	296,623
Total	**183,984**	**8,538,931**

Source: David Arnold, Colonizing the body, 1993, p. 201.

According to Arnold, during the plague there were unprecedented incidents of physical assault by the colonial power on the colonized population that was particularly witnessed in Bombay as this city was the seat of imperial authority, centre of trade and commerce with most of the Europeans reside in the city. He wrote on the significance and far-reaching repercussions of the plague epidemic:

...the manner in which it was perceived by the colonial

authorities and the nature of the sanitary and medical measures deployed against it, bubonic plague provoked an unparalleled crisis in the history of state medicine in India. The significance of plague for the political epidemiology of colonial India was far greater than that of the concurrent epidemics of malaria or influenza, even though in any given year the mortality they caused might have been considerably greater. Plague, like smallpox and cholera, dramatically restated the centrality of epidemic disease to the colonial state medicine of the period; but it also emphasized the enormous differences in perceptions and response indigenous and colonial alike between one epidemic disease and another" (Arnold, 1993, 202)

There was an outbreak of plague in Calcutta in 1898, though suspects were reported as early as 1896. The initial sporadic occurrence was declared an epidemic within couple of years in spite of the fact that a Medical Board, later called Plague Commission, was formed through Government Resolution No. 937 T-M, dated 10th October, 1896 with H.H. Risley, Secretary to Government, Financial and Municipal Department, as President of the Board, to devise measures and determine actions required to contain the spread of bubonic plague in Bengal. Of course, being a port city and center of imperial activity, Calcutta was a great concern for all as closure of port would automatically cease the export-import of agricultural and manufacturing industries, directly striking hard on the interest of banking and mercantile section of the province and subsequently, Government income through revenue. This provides the logic to understand that why the government clearly mentioned that the Medical Board, in first instance, was to deal with the spread of disease in the following areas (Plague commission, 1899, iii-iv):

i. Calcutta town
ii. Port of Calcutta

iii. Municipality of Howrah
iv. Small Municipalities adjacent to Calcutta and Howrah
v. Railway lines

It is to be noted that all the above mentioned places were commercial centers and railways, the way to connect these places. There is one very interesting incident that I came through when delved into the report. On 10th October, 1896, Government of Bengal suggested prohibiting imports of rags and second-hand clothing from Bombay. All concerned companies and authorities related to these articles were instructed not to accept cargoes of such articles. On 17th December, there was a consignment of 65 packages of rags and 15 bags of paper-cuttings from Bombay that was ordered to be destructed by fire due to threat of possible spread of plague into the port city. This consignment cost a loss of 1,367-3/- that was too high at that time (Plague Commission, 1899, 6). From this single incident, the level of fear and commercial loss to this port city can be envisaged.

After having a bitter experience of resistance in Bombay, the Government of Bengal took lesson by adopting relatively moderate segregation policy. The policy of state interventions and involvement that led to the outbreak of public unrest in Bombay was also adopted in Bengal, but the way was different. What was achieved in Bombay through force and subsequent public resistance, the same was done in Bengal with consent. This moderate attitude and respecting peoples sentiments enabled them to ward off an iota of possibility of public unrest (Chatterjee, 2005). In Kanpur, riot was witnessed in April 1900 due to execution of strict plague control measures that disturbed the normal life of people and evoked disruptions. It won't be an exaggeration to say that people were more fearful of insensitive execution of rules and measures during epidemic rather than the disease itself and this was reflected in form of common resistance in different places. A private European medical practitioner of Bombay mentioned that plague patients died more of fear rather than that of plague when taken to hospitals (Ramanna, 2006).

The cultural interventions of British under the cloak of prevention during the emergent epidemic times were not only through draconian administrative measures, as we have seen in case of plague epidemic in Bombay. They also had eye on socio-religious life of Indian people targeting pilgrimages of Hindus to holy places of Haridwar and Allahabad. The International Sanitary conferences considered these events to be the origin, from where cholera virus spread to the rest of the world. These pilgrimages were seen as *reservoirs of pandemics.* Nothing strange on such postulation, as British always held native culture responsible for every ill occurrings or crime that occurred. *Hajj* of Muslims too was seen by colonial masters as an impending threat to European nations after the opening of Suez Canal in 1869, as it dramatically reduced the time and distance of travel, resulting in sudden rise in the number of pilgrims from this subcontinent. Saurabh Mishra in his study on *Hajj* pilgrims and epidemic policy of the government states that these pilgrims were seen as *carriers of epidemics* by the colonizers. In 1882, Superior Council of Health (Constantinople) issued a notification regarding 15 days mandatory quarantine of all pilgrims from Bombay at the island of Kamran (Pati and Harrison, 2009, 3, 32). The hardships faced by Mecca pilgrims during the quarantine period is mentioned exhaustively in the travelogue of Mirza Irfan Ali Beg, Deputy Collector of Mainpuri entitled *Pilgrimage to Mecca.* This book is a diary that includes daily accounts of his travel covering span of four months from 9th April 9th July, 1894 while he was on a privilege leave for Mecca pilgrimage. He tells that all pilgrims were quarantined at Kamran island, which was a waste land with no agriculture and very less population, mainly living on export of handicraft articles. These pilgrims had to pay Quarantine tax of Rs 12/8 per head, amount that many fail to pay. Mirza gives the detail of hardships that one has to face during this quarantine period with no proper sanitation facilities and too many restrictions imposed. He narrates that in 1890 a pilgrimage ship with nearly 700 pilgrims was sent back to India, as many died of extreme heat and cholera attacked the group. After 22 days, *neither cholera ceased to spare their lives nor the quarantine permitted them to be free*". Mirza gives an emotional articulation of these hardships of his fellow brothers in form of couplet:

Mid Jaddah and the Aden way,
The quarantine at Kamran lay.
The Hafis of the Indian land
Are first tried on this sand;
If one can save his life here,
In going Haj he has no fear.
Who does not die in ten days,
Good luck has he in all his ways.
In epidemic one if die,
All the restraint hard would lie;
What Sadi said is all the truth
And all his saying does here soothe: " Of Cholera one if die, behold,
All will be doomed either young or old
You see if one be grazing found,
The total herd is sent to pound."
One death if occur here indeed
The quarantine's term must exceed.
Impossible it is to see,
One out of quarantine to be.
The damp climate and the sand,
And dangerous is the sea strand.
Fear and hope together run
In every heart they make a fun.
Kepeat 0 ! Arif, on and on,
The al-Hafiz and al-Aman.

(Mirza, 1896, 46-52).

Being center of administrative and trade activities, the town was so overcrowded that even the Plague Commission of Bengal had accepted, in its proceedings, that so much overcrowding in the wards was dangerous to public health. The level of danger could be envisaged by the fact that Ward no. VIII had a recorded population density of 1,44,640 per square mile (Plague Commission, 1899, xlix). The adverse commercial impact was not the only reason of British trepidation, they were more apprehended of their international image of racial superiority because of which they had taken the onus of their civilizing mission with the aim to bring enlightenment in all Asian colonies. Outbreak of epidemic was tarnishing this image, as public health has always been the symbol of modernity and advance civilization that enables British to legalise their stronghold rule and control over the primitive, barbarous people of the colonies. This led them to accentuate more on the role of morals and society of the Indians as the reason for spread of the disease and remained unaccountable towards their policies in different administrative departments. The port cities and commercial centers were directly linked with the world market through export-import relations. Virulent epidemic spread in these places exposed the limitations, inadequacies and failure of the government and administration that British boast of and tarnished their image of high administrative efficiency with adequate public health policy.

The most horrendous pandemic that trapped the globe in its poisonous tentacles was of influenza in 1918-19. Dubbed as mother of all pandemics, it is regarded as one of the *greatest holocausts in history"* (Waring, 1971, 33). Estimated world mortality due to influenza pandemic is about 30 million or more that is considerably more than the total caualities of First World War (Killingray, 2003). Number of famous people succumbed to this unprecedented pandemic that had infiltrated all nations across the globe. The list includes renowned sociologist Max Weber, Fredrick Trump, grandfather of former US President Donald Trump, Gandhi's eldest son Harilal's wife and son, wife of Abdul Ghaffar Khan and survivors list includes Mahatma Gandhi, Walt Disney, George Clemenceau, David Lloyd George and then US President Woodrow Wilson, who was attacked by influenza while the peace negotiations for the Treaty of Versailles was going on. The country that faced the worst trauma due to this influenza pandemic was India with an estimated mortality rate of 14 million in India, about 38 per cent of the global mortality (Chandra, 2012). The major reason of high mortality was due to World War that led to heavy military movements and mobilization and along with them the influenza virus (Coombs, 2020). While the World War was going on, this unknown invisible enemy entered the trenches and soon turned into a global calamity with staggering mortality statistics.

These epidemics were global and occurring in most of the western countries in 19th century, but the responses were different. Where imperialist rulers adopted preventive measures in their own nations as public welfare policy; in India and other colonies, these measures were used as tools to consolidate the imperial authority with features of racial discrimination, exploitation, coercive methods, no medical facilities for local inhabitants particularly rural population, and ruining the indigenous medical system. This process of ruining was completed in 1835 with the passing of new education resolution that ended oriental policy of patronizing indigenous learning and completely wrecked the existing medical system with the replacement of vernacular languages by English as medium of instruction and connecting this as mandatory provision for any Government aid and funding. It must be remembered that the British always projected themselves to be of superior race, who were on the divine mission of the God as his agents to make the whole world civilized through the military strength of troops and moral strength of officers. For strong imperial hold, they adopted the policy of cultural intervention into the indigenous system of colonies by introducing western ways and ideas on the principal of cultural hegemony. The western medicines contributed in establishing this ideological hegemony of the Raj.

The most important aspect, while we study the history of epidemics, is the intertwined relationship between colonialism and medicine, as the aims and policies of both were same in colonies like India. Western colonial powers responded vigorously to the diseases in their overseas colonies with their motives to protect their troops and administrators, maintain health to keep the productivity of native work force and deflect international criticism. J.N. Hays stated,

> ...scientific medicine provided a vehicle for thorough social and political control of fractions colonies. And the sense persisted that Western lives mattered more than those of the subject peoples; if wars on disease threatened to cost too much, the health of the "native" might be ignored (Hay, 2009, 183)

Western medicines had been one the major tool of state interventions and oppressions in the name of public health and civilizing mission with a health policy that was dictated by the imperial masters sitting in well-equipped luxurious offices in London with sheer disregard of Indian culture, society, traditions and indigenous medical system, that was so well advanced that even today western scientists are doing research studies on the details mentioned in ancient manuscripts like *Sushruta Samhita* and *Carak Samhita* written two millennium before. Under the cloak of benevolence of colonial governance, medicine, as called by Mark Harrison, was being used by the rulers as a, *colonizing discourse and instrument of social control* (Harrison, 1994). It is because of this reason that David Arnold had used the term "*colonial medicine*" and defined it stating that it was *the operation of colonial power within and through medicine in a colonial setting* (Arnold, 2000, 15). He opined that *Western medicine in India was self evidently a colonial science, moving mostly from metropole to colony and reinforcing the institutional and technical dominance of the colonizers.* (Arnold, 1993, 290). It will be apt to quote here the lines of Madhuri Sharma (2012, 5), who states: *Colonial medicine proved, in fact, to be a twin-edged weapon which cut the colonized both physically and morally. Not only the body but also the mind was conquered.*

Epilogue

In the name of medical science, western knowledge, English language and literature, advanced technology, unified political power, superior culture, organized administration, British had displayed all forms of barbarity on the inhabitants of the colonies. David Arnold regarded arrival of western medicines in India as a part of *new imperialism* of 1880s and 1890s. The unleashed coerciveness and enormities of the British rule during the times of epidemics in the name of combating measures failed to reduce the mortality rate of the Indians. This can be clearly seen in case of plague epidemic mortality rate given in Table 15.4 and 15.5. Though for every epidemic that occurred in India, be it smallpox, cholera, malaria or plague, English people had always emphasized role of social conditions, traditions, morals, low standard living conditions, bad life habits, poor sanitation, squalor surroundings of the local inhabitants with the climate conditions conducive to its culmination as an epidemic (Mark Harrison, 2002, 176). If it was so then why the people were more afraid of British medical professionals rather than the disease itself? Why the people came on the streets for violent resistance against medical practitioners in Bombay knowing that the disease was contiguous and such movement in crowd could be lethal for them and their families? If the sanitation conditions were so poor in Bombay and there was urgency to empower local officers to issue orders to bulldoze any building, then being rulers who were responsible for providing proper sanitation to the people? If the overcrowded slum was a matter of grave concern for them during the time of epidemic, then being the most civilized administrators who were responsible to plan for proper urbanization and residential place for the workers while Bombay and Bengal was being developed as the centre of trade and commerce activities in India?

These questions and administrative loopholes from the highest to lowest rung of the authority were never raised and revealed in any of the government reports on epidemic as these reports were not only a way to boast the British administrative and policy making decisions, but were also a tool to reinforce the imperial power by way of favourable documentation to be left for the posterity and future researchers. The inconvenient documentary evidences were kept under cover or might have been destroyed in many cases (Watts, 2001). In 234 pages report of Bombay Plague Committee, the riot of 9th March was not given a space of more than a small para of 8 lines. Only the goods were to be documented that may appease and sound like dulcet tone to the ears of the upper echelon authorities sitting at London in their luxurious office equipped with best available facilities of the time (of course, sponsored by the drained wealth of India) talking about the sanitation and bad life habits of the poor Indians living in slums while showing a callous indifference to their sufferings. Most of the British official records, reports, documents submitted by English scientists and administrators do not give space to such data or description that does not reinforce the self-image of the British, who were here to bring enlightenment and progress in India as this was not liked by their masters at home.

During the colonial period, medicine was something that

was not simply contained within the diameter of health, patients and diseases. It entered into the wider arenas of social interventions, containment of individual rights, oppression and racial discrimination through the whole rung of medical authoritarian structure that was destructing the indigenous medical system to establish their hegemony. This they were doing by breaking the moral power of the Indians and their faith in themselves during the epidemic times. British medicine, health and sanitation policy was a part of colonizing process that fastened up with the occurrence of epidemics in different parts of India. British always emphasized the social and moral conditions of Indians and conducive climate as the major reason for occurrence of all epidemics and endeavoured to establish the fact that it was a common phenomenon in India. They couldn't dare to accept the loopholes and failure of their own administrative system and policies that were responsible for the frequent occurrence of epidemics, speedy spread and high severity. The simple formula of colonial consciousness was—everything good that happened was the result of the benevolence and civilizing presence of the ruling race of colonizers and everything bad was due to barbarous native culture of the colonized. Seventy-four years after the withdrawal and departure of these so-called civilized colonizers, the political landscape is completely reversed. The same nation which they plundered and looted for almost two centuries and tagged as barbarous is emerging as a global leader during the twenty-first century Covid pandemic, while most of the developed nations have shattered. Under the Act East Policy, the Indian government has adopted the Vaccine *Maitri* diplomacy, wherein the government is giving millions of doses of Covaxin/Covidshield vaccine to its neighbour countries as gift. Whereas on the other hand, the British Parliament, despite facing second wave of mutant corona virus, is discussing over the recent legislations of Indian parliament, which is the par example of colonial hangover!!!

REFERENCES

1. Alam, M. (2016). White Man's 'Diseases' and White Man's 'Cures': Smallpox Vaccination in the Early Period of 'Empire' in Fiji. *Proceedings of the Indian History Congress, 77,* 777-790. doi:10.2307/26552707
2. Arnold, David, ed. (1988). *Imperial Medicine and Indigenous Societies.* Manchester: Manchester University Press
3. —— (2000). *The New Cambridge History of India: Science, Technology and Medicine in Colonial India,* volume III. Cambridge: Cambridge University Press.
4. Arnold, David.(1993).*Colonizing The Body: State Medicine and Epidemic Diseases in Nineteenth-century India.* Berkeley Los Angeles: University of California
5. Beg, Mirza Irfan Ali (1896). *Pilgrimage to Mecca.* Benares: The Chandraprabha Press Company Limited.
6. Bombay Plague Committee. (1898). *Report of the Bombay Plague Committee on Plague in Bombay, 1898.* Bombay: Times of India Steam Press
7. Burrell, S., and Gill, G. The Liverpool Cholera Epidemic of 1832 and Anatomical Dissection—Medical Mistrust and Civil Unrest. *Journal of the History of Medicine and Allied Sciences* 60, no. 4 (2005): 478-98. Accessed December 7, 2020. http://www.jstor.org/stable/24632238.
8. Chandra, S., Kuljanin, G., & Wray, J. (2012). Mortality From the Influenza Pandemic of 1918-1919: The Case of India. *Demography,* 49(3), 857-865. Retrieved November 29, 2020, from http://www.jstor.org/stable/23252674
9. Chatterjee, S. (2005). Plague and Politics in Bengal 1896 to 1898. *Proceedings of the Indian History Congress,* 66, 1194-1201. Retrieved November 29, 2020, from http://www.jstor.org/stable/44145931
10. Coombs, H. (2020). *COVID-19: NATO in the Age of Pandemics* (pp. 61-70, Rep.) (Tardy T., Ed.). NATO Defense College. doi:10.2307/resrep25148.13
11. Government of India. (1907). *Imperial Gazetteer of India: The Indian Empire, Administrative,* vol. IV. Oxford: Clarendon Press
12. Harrison, Mark. (1994). *Public Health in British India: Anglo-India Preventive Medicine 1859-1914.* Cambridge: Cambridge University Press.
13. —— (2002). *Climates and Constitutions: Health, Race, Environment and British Imperialism in India 1600-1850.* New Delhi: Oxford University Press.
14. Hays, J.N. (2009). *The Burdens of Disease: Epidemics and Human Response in Western History.* London: Rutgers University Press
15. Hobson, J.A. (1902). *Imperialism: A Study.* London: George Allen and Unwin Ltd.
16. House of Commons, Statement Exhibiting the Moral and Material Progress and Condition of India during the year 1891-92 and the Nine Preceding

Years, 24th March, 1894. London: Her Majesty's Stationary Office

17. Kidambi, P. (2004). An infection of locality: Plague, pythogenesis and the poor in Bombay, c. 1896-1905. *Urban History*, 31(2), 249-267. Retrieved November 29, 2020, from http://www.jstor.org/stable/44614117
18. Killingray, D. (2003). "A New 'Imperial Disease': The Influenza Pandemic of 1918-19 and its Impact on the British Empire." *Caribbean Quarterly*, 49(4), 30-49. Retrieved November 29, 2020, from http://www.jstor.org/stable/40654422
19. Kumar, Anil. (1998). *Medicine and the Raj: British Medical Policy in India*. New Delhi: Sage Publications
20. MacLeod, Roy and Milton Lewis, eds. (1988). *Disease, Medicine and Empire: Perspectives on Western Medicine and the Experience of European Expansion*. London: Routledge.
21. Morens, D., Folkers, G., & Fauci, A. (2009). What Is a Pandemic? *The Journal of Infectious Diseases*, 200(7), 1018-1021. Retrieved November 28, 2020, from http://www.jstor.org/stable/27794175
22. Nanda, C. (2015). Disciplining A "Pathological" Province? Epidemic Disease and Health Interventions in Colonial Orissa. *Proceedings of the Indian History Congress*, 76, 305-317. Retrieved November 28, 2020, from http://www.jstor.org/stable/44156598
23. Nicholas, R. (1981). The Goddess and Epidemic Smallpox in Bengal. *The Journal of Asian Studies*, 41(1), 21-44. doi:10.2307/2055600
24. Parkes, Edmund, A. (1866). *A Manual of Practical Hygiene*. London: John Churchill and Sons.
25. Pati, Biswamoy and Harrison, Mark (eds.). (2009). *The Social History of Health and Medicine in Colonial India*. New York: Routledge
26. Plague Commission. (1899). *History and Proceedings of the Plague Commission, Bengal 1896 to 1898*, Calcutta: Bengal Secretariat Press, 1899.
27. Plague in Bombay. (1896). *The British Medical Journal*, 2(1867), 1064-1064. Retrieved December 10, 2020, from http://www.jstor.org/stable/20247267
28. Rake, B. *et al.* (1893). *Leprosy in India: Report of the Leprosy Commission in India, 1890-91*. Calcutta: Superintendent of Government Printing India
29. Ramanna, Mridula, (July 22-28, 2006). Systems of Medicine: Issues and Responses in Bombay Presidency. *Economic and Political Weekly*, 41(29), pp. 3221-3226
30. Sharma, Madhuri. (2012). *Indigenous and Western Medicine in Colonial India*. Delhi: Cambridge University Press India Pvt. Ltd
31. Taubenberger, J. K., & Morens, D. M. (2006). 1918 influenza: The mother of all pandemics. *Emerging Infectious Diseases*, 12, 15-22
32. The Plague in Bombay. (1896). *The British Medical Journal*, 2(1871), 1402. Retrieved December 10, 2020, from http://www.jstor.org/stable/

20247652

33. Waring, J. I. (1971). *A history of medicine in South Carolina 1900-1970*. Columbia: South Carolina Medical Association.
34. Watts, S. (1999). British Development Policies and Malaria in India 1897-c. 1929. *Past & Present*, (165), 141-181. Retrieved November 29, 2020, from http://www.jstor.org/stable/651287
35. ——(2001). From Rapid Change to Stasis: Official Responses to Cholera in British-Ruled India and Egypt: 1860 to c. 1921. *Journal of World History*, 12(2), 321-374. Retrieved December 6, 2020, from http://www.jstor.org/stable/20078912
36. ——(1997). *Epidemics and History: Disease, Power and Imperialism*. London: Yale University Press

16

The Cataclysm Cliff

Re-evaluating Bubonic Plague of 1896 and Visualising the Political Dynamics

Shalini Pathak

ABSTRACT

Several research papers and writings have been concluded since the outbreak of the corona pandemic and in general all these writings have been Covid-19 centric taking into account several dimensions of the outbreak. However, in this chapter an attempt has been made to comprehend the political dynamics existing during the nineteenth century, a period when India was completely governed by the British. In the chapter, an attempt has been made to explain and analyse the reasons behind the outbreak of the bubonic plague and to make a comparative study of the bubonic plague and the outbreak of Corona with special attention to the historicity of both the disastrous outbreaks. The paper also delves into the mishandling of the plague and the modus operandi *of the British government, taking into account both the Congress and the Nationalist perception and throwing light on the circumstances which actuated the Chapekar brothers for their revolutionary action.*

Keywords: British Policy, Bubonic Plague, Chapekar Brothers, Congress, Epidemic, Nationalism, Rand, Tilak

5th June is celebrated every year as the World Environment Day, but this celebration for keeping the environment safe and secure has only observed its thickness in the form of Conferences, Summits, Seminars, Conventions, theme plays, books and conversation between people. The second decade of the twenty-first century witnessed the emanation of COVID-19, much popularized abbreviated form of Corona Virus Disease of 2019 in December 2019. The place of emanation of this pandemic was Wuhan, the capital city of Hubei province in the People's Republic of China. Wuhan is an important commercial centre, which is divided by the Yangtze and the Han River. It is not only the largest city in Hubei province, but also is the most populated one in Central China.

Pandemic is a Greek terminology, which is bifurcated into two *paen* and *demik*, which means 'all' and 'people' respectively. The word pandemic is self-explanatory in itself as it means 'all people' thus eliminating the perception that a disease outbreak in a particular country, region or a territory. It simply means an epidemic of disease without any political, social, economic, religious, cultural, geographical and traditional complexion. A disease which neither recognizes country, nor a powerful country, nor colour, age, gender, nationality or race, better said limitless or no boundaries. It is extremely hard to demarcate the difference between a pandemic and epidemic and it has already seeked adequate attention and research of several scientists across the globe but one thing which delivers a permanency to pandemic and epidemic is its course and nature, with course recognizing no international boundaries of any country and nature being completely disastrous and catastrophic. Human history has come across several epidemic and diseases like smallpox, cholera, influenza, bubonic plague and the most recent and deadliest Corona virus. Any disease or epidemic cannot be circled in the category of pandemic, besides the fact that the similarity between epidemic, disease and pandemic is quite obvious as it involves large scale deaths and intense spreadibility embracing all international boundaries, however the salient characteristic which set apart pandemic from any other disease or epidemic is its contagious and infectious trait. To come in the category of pandemic, the disease needs to be contagious and infectious.

Historic Coincidence in Outbreak of Plague

The second half of the nineteenth century was one of the most challenging decades in Indian history as what India witnessed was the outbreak of the revolt of 1857. The nineteenth century was one of the most challenging centuries as it not only witnessed the First War of Independence, but it also witnessed the outbreak of famine and simultaneously the outbreak of bubonic plague. On one, the revolt possessed its own implications and on the other, India observed the brunt of epidemic towards the closing decade. The outbreak of the bubonic plague in Bombay intertwined with the outbreak of famine hard-hited entire India. It affected the entire Indian sub-continent causing severe mortality and debility. The pre-existing compelling situation became more disastrous with the outbreak of plague.

The term Plague was coined by a Greek physician Galen, which meant any quickly spreading fatal disease. The Bubonic Plague was one of the first severe outbreaks of epidemic that India observed under the British rule. Since it broke out in Bombay, therefore the popular nomenclature which it received was the Bombay Plague. The reason for the outbreak of the plague was the arrival of thousands of pilgrims in 1896 from the Himalayan region, where the plague was already in amplified mode and their arrival exacerbated the pre-existing condition, making them potent carriers of the plague (Deshmukh, 1988).

It is important to comprehend the origination of plague

in expansion hierarchy in order to maintain the exactness of the topic. A little more in-depth study confirms that the inception of the Bombay Plague is attributed to the arrival of *Mandarin* ship from Hong Kong in 1896 and Hong Kong during this time was in throes of the outbreak. It is extremely interesting to note that the place of origination of the plague was none other than a Chinese province named Yunnan, where the plague was caused by the bite of infected fleas in rodents transferring to humans. However, the expansion hierarchy exists in a reversal order. It was in the year 1894 that the plague broke out in the Yunnan province of China from where it spread to Hong Kong which was under the British domination and it was from Hong Kong that the plague through the merchant ships made its disastrous headway towards Bombay, which too was under the British domination (BBC News, 2020).

The reports of *Indian Express* mentions, "By the end of February 1897, Pune had recorded 308 cases of plague with 271 deaths. The dread of the disease which had such a high mortality rate had caused the locals to flee the city. The municipal officials estimated that about 15,000 to 20,000 locals had left the city to escape the pandemic and had settled in the villages in the outskirts." (*Indian Express*, 2020) The spreadibility of the plague was far-reaching. From Poona the plague spread multiplied and was quickly observed in Calcutta, United Provinces, North West Frontier Province, Hyderabad, Mysore, Madras, Agra, Oudh and Burma (Malhotra, 2020). Myron Echenberg in his book *Plague Ports: The Global Urban Impact of Bubonic Plague 1894-1901*, has mentioned "Between the Plague's arrival in 1896 and 1921, an estimated 12 million Indians lost their lives compared in the 3 million of the rest of the world combined".

Measures Adopted by British Government

The magnitude of the Plague was too high and after the case

of plague was observed in Bombay, it spread tremendously to Bengal, Burma, United Provinces, Punjab and instantaneously its reverberations were throughout Northern India and Western. (Lentin, 2020). The devastation scale in the eastern India and southern India was less in comparison. Previously, the British government was blind towards the outbreak of the plague, but looking into the seriousness and the pattern of spreadibility of the Plague, forthwith a Plague Committee was formed under the chairmanship of Brigadier General W.F. Gatacre. The objective of the Plague Committee was to delve into the causes of the plague and to control its spreadibility (Malhotra, 2020). The measures which were adopted to counter the spread of plague were atrocious and disdainful. The measures included forceful entry in houses, examining the people residing there, forcibly driving them to segregation camps, severe restrictions on the mobility of people, preventing people to leave or enter Poona. The severity level of the measures adopted was unthinkable. Under the cloak of controlling epidemic the people were treated ruthlessly. There were reports which indicated that the soldiers, deployed for the pandemic management, not only mishandled the people but they were denied permission to conduct funerals until the deaths were registered. People who broke these regulations were subjected to criminal activities.

Looking onto the seriousness of the problem, the Governor of Bombay Presidency William Mansfield Sandhurst decided to appoint an Oxford educated, Walter Charles Rand, It was in February 1897, Walter Charles Rand ICS, was appointed as an Assistant Collector and Chairman of the Poona Plague Committee (*Indian Express*, 2020). The measures adopted by Rand were callous, ferocious and abominable. His unsparing behavior towards the victims and mildly asymptomatic people was so brutal in its complexion that he was criticised by then political leaders of India amongst which G.K. Gokhale and Lokmanya Bal Gangadhar Tilak were most prominent. The Epidemic Disease Act of 1897 was passed which mentioned about the power to take special measures and prescribe regulations to epidemic disease, power of Central Government, prohibition of violence against healthcare service personnel and damage to property, penalty, cognizance, investigation and trial of offences, and protection to persons under the Act. The regulations and provisions of the Act were apparently outlined, but the pattern in which the power was adroitly used was inimical and destructive (Indiacode).

Under the Act, the officer was empowered to take any decision to control the epidemic. He could take possessions of any suspected patient, controlling places of crowd and examining any individual at any place without any permission. They also possessed the power to put behind the bars suspected persons for six months if they oppose or create any sort of hindrance in the process. The ignominious and demeaning behaviour of the soldiers towards women crushed their self-esteem and dignity, which caused intense unrest amongst the people of India (*Hindustan Times*, 2020). *The New York Times* in its issue of June 1897 wrote, "Two kinds of disease and both deadly- natives dying by hundreds of hunger and overseers stealing the supplies." The measures which the British government adopted to tackle plague was completely non-compatible. People who showed even a minuscule sign or were just suspected of being infected were compelled and driven to the detention centers. The oppression and the power display by the authorities exacerbated the pre-existing grim condition. Instead of rendering a solution to the problem the non-congruent measures adopted by the government made the conditions more deteriorating. It seemed as if, by forcibly capturing people the government would eradicate the spread of plague. Dr. M.P. Manukar as mentioned, "It was the worst period Pune city has ever experienced in its history. About 300 to 400 people used to die at time and it was difficult task to cremate all the bodies." (Dey, 2020)

However, Rand in his report wrote, "It is a matter of great satisfaction to the members of the Plague Committee that no credible complaint that the modesty of a woman had been intentionally insulted was made either to themselves or to the officers under whom the troops worked." The writings of Rand did not cease here, and went a step further mentioning that a close watch was kept on the troops employed on the plague duty and utmost consideration was shown for the custom and tradition of the people (Couchman, 1897).

The Plague Warriors

The outbreak of the pandemic during the twenty-first century possesses its own trait, but the cataclysm clamp of the pandemic and the epidemic of 1896 exhibits a similarity. As Corona was being tackled sublimely by the Corona warriors, similarly the bubonic plague of 1896 too witnessed the benevolence and magnacious gesture from the plague warriors. Since India was tied to the colonial fetters and the entire medicinal treatment was to pass through the colonial scanner, therefore the protection ratio provided to the victims was not a remarkable one, but even then selfless help rendered by certain people was of utmost importance who neither took into cognizance the colonial power nor were distracted by the fact that their own life was at stake. While making a study on the bubonic plague we come across two significant persons who dedicated their life in countering to the disaster.

The first was Acacios Gabriel Viegas, a Goan doctor who served the people with his medicinal and remediable service in the most remarkable manner and diagnosed the first victim affected by plague on September 1896 (Tim Willasey-Wilsey, 2020). Born in 1856, just a year before the outbreak of Revolt of 1857, at the age of 40, he was the first to make a sincere revelation about the outbreak of bubonic plague. Although the estimated toll was too high but Viegas expedient and well-timed diagnosis, helped the people to counter the severe conditions. It was only after his diagnosis that the Governor of Bombay underwent confabulations with other medical experts and a team was constituted to deal with the situation. The ballooned deleterious condition was dwarfed by his humanitarian inputs and the selfless service which he rendered to the people of India was remarkable. With probability ratio in negative, he rendered his service to the people of India. Besides the fact that he was also the President of the Bombay Municipal Corporation he delivered his helping hand. It was due to his spectacular service that the statue of Acacios Viegas was erected in the Cowasji Jehangir Hall on his birth centenary in 1956 in Bombay (Wikipedia).

The second person who deserves a mention here is Waldemar Haffkine, a Ukrainian-Jewish scientist, who rendered his services at the age of 36. He completed his studies from the Pasteur Institute of Paris and successfully developed vaccines for cholera and the deadly plague. Recognized as the first microbiologist, he was called by Joseph Lister "savior of humanity" Dr. Waldemar Mordecai Haffkine Haffkine.

> The journey we make here upon the Earth is so short, before we know where we are, we are at the end, and called upon to answer an inner voice: Have you finished the work you had to do? Happy they are who can think, yes, they have finished their work.
>
> (H. Jhala, 2020)

Haffkine came to Bombay in 1896 after the outbreak of pandemic and passionately committed himself in developing the vaccine to counter epidemic. As a bacteriologist, he was well cognizant of the Indian environment and had already successfully developed a vaccine for cholera which erupted in Calcutta in 1893. Just after three years the outbreak of plague devastated the entire social and economic fabric of India. He worked with the JJ Group of Hospitals to develop a vaccine for plague and it was in January 1897 that the tedious task of developing vaccine was complete. Post-completion the vaccine was tried on the volunteers of Byculla jail with positive results (www.haffkineinstitute.org)

In 1898, the laboratory where Haffkine was working was moved to Khushru Palace. The owner of this Lodge was none other than Aga Khan III, who was the Head of the Khoja Mussalman community. He supported the efforts of Haffkine and offered him his Khushru Palace, situated in Mazagaon, Bombay in order to set up his laboratory and channelize his medicinal efforts. His endeavour and dedication received recognition when in 1925 the Bombay Bacteriology Laboratory was named as Haffkine Institute which was aimed at training, research and testing and is located in Parel, Mumbai. The Endeavour of both the important plague warriors cannot be

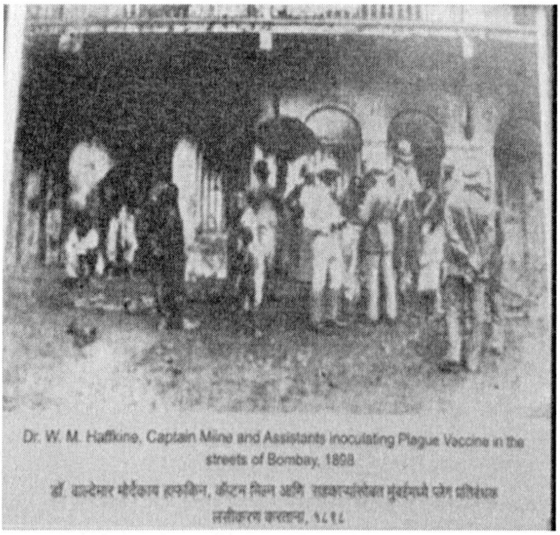
Dr. W. M. Haffkine, Captain Mine and Assistants inoculating Plague Vaccine in the
streets of Bombay, 1898

Photo 16.1: Dr. Haffkine's effort to save the people of Bombay during the Plague Epidemic of 1896-97. Photo edited by Aditya Chichkar.

Source: Retrieved on 17th April, 2016 from https://ismailimail.files.wordpress.com/2016/04/image.png?w=730&h=339

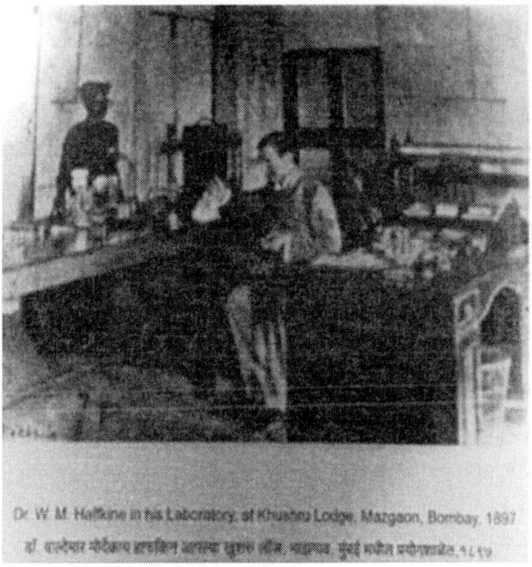
Dr. W. M. Haffkine in his Laboratory at Khushru Lodge, Mazgaon, Bombay 1897

Photo 16.2: Dr. Waldemar Haffkine at Khushru Lodge owned by Aga Khan III.

Source: Retrieved on 17th April, 2016 from https://ismailimail.files.wordpress.com/2016/04/image.png?w=730&h=339

dimmed by the mists of time and possess reminiscence through their statue and Haffkine Institute in Bombay (Willasey-Wilsey, 2020).

The Nationalist Angle

To comprehend the dreadful turbulence an in-depth study is mandatory wherein it is important to take a peek into the Nationalist angle too. The political situation during the nineteenth century was too pressing and demanding. The callous and Beplorable action taken on the part of government to cripple the rebellion of 1857, was one of the most reprehensible acts of the government, whose memories were still sharp and awake. By the time the mental mending process was shaping up, a new Act of the government triggered the nationalist feeling in the most pronounced manner. This Act was none other than the passage of the Vernacular Press Act of 1878, which outrightly exhibited the government machinations of curbing any expression of criticism of the British policies. Although the Act passed by Lord Lytton in 1878 was soon repealed by Lord Ripon, taking into account the opposition from wide spectrum of Indian populace, but all these politically-motivated act of the government worked as a catalyst to build up the nationalistic feeling.

While India was witnessing the political turbulence and also the heat of 1857, the nation was also witnessing the birth of Chapekar Brothers, Damodar in 1869, Balkrishna in 1873 and Vasudeo in 1880, who belonged to Chinchwad, a small village in the city of Poona. Determined, conservative and intolerant towards their approach, the Chapekar Brothers grew hearing Tilak and Gokhale sayings and very soon established an association called the Chapekaer Club with the objective of imparting physical and military training. Imbued with intense nationalism, very soon they associated themselves with the *Ganapati* and *Shivaji* festival initiated by Bal Gangadhar Tilak (*History of Freedom Movement Papers*). It was during this time when the bubonic plague hard-hited India in 1896 particularly, the Bombay Presidency. At this critical juncture, it is important to comprehend that the political-economic dynamics of Bombay was capital-oriented. The apprehension which blanketed the British mercantile community was a severe dip in the thriving commerce, as Bombay was the epicenter of trade and commerce during the nineteenth century. Therefore, it was obligatory for the British authorities to adopt prompt actions to curb the growth and spread of the plague, not in the interest of the people of India, but in the deep-seated commercial interest. For complete eradication of epidemic, W.C. Rand was appointed as the Plague Commissioner of Poona. The measures adopted by Rand were extremely harsh in their nature. The entrenched inhumane act of Rand stirred the mind of Chapekar Brothers and it became extremely hard for them to keep themselves aloof from the entire plague-curbing process. It was at this juncture they decided to adopt extreme step of killing Rand, whom they observed the source of misfortune, dishonor, harassment and remorse.

To implement their task, the day selected by them was the 60th year of Queen Victoria's regime. The Diamond Jubilee of Queen Victoria hegemony was decided to be celebrated on 22nd June 1897 in Pune and the venue selected for the celebrations was the Government House, which at present is the Main building of the Savitribai Phule University. The Chapekar Brothers decided to murder Rand for his vindictive, malicious and evil-intentioned measures which were operated in the most inhumane and despotic manner. The eruption of bubonic plague was in stark contrast with the ceremonial event of 22nd June 1897 with the Diamond Jubilee celebrations of the coronation of the Queen Victoria in Pune (*History of Freedom Movement Papers*). The cultural insensitivity displayed by the authorities towards the socially fragile people was a cold-blooded act of the government. The social, cultural and political abrasiveness exhibited by Rand elicited strong feelings against him, which was finally expressed in the form of his assassination. The Chapekar brothers, Damodar, Vasudeo, Balkrishna along with M.V.Ranade were sentenced to death.

Bal Gangadhar Tilak, the fiery Nationalist leader of India, wrote, "Her Majesty the Queen, the Secretary of State and his Council should not have issued the orders for practicing tyranny upon the people of India without any special advantage to be gained. The government should not have entrusted the execution of this order to suspicious, sullen and tyrannical officer like Rand" (Myron). The writings of Tilak surely made a political incision into the skeletal promises, thin views, and insubstantial functionary and of course the *modus operandi* of the government. Gopal Krishna Gokhale denounced the action taken on part of the government to curb the outbreak of Plague and claimed that the British were ignorant of Indian languages, customs and sentiments. It is interesting to note that Bal Gangadhar Tilak was charged under Section 124A for his writings in *Kesari* which was completely against the policies of the government. Tilak was convicted of sedition and was sentenced to eighteen months of rigorous imprisonment. The government immediately imposed a ban on the acclamation of *Shivaji* festival and also the *Ganapati* festival. It was alleged by the British government that the articles were intended "to attempt to excite feeling of disloyalty and disaffection to the British Government" (*History of Freedom Movement Papers*).

The Congress Angle

Before the outbreak of the Bubonic Plague, just eleven years back, one of the most important national organizations, the Indian National Congress was founded that represented entire India. *Albeit*, the aim with which the Indian National Congress was founded was to obtain a greater share in the government, but besides the political complexion the Congress was also aimed to advance the grievances of the people of India. Other than the political dialogue, it was also the supreme platform for societal and civic dialogues. One of the most astonishing facts which need a mention here is that the twelfth session of the Indian National Congress was summoned in Calcutta in 1896 under the Presidentship of Rahimtullah M. Sayani. Indubitably the session was important as it was summoned after the outbreak of the Bubonic plague but it did not addressed the outbreak of the Plague which had deeply impacted the very social, cultural, religious, political and economic fabric of India. Interestingly, President during his address mentioned about the British policy in India which stated, "It is the duty of England to study the interest, the happiness and the welfare of the people of India." It was also stated, "Policy of British rule in India should be a policy of justice, good faith and righteousness and of advancement of the people". (A.M.Zaidi). However, the entire scenario was acutely antithetical to the address delivered. The British neither took cognizance of the outbreak of Plague nor did they exhibit a pinch of empathy towards the victim patients and sufferers. The squalid behavior displayed by them was miles ahead scary.

Interestingly when the Congress was founded in 1885, and the session was to be summoned at Poona even then due to the outbreak of cholera the venue of the Congress was changed from Poona and the new venue for the Congress session was Bombay. Deprived of the mention of cholera, the session was a success, as the Congress was a nascent organisation and the entire political and social issues were to be actuated with the passage of time. But even after eleven years when not a single mention regarding the grievances of the people was addressed in the 1896 session of the Congress that was a matter of concern. When we compare the bubonic plague and the Corona virus attack, both the disasters originated in China, with Yunnan being the origination place of the former and Wuhan being the origination place of origination of the latter. The resemblance visualized in the origin has a lot to say than to up the silent quotient. This is one of the deadliest situations which have been well served to the world by China.

A peek into the last decade of the nineteenth century will exhibit certain interesting historic coincidences with respect to the outbreak of the bubonic plague. It was the same century and the same decade when Swami Vivekananda represented India in the Parliament of World's Religion in 1893 in Chicago, America. The global recognition given to India during the colonial time was tremendous. It was the same year when Mahatma Gandhi after successfully applying his political weapon of *Satyagraha* coated with *ahimsa* in South Africa came to India in 1893. In fact the last decade even witnessed the commencement of *Ganapati* festival and the *Shivaji* festival by

Tilak, who sparked the socio-cultural phenomena by giving it a national metamorphose and connecting it with nationalism, pride and honour. Thus, the second half of the nineteenth century was not only marked by revolt, plague and famine, but was historically counter-balanced by Swami Vivekananda representation of India, arrival of Mahatma Gandhi from South Africa, establishment of Indian National Congress, commencement of *Ganpati* and *Shivaji* festival and arrival of Besant in 1897. The political, social, cultural, religious and dreadful uproar was not squally, but possessed its own historic chronology. It was the time when India was observing its political manuring. The first recorded case of bubonic plague in Poona was discovered on 2nd October, the day when Gandhi was born, man who lead the Indian National Movement. It was not only the Jallianwala Bagh massacre one of the cold blooded act of the British government, infact the *modus operandi* of the government to control plague too was an cold blooded act of the government.

REFERENCES

1. Bubonic Plague: The First Pandemic. (April 25, 2019). Retrieved from https://www.sciencemuseum.org.uk/objects-and-stories/medicine/bubonic-plague-first-pandemic
2. Cynthia Deshmukh. (1988). The Bombay Plague 1896-1897. *Proceedings of the Indian History Congress*, 49, 478-483. Retrieved on 11th January, 2021 from https://www.jstor.org/stable/44148433?seq=1
3. Haffkine, Waldemar (December 11, 2020) The Vaccine Pioneer the World Forgot. *BBC News*. Retrieved from https://www.bbc.com/news/world-asia-india-55050012
4. Rashid, Atik. (June 9, 2020). The Oppressive Containment Measures during Poona Plague led to Assassination of British Officer. *The Indian Express*. New Delhi. Retrieved from https://indianexpress.com/article/research/how-oppressive-containment-measures-during-poona-plague-led-to-assassination-of-british-officer-6450775/
5. Malhotra, Aanchal. (2020). *When the 1897 Bubonic Plague Ravaged India*. Retrieved on 19 January. https://www.livemint.com/mint-lounge/features/when-the-1897-bubonic-plague-ravaged-india-11587876174403.html

6. Myron J. Echenberg. Plague Ports: The Global Urban Impact of Bubonic Plague 1894-1901, New York University Press, New York. 66-68. Retrieved on 12th January 2021, https://en.wikipedia.org/wiki/Chapekar_brothers
7. Lentin, Sifra. (2020). Lessons from the Bombay Plague. *Gateway House; Indian Council on Global Relation*. Retrieved on January 11, 2021 https://www.gatewayhouse.in/lessons-bombay-plague/
8. Indiacode. Retrieved on January 11, 2021 from https://www.indiacode.nic.in/bitstream/123456789/2326/1/A1897_03.pdf
9. *Hindustan Times*. Retrieved from https://www.hindustantimes.com/india/112-yr-old-act-brings-back-nightmares-for-pune/story-a071LT1DVhdks45oSnK7tJ.html
10. Dey, Monidipa Bose. March 24, 2020. *Lessons from the Bubonic Plague of 1896*. Retrieved from https://www.livehistoryindia.com/history-daily/2020/03/24/lessons-from-the-bubonic-plague-of-1897.
11. Couchman, M.F. (1897). *Account of Plague Administration in the Bombay Presidency from September 1896 till May 1897*, 89-100. Bombay: Government Central Press.
12. Tim Willasey-Wilsey (2020). Policy Dilemmas from the Bombay Plague of 1896. Gateway House; Indian Council on Global Relation. Retrieved on 12 January 2021, https://www.gatewayhouse.in/bombay-plague-1896/
13. Retrieved from https://en.wikipedia.org/wiki/Acacio_Gabriel_Viegas
14. Guntur, Joel and Panday, Vikas. (11 December 2020). "Jhala H. I.W.M.W Haffkine, Bacteriologist- A Great Saviour of Mankind." *Indian Journal of History and Science.* Retrieved from http://www.haffkineinstitute.org/waldemar.htm
15. Report on the Ganapati and Shivaji Festival in Maharashtra, 1897-1910. *History of Freedom Movement Papers, Region- I*, File no. 32/2, 11-13. Private Papers Section, National Archives of India, New Delhi
16. Report on the Background of the Revolutionary Cult in Maharashtra, 1897-1910", *History of Freedom Movement Papers, Region IV and V*, File no. 16/2, 134-136. Private Papers Section, National Archives of India, New Delhi
17. Zaidi, A.M., *Congress Presidential Address*, vol 1, 1885-1900, 293. Retrieved from http://www.columbia.edu/itc/mealac/pritchett/00litlinks/sayani_congress_1896/index.html

17

Exploring Pandemics and Epidemics in Colonial India and AssamThrough the Lens of a Historian

Moushumi Dutta Pathak

ABSTRACT

The outbreak of the Covid-19 or the Coronavirus in pandemic form in 2019 has resulted in an enquiry in the human mind that since when did a pandemic and epidemic begun in human civilization. India, being a third-world country, has encountered a variety of epidemics and pandemics through time. Several accounts of influenza, cholera, dengue, smallpox and others have been recorded throughout history; while we have been able to eradicate some; many diseases still continue to pose a threat to the population. The basic definition of an epidemic thus it is a disease that affects a large number of people within a community, population or region. A pandemic is an epidemic which spread over multiple countries or continents. This paper proposes to explore the pandemics and epidemics that have taken their toll in Colonial India and also in my own state of Assam. To speak of the colonial period in the sub-continent, we basically speak of that particular period that is with the onset of British rule since the Battle of Plassey and thereafter till the independence of the sub-continent in 1947from the scourge of British domination. The British colonisers reached the sub-continent and confronted a society which they perceived to be filthy, foul, dirty and contaminated with unhealthy practices and thus, being infested with diseases that were a result of the presence of mosquitoes, rats, vectors, rodents, fleas. This thereby resulted in the outbreak of severe variables of pandemic and epidemic in different parts of the sub-continent of India.

Keywords: Assam, British, Colonial India, Diseases, Epidemic, Pandemic

India, being a third-world country, has encountered a variety of epidemics and pandemics through time. Several accounts of influenza, cholera, dengue, smallpox and other diseases have been recorded throughout history; while we have been able to eradicate some; many diseases still continue to pose a threat to the population. For the purposes of this paper, an epidemic is defined as "*the occurrence in a community or region of cases of an illness . . . clearly in excess of normal expectancy*" (Porta, 2014). The basic definition of an epidemic thus, it is a disease that affects a large number of people within a community, population or region. According to Park, epidemic is an unusual occurrence in a community or region of disease, specific health-related behavior or other health-related events clearly in excess of expected occurrence (Sweta, 2019, 793). It is a sudden, severe widespread outbreak of a disease pre-existing in the community. A pandemic is defined as "*an epidemic occurring over a very wide area, crossing international boundaries, and usually affecting a large number of people*" (Porta, 2014). Pandemics are, therefore, identified by their geographic scale rather than the severity of illness. For example, in contrast to annual seasonal influenza epidemics, pandemic influenza is defined as "*when a new influenza virus emerges and spreads around the world, and most people do not have immunity"* (WHO, 2010). Thus, a pandemic is an epidemic that spread over multiple countries or continents. The death toll is usually high in pandemics than epidemics as concluded by the study comparing the mortality rate of influenza pandemic and epidemic.

Pandemics are large scale outbreaks of infectious disease that can greatly increase the morbidity and mortality over a wide geographic area and cause significant economic, social, and political disruption. Evidence suggests that the likelihood of pandemics has increased over the past century because of increased global travel and integration, urbanization, changes in land use, and over exploitation of the natural environment. These trends likely will continue and will intensify. Significant policy attention has focused on the need to identify and limit emerging outbreaks that might lead to pandemics and to expand and sustain investment to build preparedness and health capacity (Smolinsky, *et.al.* 2003)

- Pandemics can cause significant, widespread increases in morbidity and mortality and have disproportionately higher mortality impacts on LMICs.
- Pandemics can cause economic damage through multiple channels, including short-term fiscal shocks and long-term negative shocks to economic growth.
- Individual behavioral changes, such as fear-induced aversion to workplaces and other public gathering place are a primary cause of negative shocks to economic growth during pandemics.
- Some pandemic mitigation measures can cause significant social and economic disruption.
- In countries with weak institutions and legacies of political instability, pandemics can increase political stresses and tensions. In these contexts, outbreak response measures such as quarantines have sparked violence and tension between states and citizens.

This paper proposes to explore the pandemics and epidemics that have taken their toll in colonial India with special reference to the state, Assam. To speak of the colonial period in the sub-continent, we basically speak of that particular period that is with the onset of British rule since the Battle of Plassey and thereafter till the independence of the sub-continent in 1947 from the scourge of British domination. The colonizing spirit of the English East India Company was in consonance to the ideas of Industrial Revolution that had taken place in England. The British colonisers reached the sub-continent and confronted a society which they perceived to be filthy, foul, dirty and contaminated with unhealthy practices and thus being infested with diseases that were a result of the presence of mosquitoes, rats, vectors, rodents, fleas. This thereby resulted in the outbreak of severe variables of pandemic and epidemic in different parts of the sub-continent of India.

In 1763-64 the colonial government that was established as a part of the new colonial administration formed Indian Medical Service (IMS) to regulate and remedy the health concerns that the country faced in the late eighteenth century. India's public health policy during this period was primarily concerned with protecting the British officials against diseases that they might contract during their stay in India. Michel Foucault, the French Social theorist propounded that, under colonial rule, medicine and health policies too had become a tool to colonize the society and land, and not just the body. Similarly, the British government had put in place medical authorities who also behaved like social authorities while taking decisions with regards to the functioning of towns, districts etc. Anirban Chanda and Sahil Bansal reported in the *Outlook* magazine that it was on 26th September 1896 that the *Bombay Gazette* signalled the presence of "genuine cases" of bubonic plague in Bombay. The Plague claiming lives of thousands of people in Bombay itself, made its way to United

Provinces and Punjab at the turn of twentieth century. There were 20,788 deaths due to plague reported in Bombay alone in 1903. The alarmingly unhealthy state of the city of Bombay, as recorded by the British historian, Sir Sidney James Mark Low, was one of the reasons why the British thought, plague would further spread like a wildfire

> The Island city...has its palaces fit for a prince and its human kennels unfit for a dog...It is the city of Parsi millionaire. It is the city of Plague.

Plague has been perceived as a 'disease of locality' and the consequent disturbances as a 'crisis of sanitary order'. The urban expansion in high density areas coupled with poor sanitary conditions and improper ventilation had the propensity to become principal cause of disease. There was also widespread belief in official medical circles that plague was an air-borne contagion. The rat-flea theory of plague was not found to be true for a long time and it was thought safer to regard plague as contagious disease. This entailed breaking the *chains of transmission and interrupting the circulation of carriers by means of cordons, quarantines and sequestration.* Plague ravaged India seriously for two decades and sporadically thereafter from its outbreak in Bombay city in 1896 with at least twelve million lives and probably many more succumbed. The plague epidemic led to massive fatalities, they greatly disrupted ordinary people who were compelled to evacuate their homes and camp in fields during conflagrations. Historians have tried to extract the potent factor behind the spread of the virus in India and its manifestation in severe forms in the region. Plague has manifested itself in humans in several forms—bubonic or glandular and pneumonic, the only form directly communicated from one human to another and septicemic, an explosive variation of bubonic plague. The term originates from Latin means *plaga* or blow. Historically, the black rat and its frequent flea the *Xenopysllacheopis* was the most important factor for the transmission of the pestilence to humanity (Klein, 1988, 783-85).

Plague was not new to India in the 1890's; it subsisted through century in several locales, periodically causing severe outbreaks and onslaughts. Plague attacked Gujarat and Sind and ravaged Ahmedabad and other towns and villages. In the 1830's plague embers smoldered in the Pali region of Rajputana. Of Pali's twenty thousand inhabitants, one-fifth is believed to have died of plague. Plague epidemic basically stimulated with population pressure, crowding, malnutrition and insanitation that increased the human vulnerability to infection. But it wasn't just the death toll that created a dramatic ruckus around plague. The steps taken by the colonial government in response to the spread of the epidemic were equally drastic. Natasha Sarkar, writing for the Proceedings of Indian History Congress (2001), records that the Health Committee invited severe criticism on its quarantine policy. For instance, the Committee did not issue notices of quarantined areas in advance. This caused great inconvenience to the ordinary people who regularly commuted to Bombay Presidency for work. Moreover, Europeans and first-class passengers were exempted from quarantine. Newspapers of the city heavily criticised such an exemption and questioned whether the Europeans were immune to plague!

This British centrist attitude, as reflected in the Indian public health policy, was persistent for the greater part of the early 20th century, at a time when the bubonic plague had already claimed thousands of lives. Amongst the class of special groups were the Indian elites, who were of key importance to the British for the maintenance of their colonial rule, and therefore, the colonial authorities never interfered with the free movement and freedom of trade of the Indian upper class. At the height of the plague, the wealthy business class was the first to leave Bombay for their native towns while government made several attempts to confine the working class to Bombay to ensure that the infection would not spread to rural areas. This stand of the government was highly discriminatory which sparked a lot of criticism amongst the natives and ultimately culminated to the anti-colonial struggle thereby fanning the ideas of nationalism.

It was only after the international actors started placing embargoes on trading with India because of the callous attitude of the British towards the spread of plague that the colonial government passed the Epidemic Diseases Act of 1897, in addition to adopting measures like quarantine. The excerpt below was published in the *British Medical Journal* on 20th February 1897. It lists out some of the measures imposed by the colonial government under the Act in Bombay:

> Under Epidemic Diseases Act Government have empowered Municipal Commissioner of his own authority and without reference to the magistrate, (1) to prohibit the use of dwellings unfit for habitation;... (2) to require vacation of buildings and premises for cleansing and disinfecting; (3) to cut off water connections...for strict medical inspection of all passengers.

The Epidemic Diseases Act passed in 1897 has however drawn criticism from all spectrum of the society. It was taken to be enacted in *hasty ignorance of the harsh effects that would befall the country's poor and downtrodden.* The measures adopted under this Act enforced regulations that were unbecoming in a native state for its native populace. However, it was not the plague only that came to be considered a pandemic. India came to be affected by the strains of other viruses like the Spanish flu in 1918 that entered India through the soldiers of the First World War. It was in the city of Bombay again that took a toll of the disease. It ended up killing lakhs of people that led to massive socio-economic disruption. But Colonial India with the previous experience of the Plague and the Epidemic Diseases Act that followed did not enforce land quarantines this time but schools and colleges were closed and social gatherings were restricted and people were advised not to travel. This led to a considerable breakdown of the economy.

Epidemics also seem to have intruded into state of Assam in the colonial period. The establishment of the British colonial rule from the first quarter of the 19th century was a momentous development in the history of Assam. Apart from the near total disjuncture with the pre-colonial root, the people of Assam had also experienced a new kind of socio-cultural domination by colonial rule. On the other hand, the colonial authorities had also found themselves in a totally different kind of environment. In this environment they had not only encountered a completely new socio-cultural setup but also a host of epidemic and endemic diseases which threatened the base of their rule. Assam's interaction with western medical science began with the doctors and surgeons who accompanied the military and visited the region since late 18th century. The Company began to administer the region since 1820s and soon the health of their employees as well as the natives became one of its primary concerns. They realized that they were now prone to some new diseases, which they did not suffer in their homeland owing to the climatic and sanitary condition of the region. On the eve of and beginning with British administration in Assam, Captain R.B. Pemberton, who was the Joint Commissioner of Manipur, had termed Assam as the third most unhealthy place after Araccan and Rangoon (Goswami, 2011, 978). References of unhealthy climate had been also found in the *Fatiyah-i-Ibriyah* by Shiabuddin Talish during his visit in the medieval period as a part of Mirjumla's invasion.

During the nineteenth century, smallpox was one of the chief epidemic diseases in Assam. Mortality rate with this disease was very high and it mainly affected the poorer section of the society. In 1832, smallpox occurred in the Nagaon district in an epidemic form. In the second half of the nineteenth century, the epidemic form of smallpox became more frequent in every district of Assam. In the traditional Assamese society, smallpox was widely identified with the Hindu Goddess *Sitala*, whose awesome presence conflagrated fever and eruption. A benign Goddess was sought through songs, prayers, cooling potions. Apart from it smallpox was sought to be cured through the process of variolation. This involved inoculation by the *Tikadars* with live smallpox matter. More concrete steps to curb the practice of variolation were taken in Vaccination Act of the 1870s and 1880s by making variolation illegal and vaccination compulsory. All these regulatory provisions had completely undermined the indigenous system of variolation, which set off controversies exploding old myths and often creating new ones. The local society was averse to the medical regulations that set in through the introduction of western medicine.

Another chief disease which needs special mention is malarial fevers. It was the most common disease among the ethnic communities with far-reaching consequences. As it was almost impossible in the nineteenth century to distinguish the characteristic of one fever from another, government records clubbed together different fevers including *Kala-azar* under same label. An investigation about *Kala-azar* was carried out by G.M. Giles, Surgeon, IMS, on special duty in Assam in 1898. He concluded that the disease was *anchylostomiasis* with slightly different symptoms. In 1899, Surgeon Major Ronald Ross investigated the disease and reported that Kala-azar was an epidemic and communicable disease with symptoms resembling those of malaria except *hepatomegaly* and *spleenomegaly*. Spleen and liver enlargement observed in these cases by Ross was not a character of malaria. *Anchylostomas* were found but these do not cause such symptoms. Ross concluded that it was not a malarial fever, but a disease microscopically and macroscopically similar, except for the absence of parasites and melanin; and the presence of visceral invasion especially that of spleen and liver (Giles, 1890). However, after 1898 the colonial government started to mention kala-azar as a separate category. Up to the nineteenth century the answer to malaria in western medical discourse was quinine.

Unlike smallpox, malarial fever, and to great extent cholera, as highly political disease, seemed to threaten the slender basis of British power in India, and stand at the critical point of interaction between the colonial state and indigenous society. In contrast to the cheap, simple, and to some extent successful smallpox vaccination, which became emblematic of the colonial state's self declared benevolence and humanity towards the people of India, cholera as well as malarial fevers was an unsettling and incomprehensible disease that mocked western medicine's effort to understand it. Throughout the nineteenth century, cholera leaped across all the preventive hurdles and caused epidemic havoc all over Assam. As colonial rule was unable to control the disease, they frequently blamed the natural obstacles and opium-eating habit of the 'native' population for the occurrence of the disease. This inability of the colonial authorities to control cholera had demonstrated the limitations of western medicine and the prevalence of indigenous way of health-care systems among the ethnic communities (Goswami, 2011, 979). During the cholera outbreak in the nineteenth century, the colonial government failed to depend on the western medicine and accused the opium eating habit of the native populace to be the main factor behind the disease. They seemed to have sought to establish a relation between the Hindu pilgrims and the disease because of the *prasad* that was being distributed among the devotees. This thereby led to the closure of Jagganath temple temporarily. The first case was reported on 23rd August 1817 by a civil surgeon of Jessore. The overall estimation of the mortality is not available as the data collection in India began much later, probably in the late 1860s.

As for the geography, it is important to note that the year 1817 had brought a very heavy rainfall leading to flooding which could have been the cause for such a rapid spread. While the Europeans living in India then and the elite were not seriously affected, the slum dwellers and rural poor people were the worst sufferers. This was probably due to the differences in living conditions, personal hygiene and practices. The second outbreak started around 1826 from Bengal and spread through the rivers to various parts of northern India. After affecting the United Provinces (UP), its impact was huge on areas around Punjab and Delhi, but most significant is its pandemic spread to countries like China. Cholera spread far and wide, all along the trade routes from China affecting several cities and villages alike. In each place, it lasted for a few weeks and killed hundreds of people every day. The *Kumbh Mela* at Hardwar in April 1867 has also been considered responsible for the epidemic spread of cholera in northern India. Madras Presidency in 1877 was the worst hit and the cholera epidemic was responsible for about 10% of the annual mortality then (Sweta, 2019, 976).

Colonial India was thus ravaged not only because of the epidemics and pandemics but also because of the consequences that followed thereafter. They set in a life of the 'new normal' with social distancing and quarantined life. It had its effect on the economy. We also cannot ignore the pattern of migration that followed with the pandemic. Of course, as citizens of independent India we have experienced our share of the pandemic through the Covid-19 and masked life that was enforced hereafter with regulations that were chalked with the pulling in of the 123 year old Epidemic Diseases Prevention Act.

REFERENCES

1. Giles, G.M.J.(1890). *A Report of an Investigation into the Causes of the Diseases known in Assam as Kala-Azar and Beriberi*. Shilong (India): Assam Secretariat

Press.

2. Goswami, Kishore. (2010). Disease and Medicine in Colonial Assam: British Health Policies, Objectives and Social Impact. *Indian History Congress Proceedings,* 2010.
3. Klein, Ira. (1988). Plague, Policy and Popular Unrest in British India. *Modern Asian Studies,* 22(4), 723-755.
4. Porta M., (Ed.) (2014). *A Dictionary of Epidemiology*. (6thedn.). Oxford: Oxford University Press.
5. Smolinsky, M S., Hamburg, M.A, Lederberg, J. (eds.) (2003). *Microbial Threats to Health: Emergence, Detection, and Response*. Washington DC: National Academies Press.
6. Sweta, G., Anantha, Eashwar V M, Gopalakrishnan. (2019). Epidemics and Pandemics in India throughout History: A Review Article. *Indian Journal of Public Health Research & Development,* 10(8).
7. World Health Organization.(2010). What Is a Pandemic? WHO, 24th February.

18
Epidemics and Pandemics: The Chronicle of Colonial India

Punita Pathak

ABSTRACT

During the colonial era, India was changing socially, economically and demographically as industrialization and commercialization was taking place. This gave impetus to migration towards urban areas leading to water scarcity, pollution and filth due to overcrowding. Rural areas suffered from unhealthy sanitary conditions due to lack of proper drainage, unhygienic environment, ventilation etc. The population in old India had all socio-economic factors favourable to rise of epidemic diseases such as extreme poverty, multiple famines, food shortage, undernourishment and malnutrition etc. The inhuman insensitivity of colonizers and the oppressive nature of British imperialism in India resulted in the miserable condition. Some social factors as illiteracy, ignorance and superstition also contributed to the prevalence of disease and illness among the people as the women and children are the most vulnerable section of the society. Several epidemics like cholera, malaria, smallpox and plague occurred in that period with high mortality.

To control and curb fatalities, the vaccination and

immunization policies were adopted to prevent epidemics, role of local self-government were improved to formulate new and effective health policies. Apart from these measures, the socio-religious reform movements, organizations, Indian press and political platforms also contributed their maximum for the improvement of health services. By the beginning of 20th century the medical science also improved. Gradually the emphasis was imposed onimprovement of rural health services, health education, organising health camps, awareness etc. On January 28, 1897, the Epidemic Diseases Bill was passed to ensure that some measures should be promptly taken to control the epidemic. The Bill also noted that several municipal bodies and other local governments had the power to deal with such situations. Some modifications were later done, that commission or abetment of acts of violence against healthcare service personnel shall be punished with imprisonment for a term of three months to five years with a fine of Rs. 50,000 to Rs. 2 lakh. The colonial India has witnessed an era in which several epidemics and pandemics took place causing a heavy toll to the people but have we evolved into enlightened beings and are we willing to learn from history? The history itself and the current crisis clearly indicates that not only do we need much better medical infrastructure and legal instruments but, more importantly, the development of a specialised educational programme that aims at preconditioning the people's responses and eliminating the cognitive bias during pandemics.

Keywords: Demographic, Eliminate, Endemic, Health education, Medical infrastructure, Pandemic.

An epidemic is defined as *an outbreak of a disease that occurs over a wide geographic area and affects an exceptionally high proportion of the population* (Clendening, 1960). It is an event in which a disease is actively spreading or an outbreak when there is a sudden increase in the number of cases of a specific disease such as the cholera in 1817–1821 (Martin and Martin,

2006).Whereas the term pandemic relates to wide geographic spread and is used to describe a disease that affects a whole country or the entire world. Hence, a pandemic is an epidemic on a national or global level. For example, the bubonic plague of 14th century or flu pandemic of 1968 (Saunders and Krewski, 2016). A pandemic affects a wider geographical area, often worldwide, infecting a larger number of people. It is often caused by a new virus or a new strain of virus that has not circulated among the people for a long time. It is observed that humans have little or no immunity against the virus and it spreads quickly. It also causes more deaths and often creates social disruption and economic loss (Hays, 2005).The terms pandemic and epidemic are never used to indicate the severity of the disease, but only the degree at which the disease is spreading.

The history of pandemics and epidemics is as old as the history of mankind. Surprisingly, initially our ancient ancestors were actually exposed to far fewer infections and diseases than us. But around 10,000 years ago, people started evolving culturally and establishing a society primarily based on agriculture. It was though very pivotal and revolutionary as these settlements were shaping the future of human civilization, but they also brought new diseases and epidemics with them. People were now living close together in unsanitary communities that were conducive to prevalent animal diseases to jump species and cause an outbreak (Cartwright, 2014). During the period of nineteenth century, India was also witnessing industrialization and commercialization as the rest of world. Due to urbanization and commercialization, huge migration started to the urban areas came into existence. Those areas started suffering from water scarcity, overcrowding and filth. On the contrary the rural areas suffered from unhealthy sanitary conditions due to lack of proper drainage, houses without proper ventilation or litter management facility. The population and environmental factors in India had all social and economic factors favourable for the rise of epidemic diseases. The Indian provinces were extremely poverty-stricken, sunken in debt and suffered from serious food shortage and malnutrition. The survey done by various researchers from Harvard, such as Francis Buchanan, Montgomery Martin, Major John Butler, and Donald Butler, suggested that chronic poverty among the people lead to very poor health conditions (Kawachi et al, 1997). It has been argued that the economic exploitation of the people and ruthless use of natural resources by the colonial rulers was responsible for growing poverty and environmental changes. People were forced to migrate from their native places in search of work, when their ancestral handloom, cottage industries, pottery works and animal husbandry were ruined. Their uneven settlements around port cities and industrial areas created unsanitary conditions that contributed to the spread of diseases. It was actually due to the inhuman insensitivity of colonizers and the oppressive nature of British imperialism in India that resulted in the miserable condition of the masses (Stanley, 2020). The general poverty, malnutrition and undernourishment in that era were the main reasons behind the epidemics. The people were not getting enough nourishment for maintaining average health. Consequently, their general health deteriorated gradually and became susceptible to diseases. Along with this, the export of food grains kept prices high and impacted on food availability. This in turn influenced mortality and just not the death rate, even birth rate was affected by scarcity. This was a chronic problem which existed not just in officially declared famine years but in general all the time (McAlpin and Michelle, 1983). Causes for mortality in either famine or non-famine years were always the same, i.e. high prices, scarcity of grains, contaminated water, filthy living condition, poverty and negligence towards hygiene and health. Some social factors such as illiteracy, ignorance, superstition also contributed in the prevalence of disease and illness among the people (Arnold, 1993).

The social development in the form of expansion of roads, railways and the construction of canals exploited the environment, which was exacerbated with the changing environmental and climatic factors responsible for the multiple diseases and ill health. The most vulnerable section of the society consists of the women and children and was mostly engulfed by under-nourishment and/or malnutrition. It was observed that more number of females were dying in colonial India than males and most of them were in the reproductive age group. The epidemics like cholera and malaria took heavy toll of lives and most of them were children and women especially pregnant women due to lack of resistance in body. The people due to ignorance, did not have any concern for their health, especially women during their pregnancy period were not cared properly and thus female mortality was higher than that of males. The children were often vulnerable to multiple ailments on account of absence of proper medical care. Death and desolation, want and suffering that had been ever present were also a characteristic feature of the epidemics. As the severity of the epidemics increased, the agricultural labourers and the landless were the next worst victims.

Every colonial epidemic report is consistent with one basic fact that high mortality was due to poverty and want in the general population. But, in fact, most of the epidemic and distress relief in the country was not provided by the colonial establishment but by the private charitable relief organizations and individuals. The colonial relief measures given by the British government was only a small fraction for the sufferers. The colonial government did not bother to employ properly conversant people of local areas to detect diseases and mortality. This was also one of the reasons for such high death rates from various diseases in all the provinces of India. The local authorities were asked to implement epidemic measures that were inadequate without any backup of the government officials. Smallpox vaccination was never popular in some regions of colonial India because of its association with the colonial state. Therefore colonial vaccination made very little impact in addressing the problem of disease. Colonial medicine remained unfamiliar to local culture and never acquired roots in the society of the colonized. It failed to win the trust of the local populace. It is important to understand here that charitable institutions and philanthropic individual's spent more money on public medicines than the colonial state. And the general mass used a wide variety of traditional medicines to counter colonial epidemics on the face of the failure of colonial medicine and the state in providing relief. And thus durimg 19th century, acute indifference of the common people towards colonial government and its health policies was seen. People did not show their enthusiasm to avail the medical facilities.

Though by the end of 19th century the number of people increased who availed medical facilities provided by colonial state. The social workers and the press played a vital role in making people aware towards health and medical measures. Various medical colleges, government and charitable hospitals were initiated for better healthcare. The vaccination and immunization policy were adopted to prevent smallpox, cholera, plague and other epidemics, role of local self government were improved to formulate health policies (Arnold, 1986 and General Department Bombay, Government Central Press, 1896). Apart from these the socio-religious reform movements, organizations, Indian press and political organisations also contributed their maximum for the welfare of Indian society. By the beginning of 20th century, after the end of First World War, the government realised that to maintain its colonialism, they have to give better healthcare (Mushtaq, 2009). Meanwhile, the medical science was also advancing leaps and bound by various researches, studies and guidelines, which realized that poverty and poor sanitation are closely linked to ill health and social factors (Armold, 2012). The starvation and malnutrition can weaken the human body that was widespread in 19th century colonial India due to unplanned and selfish economic policies. To strengthen the health status of Indian population, several health camps and rural health services were started for community welfare, particularly in rural sector (Harrison, 1994).There are few epidemics to be mentioned that were very deadly and so malignantly spreading that they remained imprinted in the chapters of history.

Bubonic Plague is a deadly infection caused by the bacteria *yersinia pestis*, also referred to as the Black Death. For centuries, plague has been synonymous of disaster for the people of Asia, Europe, and Africa, claiming a significant proportion of the population. As the situation worsened, things became so terrible that historians reported, on occasions there were not enough survivors to bury the dead. The spread of Plague in India has a long history. There are reports of various plague outbreaks in India, but trustworthy information is present about 1812 outbreak in Kutch that spread to Gujarat and Sind and lasted for approximately 10 years. Further, it was reported in the year 1828 and 1929 in Hansi in the Hissar district of Punjab. In 1836 and 1896, it was reported to be prevalent in the Marwar state of Rajputana and Bombay respectively. Initially, it was reported in the port cities of Bombay, Pune, Calcutta, and Karachi. In the first year, it was confined to Bombay except for minor occurrences in other parts of the country (Gatacre, 1898). In the second year, epidemics were reported in Bengal, Madras, United Provinces, Central Provinces, Punjab, Mysore, Hyderabad, and Kashmir. It devastated almost the whole of India until about 1899. By the end of 1903, deadly epidemic took lives of about 2 million people according to state records, but the actual figures might be much more. Being on the international trading route, there was immense pressure on the British imperial government of India to control this emergency. The Plague Commission was constituted in 1896 under the chairmanship of Prof. T.R. Frasor, Professor of Materia Medica at the University of Edinburgh that comprised of several members from various departments. The report of the Plague Commission in 1904 concluded that the disease was highly contagious and considered human transit as an important source of spreading the disease as they carried the germs with them (Lmb, 1908). The Commission recommended strongly that necessary preventive measures should be taken to disinfect and evacuate infected places, to put a control over mass transit, and to improve sanitary conditions. The Commission also suggested strengthening of public health services and development of laboratories.

Leprosy was also a big problem in British India and remained endemic in various zones. H.V. Carter of the Bengal Medical Department gained an authority over leprosy control in India. He earned great recognition in the Central Imperial government of India and suggested isolating lepers. He urged to establish Leper Asylums in India as these were formed in Norway in those days. After the 1889 Leprosy Bill, the National Leprosy Fund was constituted by the British Empire under chairmanship of the Prince of Wales (National Leprosy Fund, 1893). A Leprosy Commission was formed to investigate the etiology and epidemiology of leprosy. The Leprosy Commission concluded that leprosy is a disease *sui generis* caused by a bacillus having striking resemblance to tuberculosis. It is not a hereditary disease, there is spread by contagious means but the chances for that are very small. However, its spread is indirectly influenced by poor sanitation and malnutrition. The Commission suggested that segregation might not be fruitful in India. It suggested a prohibition on the sale of food articles, prostitution, and other occupations involving direct interference with people like barbers or watermen by the infected people. It insisted on the improvement of sanitary and living conditions (Carter, 1877-1887). However, the government of India passed the All-India Leprosy Act in 1898 and Leper Asylums were established in major parts of the country and forcible segregation of lepers was carried out. Different provinces furnished various surveys and reports. Excessive surveillance and research work was carried out on the distribution of lepers, hereditary transmission, and predisposition possibilities, contagiousness, and relation of disease with sanitation and diet.

Cholera was not known to the officers of the British East India Company. Before 1817, cholera was confined to Bengal but the 1817–1821 cholera epidemic in India shocked the company (Bellew, 1884). By the 1830s, cholera was known to be a life-threatening disease to the western world. In India, it gained the focus of medical services due to its serious impact on the troops and officers of the Company; otherwise, it was a disease of poor people. Due to the lack of effective treatment for cholera in that period, the main focus was set on its prevention. The British Indian government stuck to metrological theories about cholera after the Constantinople International Sanitary Conference of 1868, believing that atmospheric conditions are the basic cause of spreading the disease. After the 1868 cholera epidemic in India, the Cholera Committee was set up to investigate the causes of the disease. It comprised of the Principal Inspector General of the Indian Medical Department, Sanitary Commissioner for Madras, and Col. A.C. Silver. The origin and generation of cholera, the epidemicity and endemicity of the disease in India, transmissibility and propagation of cholera, and measures necessary for its prevention were studied (Cornish, 1871). The Committee concluded that cholera was frequent spreading especially at religious festivals and fairs. Epidemics were attributable to the importation of disease by pilgrims, travellers, and troops. The Committee suggested for improving sanitation, ensuring proper management of festivals, and developing hygienic conditions in institutions like hospitals, jails, and military cantonments. In the 1860s and 1870s, Dr. James L. Bryden, India's first epidemiologist and government's chief advisor on epidemic cholera, studied cholera extensively. John Murray, who served as Inspector General of Civil Hospitals in North Western Provinces and Bengal, conducted detailed studies on cholera and gave valuable treatment guidelines for cholera in that period (Murray, 1869). New treatment options evolved along with better prevention methods resulting in the marked decrease in cholera mortality.

Malaria fever was one of the leading causes of deaths in India. The situation worsened in early 19th century. One of the contributing factors was the establishment of the railways and irrigation network by the British government of India without keeping in view the efficient drainage systems for floods and rainwater collection. This created many fresh water reservoirs for the propagation of mosquitoes. Due to the heavy death numbers, economic losses and risk to the lives of British officers, serving in vulnerable areas, a lot of research was done for malaria control. In the 1840s, attention was paid to improve drainage system, prevent water logging and chemoprophylaxis with Quinine. Surgeon Major Sir Ronald Ross, a British national, joined the Indian Medical Services in 1881 and devoted to research for nearly two and half years. In August 1897, he demonstrated the lifecycle of the malaria parasite stating that female anopheles mosquitoes carried the protozoan parasites called "plasmodia" (Ross, 1898). He was later knighted and given a Nobel Prize in Medicine in 1902. This discovery opened new horizons in malaria research and shaped the malaria control programs toward a new direction mainly focusing on the eradication of mosquitoes. Capt. S.R. Christopher and Dr. C.A. Bentley further investigated the malaria and reported that the area of malaria hyper-endemicity consists of an endemic index of 50–100% in the district (Christophers and Bentley, 1911). Large-scale tropical aggregation of labor had an important role in the epidemiology of malaria in the tropics. They found that a lack of registration of vital occurrences; malnutrition, differential labour system, poor sanitation, and the formation of *foci* with infected immigrants were responsible for epidemicity in that region. The discovery of quinine changed the statistics of malaria related mortality and morbidity. In high-risk areas, the tropics and at special institutions like jails and post offices quinine was made available in small packs that contained 5–7 quinine granules with a price of only quarter-anna. However, it remained so until the introduction of chloroquine and WHO guidelines.

Kala-azar was first reported in the province of Assam where the Indian Officers faced a strange disease endemic called Kala-azar and Beriberi by the natives. G.M. Giles a Surgeon on special duty in Assam in 1898 and Surgeon Major Ronald Ross in 1899 investigated the disease and reported that *Kala-azar* was an epidemic and communicable disease with symptoms resembling those of malaria (Giles, 1890 Ross, 1899). This initial research provided a base for future researchers and the disease was later proved to be *visceral leishmaniasis* caused by a protozoan *Leishmania donovani*.

Tuberculosis had long been recognized as a lethal disease caused by the bacteria *Mycobacterium tuberculosis*, an organism whose existence predates even the first human settlements. One would think that modern-day sanitation and medical advances would be more than enough to curb diseases like tuberculosis, but even now, there are more than two million deaths every year from tuberculosis, mainly in developing countries such as India. It was present in India especially in lower socio-economic class long back. In 1939, the Tuberculosis Foundation of India was established to identify the sources, motivate for treatment and prevention and awareness. As there was no clinically effective treatment available for tuberculosis at that time, tuberculosis sanatoriums were formed in hilly areas to provide a healthy environment and segregation. With time, anti-tubercular drugs were discovered which were highly effective in treatment and various regimens were instituted at grass root levels (Mahadev and Kumar, 2003).

One of the commonest and earliest epidemics observed in early India was chickenpox. It was caused by the *varicella zoster virus*, which is usually seen in paediatric population whereas in some cases it is seen in adults too. The first case of chickenpox and its subsequent epidemic outbreaks date is as far back as one would think. Many people in the early 1500s actually thought chickenpox was a type of scarlet fever. Even though a vaccination is now available, only a natural recovery from chickenpox provides lifelong immunity.

Along with all these epidemics that occurred in India, there were several pandemics which engulfed whole world including India. In 1910-11,the sixth cholera outbreak began in India, subsequently spreading to the Middle East, North Africa, Eastern Europe and Russia which killed nearly 8,00,000 people. In 1918-20, Spanish flu was spread due to World War I in the whole world which was caused by the deadly strain of avian influenza. Influenza is a disease which is more than thousand years old and still infecting in the same virulence as previously. The Indian soldiers who were a part of World War I became the carriers of this disease and brought the disease into India. It killed between 17 and 18 million Indians which were more than all the casualties in World War I. The pandemic is believed to have infected a third of the world's population and claimed between 50 and 100 million lives (Taubenberger and Davis, 2006). In fact, the death toll caused by the epidemic was so high that significantly more lives were claimed by the epidemic than by World War I.

The management of epidemics in colonial India was not easy, as the participation of the British company was not adequate along with the large population with varied geographical area served as propagating factors for epidemics. One of the important social factors was concealment to evade intrusive state medical and sanitary measures. The people opposed the governmental interference during epidemics and led to an aggravation of the crisis. Interestingly, it was the fear of forced isolation and the stigma attached to being a carrier of the disease-induced people to smuggle out their symptomatic relatives to safer areas, hide them in attics, inside cupboards, under furniture, or in secret rooms whenever the search parties showed up. The response was also seen accordingly to the religious belief such as orthodox muslims feared that "surrendering" to anti-epidemic measures was against the principle of *taqdeer* (predestine); Brahmans feared for their caste; Rajputs and Muslims could not let their women be seen without *pardah*; Jains, with their utmost belief in *ahimsa*, loathed the idea of killing rats during Bubonic plagues. *The mishandling of the corpse by the colonial troops was also very much evident during those days.* As the inspection of corpses by health officials required their detention for a long time, so it was as condemned by religion too. Several rumours were spread such 'destruction of sexual powers' and the colonial state wanted to emasculate and enslave them and riots occurred in some plague-hit pockets to oppose compulsory hospitalisation and quarantine.

On 28th January, 1897, Council Member J, Woodburn tabled the Epidemic Diseases Bill during an outbreak of bubonic plague (Paul, 2020). The plague that rooted in Bombay gradually extended to other parts of the country and seemed to the government expedient that some measures should be promptly taken before the disease has attained large proportions elsewhere to hold it in check (Public Health Report, 1910) . The Bill also noted that several municipal bodies and other local governments had the power to deal with such situations but felt those were "inadequate". The then government was also concerned that several countries were alarmed by the situation in India, and Russia had speculated that the whole subcontinent might be infected. This Bill later called for special powers for governments of Indian provinces and local bodies, including checking of passengers of trains and sea routes. A Select Committee, headed by James Westland, submitted its report the very next week, on February 4, 1897, and the Bill was passed the same day, after a series of discussion. The lockdown challenge and the poor need to cope with education about the epidemic was the mainstay when the Epidemic Diseases Bill was passed amid concerns of spreading the diseases, with crowds from Bombay having reached places all over India. There were some modifications done on 22nd April, when an ordinance was called in where the Cabinet amended the Act to say that commission or abetment of acts of violence against healthcare service personnel shall be punished with imprisonment for a term of three months to five years. It also imposed fine of Rs 50,000 to Rs 2 lakh. In case of causing severe hurt, imprisonment shall be for a term of six months to seven years and with fine of Rs one lakh to Rs five lakh.

The colonial India had witnessed several epidemics and pandemics. The government at that time was not too enthusiastic regarding the Indian citizen's health and well being and it led to mass casualties, desolation of villages etc. If anything, the historical evidence and the current crisis has conveyed the message that not only do we needed much better medical infrastructure and legal instruments but, more importantly, the development of a specialised educational programme that aims at preconditioning the peoples' response and eliminating the cognitive bias during pandemics.

REFERENCES

1. Arnold, D. (1986). Cholera and Colonialism in British India. *JSTOR*. 113, 118–151.
2. ——(1993). Social Crisis and Epidemic Disease in the Famines of Nineteenth-century India, *Social History of Medicine*. 6(3), 385–404.
3. ——(2012). "The medicalization of poverty in colonial India." *Historical Research*. 85.
4. Bellew, H.W. (1884). Cholera in India, 1862 to 1881: Bengal Province, 1862 to 1881, and review. Calcutta (India), *Bengal Secretariat Press.*
5. Brief history of tuberculosis. (http://www.umdnj.edu/<"ntbcweb/history.htm, accessed on 1 March 2010). [Google Scholar]
6. Carter. HV. (1877). Observations on the prevention of leprosy by segregation. *Bombay General.*
7. ——(1887). "Memorandum on the prevention of leprosy by segregation of the affected." *Bombay General.*
8. Cartwright Frederick F. (2014). *Disease and History*. England, Sutton Publishing.
9. Christophers, S.R., Bentley C.A. (1911). Malaria in the Duars: Being the second report to the advisory committee appointed by the Government of India to conduct an enquiry regarding black water and other fevers prevalent in the Duars. *Simla: Government Monotype Press.*
10. Clendening, L. (1960).*Source Book of Medical History*. New York: Dover Publications.
11. Cornish, W.R. (1871). Cholera in southern India: A record of the progress of cholera in 1870, and resume of the records of former epidemic invasions of the Madras Presidency. Madras: Government Gazette Press.
12. Gatacre, W.F. (1898). Report on the bubonic plague in Bombay: 1896-97. Bombay: Times of India.
13. General Department Bombay, India: Presidency (1896, September). Supplement to the account of plague administration in the Bombay Presidency from till May 1897. *Mumbai:Government Central Press*
14. Giles, G.M.J. (1890). A report of an investigation into the causes of the diseases known in Assam as Kala-Azar and Beriberi. Shilong (India): Assam Secretariat Press.
15. Great Britain. National Leprosy Fund. Leprosy Commission in India. (1893). *Report of the Leprosy Commission in India,* 1890–91. Calcutta: Superintendent of Government Printing India.
16. Harrison, M. (1994). *Public Health in British India: Anglo-Indian Preventive Medicine 1859-1914.* Cambridge: Cambridge University Press.
17. Hays, J. N. (2005). *Epidemics and Pandemics: Their Impacts on Human History.* Santa Barbara, CA: ABC-CLIO.

18. India: Bombay. Plague, Cholera, and Smallpox in 1909. (1910). *Public Health Reports (1896-1970)*, 25(47), 1731-1733.
19. Kawachi, I., Kennedy, B. P., Lochner, K., Prothrow-Stith, D. (1997). Social capital, income inequality, and mortality. *American journal of public health*, 87(9), 1491–1498.
20. Lamb, G. (1908). *The etiology and epidemiology of plague: A summary of the work of the Plague Commission; issued under the authority of the Government of India by the Sanitary Commissioner with the Government of India*. Calcutta: Superintendent Government Printing India.
21. Mahadev, B. Kumar, P. (2003). History of tuberculosis control in India. *J Indian Med Assoc*, 101(3):142-3.
22. Martin, P.M., Martin, G. E. (2006). 2,500-year evolution of the term epidemic. *Emerg Infect Dis.*, 12(6), 976-980.
23. McAlpin, Michelle B. (1983). "Famines, Epidemics, and Population Growth: The Case of India." *JSTOR*. 14, (2), 351–366.
24. Murray, J. (1869). *Report on the treatment of epidemic cholera: From information collected by the governments of Bengal, Madras, Bombay, N.W. Provinces, Punjab, Oudh, and Central India, by order of the Government of India*. Calcutta: Superintendent of Government Printing.
25. Mushtaq, M.U. (2009). Public health in British India: A brief account of the history of medical services and disease prevention in colonial India. *Indian J Community Med*, 34:6-14.
26. Paul, Rudrajit. (2020). Epidemic Act of India. *Journal of the Indian Medical Association*, 118(07).
27. Ross, R. (1898). *Report on the cultivation of Protesoma, Labbe, in grey mosquitoes*. Calcutta: Office of Superintendent of Government Printing India.
28. ——(1899). *Report on the nature of Kala-Azar*. Calcutta: Office of Superintendent of Government Printing India.
29. Saunders-Hastings, P.R., Krewski, D. (2016). Reviewing the History of Pandemic Influenza: Understanding Patterns of Emergence and Transmission. *Pathogens*, 5(4):66.
30. Stanley, A. (2020). *British raj, Indian and Pakistani history*. Wolpert, Encyclopaedia Britannica.
31. Taubenberger, J.K. and David M.M. (2006). 1918 Influenza: The Mother of all Pandemics. *Emerging infectious diseases*, 12(1), 15-22.

19

Epidemics and Diseases: Community Perspectives and Government Interventions in Arunachal Pradesh Till 1950

Tajen Dabi

ABSTRACT

Before modern medicine and healthcare facilities were made available through government initiatives, epidemics used to be a dreaded phenomenon among cultures in Arunachal Pradesh. Within the context of a broad animistic-shamanistic worldview, subsistence economy and a fluid tribal polity epidemics created a wider set of actions and ramifications within and beyond an affected group. Even state approaches to reach out to the tribes of the state were marked by use of medicines and vaccines as part of diplomacy. This process started in the pre-independence and was incorporated in the post-independence period's NEFA policy. Contemporary ideas on disease and epidemics amongst the tribes have since changed a lot due to various factors. This paper provides a brief outline of the indigenous perceptions related to diseases and epidemics and the nature of state interventions in mitigating diseases and epidemics in Arunachal Pradesh.

Keywords: Arunachal Pradesh, Epidemics, Indigenous Perceptions on Epidemics and Diseases, Medical Sociology.

Across cultures, famines and scarcities were often reported which were accompanied by the outbreak of epidemics. Smallpox, that is considered a medieval disease in origin, was for the first time recognized in China before AD 500, is reported to have ravaged France in AD 580, and entered medical literature in Sanskrit in the seventh century. In India also epidemics have been reported. Ibn Batuta described a dreadful epidemic resembling plague or cholera that raged Madurai in c. 1345. Jahangir is reported to have given a careful description of the plague which spread from Punjab to Kashmir, Delhi and Agra from 1615 to 1619 (Habib 2011, 84-87). That the disease attracted the attention of the Emperor reflects the gravity of danger posed by epidemics to general public health and safety of the empire. During the colonial rule in India diseases like smallpox, cholera, plague, influenza, malaria and tuberculosis were commonly reported. The climatic conditions and diseases in India posed a challenge to the English conquest of India. During the eighteenth century, diseases were sought to be explained through 'miasmatic' theories which were replaced by tropical medicine in the late nineteenth century (Kumar, 1998, 11). With the advancement of science, the germ theory of disease finally got established in the twentieth century. Cultural perception as well as technological advancement influenced the disease etiology and the curative methods.

Chronologically, the Portuguese were the first to introduce Western medicine in India. In 1510, Albuquerque founded the Royal Hospital in Goa which after being handed over to the Jesuits, was converted into a medical school in 1842 (Kumar, 1998, 17). But the French and later the British established and consolidated it in India widely and firmly (Keshwani, 17). The motive behind these developments is explained by Anil Kumar in these lines:

Health concern has been an important feature of all

> historical processes, and more so in a process like colonization. Every naval dispatch from Europe had a surgeon on it, he not only looked after the sick on board and land, but was the first to report on the flora, fauna and resources of the new territory...Preservation of European health in new and 'hostile' lands was colonial medicine's first responsibility. Gradually the colonial doctors developed into a cultural force. Their work encompassed not only the understanding and possible conquest of new diseases but also the extension of Western cultural values to the non-Western world (Kumar, 1998, 11-12).

Thus, the composition of medical service also reflected the larger colonial policy. Doctors were strictly recruited and employed to serve imperial interests. A recent work has summarized the British medical policy in India and its nature thus:

> "The development of medical care in India...took a peculiar trajectory which was shaped by its colonial context. The hospitals and dispensaries that were part of this network were considered 'charitable' institutions, to be maintained primarily from voluntary subscriptions; for the benefit of those sections of the population unable to pay for medical care-other were to be provided medical care by private practitioners. The relationship between health and governance thus involved the larger politics of colonial domination. The nineteenth-century initiative to establish dispensaries in India was borne of the reconfiguration of the relationship between state and medicine in post-Enlightenment Europe (Sehrawat, 2013, xx).

These medical policies were extended in Assam also soon after the province was annexed in the first half of the nineteenth century. Thereafter, dispensaries were gradually opened in the hills, and in the case of Arunachal, in the foothill stations. The ethnographic diversity of Arunachal Pradesh is so vast that unless supported by insights from linguistics it will impossible to grasp even the representative vocabulary of all existing languages relating to epidemics and diseases and its social perception in a single essay. For example, in Galo language, epidemic, generically called *Chili-Rampen,* became *Nyi-Sili* (literally 'man mass-death') when casualties rose. Extant ethnological data show that amongst the shamanistic communities the worldview and approach to diseases and epidemics is similar. Among the mobile, migrating communities- which was the case with most of the animistic communities of the state until now-epidemics set in motion a further set of events. Epidemics, along with famine (*Dirii*), used to be a dreaded phenomenon. Aside from the loss of life and crops, it led to migration, inter-clan feud and murder. Epidemics were viewed to have been spread by a random visitor to the village. 'Sickness-carrying raids' were organised against the person believed to have spread the disease to avenge the loss of life when the negotiation for compensations failed. Some incidents of such nature were reported from the Kameng area by the local authorities as late as in the 1940s (letter from Lightfoot to Secretary to Governor of Assam, 1941). Within a particular speech group also, such practices led to social disharmony and inhibited the growth of a larger cohesive society. The more systemic and rational response to epidemics was to perform rituals, observe restrictions on food and movement of people, and to quarantine the affected. This approach was seen across the state in the recent COVID-19 pandemic also.

In the 1930s and 1940s, we have information about the response of the colonial authorities to epidemics. In March 1935, an outbreak of smallpox epidemic was reported from the hills beyond Denning in Lohit Valley; at Chowkham in

Khampti area in April; and at Mime-Sipo in Siang in May. About 100 deaths were reported from Chowkham, Munglang, Latao, Mumong in the Khampti areas in July the same year (Tour Diary, 1935). The epidemic spread to the un-administered Mishmi area. Sadiya, the most easterly colonial outpost in Assam, and an important trade outpost for the tribes became vulnerable. Accordingly, a vaccinator and a guard were placed at the Deopani crossing to ensure that people coming from the infected Mishmi area were vaccinated and no infected cases entered Sadiya. Orders were issued in this effect by the colonial authority by which the Adis and the Mishmis were prevented from entering Sadiya unless they were vaccinated priorly. In response to this order, a deputation of people from Dambuk and Bomjur Adi villages requested a vaccinator for their areas. The above petition was received by the Political Officer W.H. Calvert who then commented that the perception of the people was different a few years back when it was not uncommon for Government Vaccinators to be chased out of their village (Tour Diary, 1935). The above order, which required compulsory vaccination for entering the town of Sadiya during the period of the epidemic, is an example of the use of economic blockade to quarantine the infected populace during epidemic to secure the population of the administered areas. Thus, epidemics along with raids became a legitimate excuse for imposing an economic blockade on the tribes of the hills of Arunachal Pradesh by the colonial authorities of the plains.

Some relief aspects are also to be found. In July 1945 dysentery epidemic affected the villages of Koni-Yogeng, Simong, Riga, Pareng, Yeksing, Pangin and Rotung in the right bank of Siang River (Medical Department, Itanagar, 1945). Medical relief was immediately provided and as a result, no casualty was reported. In September 1946, Lohit Valley witnessed a dysentery outbreak; the tally was ninety-five cases, thirty-three deaths, and sixty-two cured (Medical

Department, Itanagar, 1946). It can be observed from the above information that medical relief was provided in a reasonably quick manner as a result of which about two-thirds of the patients' were saved. The urgency and dedication with which the relief measures were carried out bears testimony to the colonial authorities' object of winning the confidence of the people through medicine. We have a record of a more interesting cases related to an individual. The Tashigong Dzongpen of Bhutan, down with painful syphilis, sent a messenger to Lt. Thantluanga, Medical Officer of the Dirang Dzong Dispensary, requesting for treatment. The Political Officer promptly authorised the treatment citing the importance of the friendly Dzongpen to maintain the post at Dirang Dzong (Advisor to Governor of Assam to Niazi, 1945). Tashigong Dzongpen had priorly supplied the outpost at Dirang Dzong with 150 mounds of rice at a low price and the British administrators at Charduar considered that the Dzongpen's goodwill was crucial in the long term colonial strategic interest in the Mon area.

The foothill areas of Arunachal Pradesh were prone to malarial outbreaks. Anti-malarial measures were undertaken in Pasighat and Charduar again during the years 1945-47. To tackle the situation standard manuals on the control of malaria-like that of Brigadier G. Covell's *Anti-Mosquito Measures: with Special Reference to India* were consulted and all necessary steps were taken (APO Pasighat to APO Sadiya, 1945). In Charduar and Lokra an anti-malaria expert Major Kar, Assistant Director of Public Health (Malariology) in the Provincial Government of Assam, was entrusted to make an investigation and submit a comprehensive report on malaria cases on the matter. The report of Major Kar on malaria case in Charduar and Lokra is shown in the Table 19.1 (Office of the Advisor to the Governor of Assam, 1948):

Table 19.1: Total Malaria Case in Charduar Dispensary and the 5th AR Hospitals, Lokra

Year	Charduar Dispensay	AR Hospitals, Lokra
1944	160	NA
1945	245	277
1946	192	81
1947	166	236
1948	202	520

It is evident from the above report that the actual threat of malaria, and thus the heightened response to it, was on the military men who fell sick after coming back from tours in the hills. In the years 1945, 1947 and 1948 the number of Assam Rifles patients was more than that of Charduar Dispensary and this was the reason why a special malaria officer was engaged to make an investigation on the threat of malaria.

We can offer a brief conclusion that before modern medicine and healthcare facilities were made available through government initiatives, epidemics used to be a dreaded phenomenon among the communities of Arunachal Pradesh. Within the context of a broad animistic-shamanistic worldview, subsistence economy, and a fluid tribal polity epidemics created a wider set of actions and ramifications within and beyond an affected group. Even state approaches to reach out to the tribes of the state were marked by the use of medicines and vaccines as part of diplomacy. This process started in the pre-independence and was incorporated in the post-independence period's NEFA policy, an aspect outside the scope of this essay. Contemporary ideas on disease and epidemics amongst the tribes have since changed a lot due to various factors.

REFERENCES

1. Habib, Irfan. (2011). *Man and Environment: The Ecological History of India,* (2nd edn.). Aligarh Historians Society, New Delhi: Tulika Books
2. Kumar, Anil. (1998). *Medicine and the Raj.* (1951, Reprint). New Delhi : Sage Publication
3. N.H. Keshwani, "Medical Education in India Since Ancient Times" as cited in Anil Kumar, *Medicine and the Raj.* New Delhi: Sage Publication.
4. G.S. Lightfoot, P.O. Balipara FT, Charduar to the Secretary to the Governor of Assam, dated Charduar the 7th June 1941, *Governor's Secretariat,* Tribal Branch, NEFA, File No. TR/24/44-Ad.
5. Tour diary of the P.O. Sadiya for the year 1935, *Assam Secretariat, Excluded Area Records,* Pol-B, September 1936, Nos. 566 592, SAGAP, Itanagar.
6. *Medical Department,* NEFA Branch, File No. 13/29 of 1945, SAGAP, Itanagar.
7. Abridged from File No. 129/29 of 1946, *Medical Department,* NEFA Branch, SAGAP, Itanagar.
8. Adviser to the Governor of Assam to Niazi, *Medical Department,* NEFA Branch, File No. 15/29 of 1945, SAGAP, Itanagar.
9. APO, Pasighat to PO, Sadiya, Memo No. 201 SD, dated 22nd June/45, *Medical Department,* NEFA Branch, File No. 15/29 of 1945, SAGAP, Itanagar.
10. Abridged from Office of the Adviser to the Governor of Assam on Tribal Areas, File No. Med- 45/48 of 1948, SAGAP, Itanagar.

20

Environment and Pandemics

Historical Connection and Future Perspective

Squadron Leader Toolika Rani (Retd.)

ABSTRACT

From a mere unit of the universe to the most dominating species of earth, the entire saga of human evolution is a paradigm of resource utilization to resource exploitation to over-exploitation. The threshold breached and the equilibrium disturbed, it has been reflecting in the form of climate change and more frequent natural disasters. The latest pandemic has brought the focus on zoonotic diseases, which owe their origin and spread to a large extent to human activities such as landuse change, habitat fragmentation, reduced buffer between human and animals, illegal wildlife trade, pollution and unplanned urbanization etc. While the lockdown has given a glimpse of a better world sans anthropogenic disturbances in terms of improved environmental indicators, it is also an opportunity to revise the developmental strategies and make a transition for a more sustainable economic and social way of life. The chapter delves into the historical connection between environment and epidemics, climate change and diseases, the significance of environment protection, steps already taken in this direction, the policy shift required and the way forward to restore the ecological balance, highlighting the interdependence of various components of an ecosystem, including the human beings.

Keywords: Anthropogenic, Climate-Change, Ecosystem, Equilibrium, Interdependence, Pandemic, Resources, Urbanization.

Spurred by the wave of industrial revolution the world was fast on its way to mechanization. Inventions like artificial intelligence, big Data, internet of things, 3D manufacturing, virtual reality seemed to suggest that human race was launching into an altogether different trajectory; assuming the basics had long been mastered, and it was time to build colonies on other planets and extract resources from space. However, nature has its own way of reminding that humans are but a part of the universe which also encompasses other beings and that their existence is interdependent. Unsustainable extraction of natural resources by just one species. i.e. the homo sapiens has disturbed the fragile equilibrium on the only planet conducive for life. This was already being reflected in the form of climate change. The rising temperature, the frequency of floods and droughts and diseases was a warning the world had taken heed of. Thus emerged the Paris Climate Agreement in 2015 where the world had pledged to take steps to keep the average temperature rise in 21st century to below 2^0 Celsius of pre-industrial levels through comprehensive interventions. The Covid crisis has brought renewed focus on the significance of this pledge. As rivers became cleaner, the air felt purified and the birds and wildlife reclaimed their lost space during the world wide lockdown, the crisis has indirectly provided a glimpse of a better world that can be created and sustained with more consciousness towards our carbon imprint, and concerted efforts in the direction of reducing it. As countries strive to rebuild economies, the time is ripe to make a transition towards a more sustainable future and restoring the ecological balance.

Historical Linkage between Epidemics and Environment

Numerous examples from history reveal that environmental conditions played a vital role in origin and spread of various diseases. The way human beings treated their natural surroundings had an implication for their own health. Physicians had been stressing upon this linkage since long. In early modern England, fundamental to the understanding, treatment, and prevention of malaria was this crucial distinction between "good" and "bad" airs. Whether found on the shores of the *Ganges* or Thames Estuary, malaria has long been thought of as indivisible from the "hazardous" climatic conditions in which it prospers. The cause of *mal-aria* (literally: "bad air") was unquestionably attributed to noxious vapours deriving from unwholesome, stagnant climates. To dwell within a "bad air" was to embody a range of negative virtues: physically, mentally, and spiritually. Physician Tobias Venner (1577–1660) claimed, *all such are ingenious, generous, and desirous of perfection, both in mind and body endeavour to live in a pure and healthy Ayre* (Tayler, 2017).

Another example of it was Epidemic Fevers in late eighteenth century Barcelona, which affected one million people and caused 100,000 deaths. The development of intensively irrigated agriculture, the presence of textile cotton factories on Barcelona's periphery, and the existent hydro-geomorphological conditions strongly favored the proliferation of unhealthy areas. Malaria is sensitive to changes in temperature and precipitation, and these changes probably had a direct impact on the presence of epidemic malaria. A municipal proclamation (*bando*) issued by the governor of Barcelona, on 8th April, 1780 which contained new sanitation policies included systematic cleansing and drainage of fields, paths, ditches, riverbanks, and streams. Another proclamation on 31st March, 1787 proposed maintaining good water quality in local rivers and creeks and systematic planting of trees along the surrounding basins and the Llobregat rivers. In a medical report, the epidemic focus was clearly identified: *It is not difficult to find the origins of insalubrity because the marshlands are unclean.* (Kevin, 2017)

Climate Change and Disease

Human health is directly regulated by the environment around. Covid-19 shows that the health of people and the planet are one and the same. Human activity has altered virtually every corner of earth, bringing humans into contact with new vectors; seventy-five per cent of all emerging infectious diseases in humans come from animals. The long-term threats of climate change and ecosystem and biodiversity loss also spring from the destruction of nature (Anderson, 2020, 1). With increasing population, and lopsided development, landuse changes have given rise to unplanned urbanization, which in turn has reduced the buffer between the human and animals. The enhanced contact has increased the probability of zoonotic infections spread. The high density population clusters in peri-urban areas drastically increase the transmission rate; unhygienic conditions give rise to vectors that thrive in the high temperatures triggered by global warming. Thus, the chain reaction begins with destructive anthropogenic activities and ultimately comes back to haunt human beings in the form of pandemics. Realizing this, World Health Organization has propounded the 'One Health Approach'. It is a collaborative, multi-sectoral, and transdisciplinary approach—working at the local, regional, national, and global levels—with the goal of achieving optimal health outcomes recognizing the interconnection between people, animals, plants, and their shared environment (Centers for Disease Control and Prevention, 2018).

Covid-19 and Environment

The call for environment preservation isn't new. The alarm was raised as early as 1990s with the Earth Summit, 1992 when the term 'Sustainable Development' was first used in the Brundtland Commission report prior to the summit. Since then various global mechanisms have been established such as UNFCCC, Montreal Protocol, Kyoto Protocol, Paris Agreement, The 2030 Agenda and the UN Sustainable Development Goals (SDGs). However, the need to expedite climate action on a priority basis has been highlighted by Covid-19. Had we made faster progress on these processes, the world would have been better equipped to face it, with stronger health systems, fewer people living in poverty, less gender inequality, a healthier environment and more resilient societies. Covid-19 does not provide a 'silver lining' for the environment, but it provides the impetus to revisit our relationship with nature and build a better world. Governments should respond to the crisis by making policy and investment decisions that also address crises such as air pollution and the climate emergency (Anderson, 2020, 2).

Immediate Response and Long Term Policy Changes

Since Covid-19 has brought in a health emergency of extreme magnitude, the immediate challenge to environment is of medical waste disposal. The urgent need is to educate the frontline workers on the ways to dispose medical waste such as PPE, electronics, blood bags etc. Steps such as segregation, sorting, storage, stockpiling need to be strictly adhered to, in addition to not burning or dumping these wastes in open, otherwise it may lead to further environment and health damage. For long term goals, nations need to incorporate strategies to deal with pandemic medical waste into preparedness and response strategy, enact appropriate legislations, and create adequate infrastructure to implement the same. Research on better understanding of zoonotic diseases in order to be able to design a risk and response programme which takes into consideration its impact on nature is required. Evidence based policies, utilizing science tools to reveal the interconnection between unregulated wildlife trade and zoonotic diseases and impact of habitat fragmentation and biodiversity loss on human health will spur action in the direction of preserving the same.

Biodiversity: Our Shield

In the blind race of economic development, biodiversity has been the ultimate victim, as anthropogenic activities have led to the sixth mass extinction. As per Intergovernmental Science-Policy Platform on Biodiversity and Ecosystem Services (IPBES) Report, 2019, the average abundance of native species in most major land-based habitats has fallen by at least 20%, mostly since 1900. More than 40% of amphibian species, almost 33% of reef-forming corals and more than a third of all marine mammals are threatened. Tentatively 10% of insect species are threatened. At least 680 vertebrate species had been driven to extinction since the 16th century and more than 9% of all domesticated breeds of mammals used for food and agriculture had become extinct by 2016 (UN Report). Ironically, the perpetuator of this mass extinction is himself in danger now. Research has shown that in terms of diseases, biodiversity is key to maintaining the health of people, animals and the environment. Nature conservation and existence of multiple host species reduces the risk of transmission of a pathogen through what scientists call "dilution effect". This is because in a mixed population of hosts, some would be "dead end" hosts, which don't allow an infection to occur; hence conserving nature is a way to mitigate disease transmission (Bett, 2020).

Green New Deals: Ecology in Economic Development

Generally, economic development is considered to be an antithesis to environment conservation. However, for this to change, there is a need to adopt a policy shift. Utilization of natural resources does not necessarily have to lead to ecological disasters. Mindful planning, incorporation of indigenous traditional wisdom, involvement of local communities and region-specific policy-making can bring in the element of sustainability, and ensure more equitable development. Technology can be used to minimize the impact of developmental projects on nature and to device newer ways to harness the renewable.

What is required is fundamental restructuring of our economies, which is needed to stay in line with planetary boundaries. To initiate this, various world regions have been discussing different versions of "Green New Deals". The European Union, for example, aims to reduce net greenhouse gas emissions to zero by 2050 and decouple economic growth from resource use, while leaving no person and place behind. South Korea has used part of its recovery funds to restructure the economy towards green growth, and has recently renewed its ambition by pledging to reduce greenhouse gas emissions to net zero by 2050. The disruption that is part and parcel of a deep crisis may also open windows of opportunity to radically restructure our economies. Some parts of a Green New Deal may even be easier to implement now than before the crisis. Green public works programmes, for example, can go a long way to ensuring basic levels of income while benefitting the environment. Energy and resource efficiency, in particular in buildings, remain worthwhile investment opportunities in most country contexts, and less car traffic and an increase in bicycle use during lockdowns may have given us a glimpse into a more sustainable mobility in future.

As travel restrictions abound, local tourism holds the potential to create economic benefits at home and can help avoid emissions at the same time (Pegels, Brandi and Altenburg, 2020).

India's March on the Path to Sustainability

Indian way of life by default embraces and incorporates nature conservation in the day to day life. The worship of certain trees, such as *peepal*, basil, mango leaves, concept of sacred grooves, feeding the crows and pigeons, local community's affinity with certain flora and fauna such as *Bishnoi* community's belief about the *Chinkara* (Indian gazelle) are a few examples of indigenous ways of harmonious co-existence with nature. However, as a developing country India's energy and food needs are rapidly increasing, population explosion has put an unprecedented pressure on land, and water bodies. Despite these obligations, and financial and technological constraints India is at the forefront of climate action. In 2009 it adopted the National Action Plan on Climate Change (NAPCC) which includes eight missions, i.e., sustainable agriculture, solar mission, sustainable habitat, energy efficiency mission etc. Under the Paris Climate Agreement India has set following three NDCs (Nationally Determined Contributions):

- To improve the emissions intensity of its GDP by 33 to 35 per cent by 2030 below 2005 levels.
- To increase the share of non-fossil fuel-based electricity to 40 per cent by 2030.
- To enhance its forest cover that will absorb 2.5 to 3 billion tonnes of carbon dioxide by 2030.

It has also established International Solar Alliance with France to promote solar energy production and has recently enhanced its renewable energy target to 275 GW by 2027. In order to secure its energy future as well as fulfill its environmental promises, India is looking forward to diversify its energy basket by promoting biogas and second generation biofuels. For faster adoption and manufacturing of electric vehicles, FAME scheme is being run. India's UJALA scheme to install LED bulbs is world's largest domestic lighting scheme. India has accepted challenge to restore degraded land. A Mangrove restoration program is being run in Gujarat. However, 15 out of the world's 20 most polluted cities are in India and improving air quality is of utmost importance. In Covid-induced economic restructuring India is showing focus on agriculture, supporting micro-food enterprises, cluster based approach, organic farming and programs for water efficiency are already being run. Agro-forestry needs to be supported further.

An Illusionary Respite

In a curious mixture of misery and miracle, the lockdown brought an unexpected delight. The temperatures remained moderate, the breeze blew in the erstwhile sultry plains, the wildlife gave regular appearance in the neighbourhood and the serene quietness of absence of vehicular noise, the pleasant trill of birds created a world many had only imagined. Rescued from human assault for a while, the environmental indicators showed positive signs. However, this dream world can be short-lived as its foundation is not based on restraint but restriction.

Though it was expected that during lockdown green-house emission would decrease, as per data from United States National Oceanic and Atmospheric Association (NOAA) in April 2020, average concentration of CO_2 in the atmosphere was 416 ppm, the highest in 8 lakh years. While it is true that vehicular and air traffic, as well as industrial activity, has reduced sharply in most parts of the world since January 2020, this is not the case with electricity supply: 64 per cent of the global electricity energy mix comes from fossil fuels (coal: 38

per cent, gas: 23 per cent, oil: 3 per cent), according to the World Energy Outlook, 2019. Heating systems have been functioning as before COVID-19. None of the fundamentals have changed (such as the shift to renewable energy, public transport, deforestation). Forest fires and wildfires which raged recently have increased the CO_2 concentration. "Without fundamental shifts in global energy production, we should have no reason to expect a lasting reduction in emissions," says UNEP climate change expert Niklas Hagelberg (UN Environment).

Way Forward

Covid-19 has forced the humans to pause and rethink their development strategies. The recurrence of pandemics like Covid-19 reveals that keeping environmental concerns in centre is not an option but a necessity to ensure human survival. Though at a high cost, the pandemic is a trigger to restructure our way of life and a reminder to respect the basics. United Nations Environment Program (UNEP) has issued the following guidelines:

- **Investment in nature for improved human health, sustainable socio-economic recovery, poverty reduction and livelihood recovery** – Promoting expanded opportunities for valuing and investing in nature as part of the response to the COVID-19 crisis.
- **Science, technical support and advocacy to ensure progress on environmental issues through global processes** – Supporting nations to deliver stronger commitments under the Paris Agreement, agree on the post-2020 Global Biodiversity Framework, and adopt the Post-2020 Chemicals and Waste Management Framework. Supporting them to deliver on commitments made to these and other processes.
- **Raising awareness of the links between nature, health and sustainable living** – Raising public awareness of

environment and human health links, creating public support for green growth opportunities within economic recovery, and advocating sustainable living and smart choices through communication campaigns and educational platforms.

- **Continued learning** – With over 1 billion students no longer able to attend school, UNEP has been working with leaders in environmental education to create "Earth School," an innovative set of lessons hosted on TED-Ed. UNEP will also collaborate with other UN agencies, educators and governments to integrate environmental themes across curricula to help the world "learn back better" (Anderson, 2020).

The learning from pandemic shall also include instilling the value of nature conservation in the youth in order to prevent pandemics and to inculcate a more sustainable and harmonious way of life. In this context, "Earth School" is a good initiative which provides free, high-quality educational content to students through a 30-day "Adventure" into the natural world.

Role of Religious Institutions

In every part of the world behavioral patterns and daily habits are deeply connected with religious beliefs. Therefore, tapping into the potential of this mass influencer can be helpful to preserve nature. Environment conservation demands a coordinated response from policy-makers, scientists, experts, society and religious leaders. In this direction, UNEP's Faith for Earth initiative, in association with Yale Forum is a right step to inspire people and communities to preserve, protect, and restore ecosystems and biodiversity. Healthy, functioning ecosystems, and environmental law, are central to a post-COVID world, and religious institutions can help push for progress on strengthening policy frameworks to bring about necessary change (UNEP, 2020).

Conclusion

Earth- the most beautiful planet due to its capacity to sustain life needs to be handled carefully. Like every setback, Covid-19 shall also trigger a soul-searching process which results in a deeper understanding of life, the universe and the place of human species in the universe. As a unit of the earth ecosystem, the human health is intricately dependent on the health of the planet and all its inhabitants. Therefore, the erstwhile practice of overexploitation of natural resources, domination of human beings at the cost of other natural components, and the sense of supremacy over nature requires a serious pondering over the issue and revision. As a revered leader His Holiness the Dalai Lama puts it on Earth Day, 22nd April 2020:

> This blue planet is a delightful habitat. Its life is our life; its future, our future. Indeed, the earth acts like a mother to us all; as her children, we are dependent on her. We Buddhists believe that the entire world is interdependent. Our mother earth is teaching us a lesson in universal responsibility.

In Covid-19, the planet has delivered its strongest warning to date that humanity must change. Shutting down economies is a short term response to this warning. It cannot endure. Only by building functioning economies that work with nature, not against it, the world can thrive (Anderson, 2020, 1). Addressing the current pandemic and protecting ourselves against future global threats requires sound management of hazardous medical and chemical waste; strong and global stewardship of nature and biodiversity; and a clear commitment to "building back better", creating green jobs and facilitating the transition to carbon neutral economies. Humanity depends on action now for a resilient and sustainable future (UNEP, 2020). United Nations has declared the decade 2021-30 as the UN Decade of Ecosystem Restoration. Let this be an opportunity to restore the balance between excess and abstention, restraint and restriction, individualism and communism, greed and need. Let this be an opportunity to adopt Aristotle's 'Golden Mean' and Buddha's 'Middle Path' for an existence of involvement but not indulgence.

REFERENCES

1. Anderson, Inger. Working with the Environment to Protect People: UNEP's Covid-19 Response. *UNEP*, United Nations Environment Programme, Retrieved on 15th May, 2020 from https://wedocs.unep.org/bitstream/handle/20.500.11822/32218 UNEP_COVID.pdf? sequence= 1& isAllowed=y.
2. Bett, Bernard. (2020, 23 April) For Better or for Worse: The Delicate Relationship between People and the Wildlife around Them. *UN Environment*. Retrieved on 15th May, 2020 from
3. Centers for Disease Control and Prevention. (2018, 5 November). One Health Basics. *Centers for Disease Control and Prevention*, 5 Nov. 2018. Retrieved on 18th May, 2020 from www.cdc.gov/onehealth/basics/index.html.
4. His Holiness the Dalai Lama's Message for Earth Day, Wednesday, 22 April 2020. Retrieved from https://www.dalailama.com/news/2020/his-holiness-the-dalai-lamas-message-for-earth-day
5. Meredith, Tayler. (2017). The Good, the Bad, and the Ague: Defining Healthful Airs in Early Modern England. Environment & Society Portal, *Arcadia*, no. 12. Rachel Carson Center for Environment and Society. Retrieved from https://doi.org/10.5282/rcc/7895.
6. Pegels, A., Brandi, C. and Altenburg, T. (2020, 30 April). Can the Global Green New Deal Movement Survive the Pandemic? *Green Growth Knowledge Platform*. Retrieved on 15th May, 2020 https://www.greengrowthknowledge.org/blog/can-global-green-new-deal-movement-survive-pandemic
7. Pometti, Kevin. (2017) Marshlands, Sanitation Policies, and Epidemic Fevers in Late-Eighteenth-Century Barcelona (1783–1786), Environment & Society Portal, *Arcadia*, no. 28. Rachel Carson Center for Environment and Society. Retrieved from (link is external).
8. UN Environment. Record Global Carbon Dioxide Concentrations despite COVID-19 Crisis. *UN Environment*. Retrieved on 15th May, 2020 from

www.unenvironment.org/news-and-stories/story/record-global-carbon-dioxide-concentrations-despite-covid-19-crisis.

9. UNEP. (2020). "Faith-based organizations can help the transition to a more sustainable post Covid-19 World, Ecosystems and Biodiversity. *UNEP*. Retrieved on 15th May 2020 https://www.unenvironment.org/news-and-stories/story/faith-based-organizations-can-help-transition-more-sustainable-post-covid-19
10. United Nations. UN Report: Nature's Dangerous Decline 'Unprecedented'; Species Extinction Rates 'Accelerating' – United Nations Sustainable Development. *United Nations*. Retrieved on 18th May, 2020 from www.un.org/sustainabledevelopment/blog/2019/05/nature-decline-unprecedented-report/.

21

Sustainability of Museums

Accommodating and Convertible Phase During Pandemic Times

Jawa Madhur

ABSTRACT

With the occurrence of Covid-19 pandemic, the world is facing one of the major challenges. Not only communities, but institutions are also not left untouched. During this pandemic, museums around the world have come up with new ideas of serving visitors. Some are distributing information and ideas to deal with this pandemic, while others are opening their collections virtually and hosting webinars. A new concept of virtual exhibition and tour has developed. Museums in India are also playing a major role by connecting with their audiences through social media. Recently, National Museum of India hosted a talk show "#Meet our Curators". ICOM-India has also hosted a webinar on topic "Museum Inclusion in times of Social Isolation". These activities give us a glimpse about how museum professionals are still working in lockdown. Digitization has created immense opportunities for museums to connect with their audience not only at local level but globally and get direct feedback from them. Social media has helped museums to connect with younger generations who are least aware of museum activities and making them 'museum- minded'. History is full of examples on how museums have come up to fight various epidemics like Tuberculosis in the early 1900s, Spanish Flu in 1918, and AIDs in 1990, where health workers reached out museums for help. Museums like The Smithsonian's have also held an exhibition on "Outbreak: Epidemic in a Connected World" to combat misinformation about Covid-19. Museums are responsible, creative and empathic in a time when everyone could use a good old-fashioned dose of perspective.

Keyword: Digitization, e-Museums, Museum inclusion, pandemic, virtual exhibition

International Council of Museum (1959) says, "Museum is a non-profit, permanent institution in the service of society and its development, open to the public, which acquires, conserves, researches, communicates and exhibits the tangible and intangible heritage of humanity and its environment for the purpose of education, study and enjoyment". With this definition we can say that Museums convey colossal jobs and the most critical is to enable us to comprehend the crossroads of history as they are overseers of the history of humankind. Pandemic is one such occasion that has changed history and its repercussions has given a new direction and perspective to our lives. W.H.O. through its article *What is a Pandemic?* defines pandemic as "the worldwide spread of a new disease". It is contagious from human to human interaction and communicable mainly to persons with weak immunity. These typical viruses are generally originated from animals (Doshi, 2011). Corona virus first originated from Wuhan province of China in December 2019 from where it progressively spread far and wide. The first case in India was accounted on 30th January, 2020, and today we have approx. 5,562,663 affirmed instances of Covid-19 and 88,935 deaths as reported to W.H.O till 22nd September, 2020,12:10 pm CEST. Globally, as of 12:10 pm CEST, 22 September 2020, there have been 31,132,906 confirmed cases of COVID-19, including 962,008 deaths, reported to WHO and numbers are still increasing (WHO, n.d.).

Considering the past, it isn't the first occasion when we have experienced any pandemic which has affected our social, political and monetary life. The worst setbacks are faced by the cultural and public institutions like Museums. However, models can be sited from past epidemic where museums have played a significant role in countering the pandemic situation. In 1900s when tuberculosis was at its stature and ending the lives one out of seven people, museums in the USA were called for assistance to spread awareness and make people comprehend the situation. In 1905 and 1909, the American Museum of Natural History and the Smithsonian Museum facilitated two exhibitions on tuberculosis, which came up as the first blockbuster in the history of US museums. In 1918, when Spanish flu spread, the role of Oakland museum, California is worth noting, where its auditorium was converted into an emergency hospital. Museum staff offered emergency instructional activities for children in the emergency ward. In 1991, when AIDs occurred in U.S.A., the centre of disease control partnered with eight science museums and the American Medical Association to form the National AIDS Exhibition Consortium. The underlying thought was to develop an exhibition which provides safe preventive practices that would connect countless individuals (Schwarzer, 2020).

Today, the world is confronting a grave challenge in the form of Covid-19 pandemic which has disturbed the activities in every facet of life. Cultural and tourism sectors are suffering threat to the livelihood and economy of thousands of professionals are jeopardized. Numerous museum organisations around the globe started taking several measures to address the global issue by conducting webinars, virtual debates and surveys to help museums cope up with this challenging time. International Council of Museums (ICOM) responded rapidly to this emergency and provided eight steps recommendations for best ways to manage the emergency. It urged policy and decision-makers to rapidly release funds to ensure the sustainability of museums (ICOM, n.d.). ICOM also launched a global survey to analyse the impact of lockdown. The survey secured five themes: 'the current situation for museums and staff', 'expected economic impact', 'digital resources and communication', 'museum security and conservation of collection', 'freelance museum professionals'. The conclusion was drawn on the basis of responses of 1600 museums from 107 countries across five continents. This survey was conducted between 7th April to 7th May 2020. (ICOM, 2020). Correspondingly, a study was additionally conducted by UNESCO to access the impact of Covid-19 on museums. On the occasion of Museum Day, on 18th May 2020, these two studies revealed a staggering fact that nearly 13% of the museums around the world may never re-open and 90% of them globally have to close their doors due to lockdown (UNESCO, 2020).

On 15th April 2020, World Art Day, UNESCO launched a global movement named ResiliArt, which aimed to conduct virtual high-level exchange between international professions and draw support for the cultural world during the crisis (Azoulay, 2020). On 23rd July 2020, UNESCO and International Centre for the Study of the Preservation and Restoration of Cultural Property organized a webinar on Museums after the pandemic and invited experts from different regions of the world. The findings of the report were divided into three sections. The first survey was conducted on 'Museum around the world in the face of Covid-19'. The second survey was conducted on 'How much Heritage Collections matters to people and why?' The third session focussed on 'The future of the museum and the post-COVID period'. The expert stressed that museums should focus on digitization, mobile application and exhibition involving communities (UNESCO, 2020).

Considering these reports and surveys, museums and museum professionals around the world have blended supposition with these circumstances. Some accepted this pandemic as an opportunity to document a period that would be reviewed in history and looked upon to take lessons in future. They started collecting everyday experience of the people, while some attempted to discover creative ways to approach wider audience. Museums as knowledge repository have a binding responsibility to convey the correct information. So, some museums started a campaign to spread awareness about Covid-19 and help people counter their fear.

Models of Victoria and Albert Museum, London, can be referred that opened a Rapid Response Gallery in 2014 for making the museum more outward and engaging with the current topic. Covid-19 is one such event. They started documenting the everyday experience of the people. This sort of collection consisted of a wide range of materials like personal stories, crafts and artwork made during the lockdown, face masks and PPE kits and even screenshots of zoom home meetings (Victoria and Albert Museum, n.d.).

Museums like the National Museum of American History, The National Museum of African American History and Culture and the Anacostia Community Museum are aiming to document the pandemic. The Smithsonian Museum is also developing an exhibition on the theme of pandemic, "Outbreak: Epidemic in a Connected World"[see figure 21.1]

This exhibition was first proposed by Daniel Lucey, who asserted that the public needs a better comprehension of the infectious disease. The exhibition is currently joining efforts to combat misinformation about Covid-19 on multiple fronts like through volunteers, public programmes and content updates on their websites. They are also providing a platform to directly interact with scientists from CDC, NIH, USAID, Eco health and numerous other supporting organizations to provide

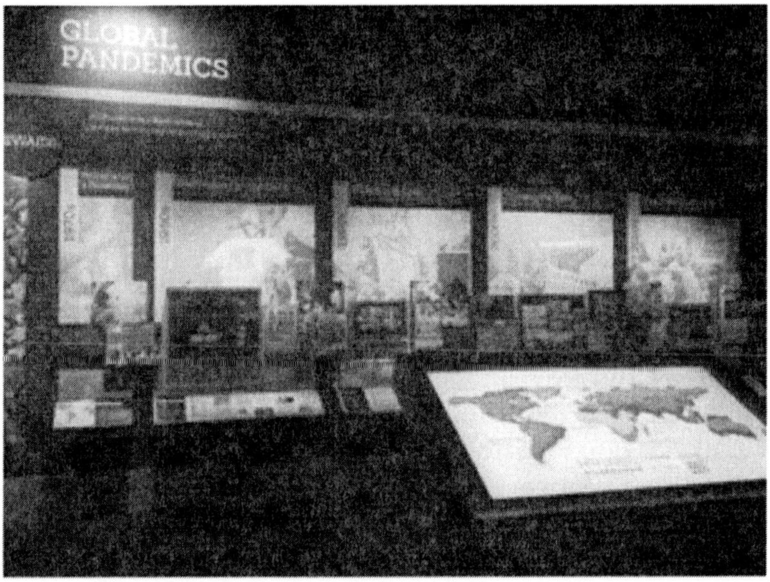

Fig. 21.1.: Outbreak: Epidemic in the Connected World
Source: https://www.smithsonianmag.com/smithsonian-institution/how-museums-can-help-public-make-sense-pandemics-180974281/

information about Covid-19 which would be otherwise difficult. They mooted an idea of 'Do-it-Yourself' version using science to guide people about their actions against pandemic and threats in present and future. This awareness programme has been embraced and customised by various countries and institutions worldwide. "Outbreak: Epidemic in a Connected World" will be on view at the Smithsonian's National Museum of Natural History from 2021 (Sholts, 2020). Similarly, museums in Canada, Germany and Europe are gathering testimonials, objects and photographs to document various aspects of life during the pandemic. Museums and heritage institutions in Normandy, France are donating mask to health professionals. Some are offering open- source templates for making face masks from promptly accessible materials and some museums like Museum of Homelessness in the U.K. are activating volunteers through its websites to provide food and care packages to the destitute (Atkinson, 2020).

Regarding documentation of Covid-19, the Museum Association issued guidelines that recommended that museums should be empathic, transparent and respectful towards interpretation and care of the collection as it presents the emotions of the people facing the pandemic. Staff and volunteers should also be respected (ICOM, n.d.). While some museums are enthusiastic about documenting this crisis, another section of museum are focussed on discovering better approaches to reach their audience with the purpose to mitigate the crisis and fear among people. On this part, our Indian museums have adopted new strategies on social media trend # or Facebook, YouTube or Twitter. Our curators availed every viable option to meet and actively engage their audience. Social media has become a medium for Indian museums to have one to one interaction with their audience and create awareness about the pandemic.

On 18th May, on the event of International Museum Day, ICOM-India organised a webinar on the topic 'Museum Inclusion in times of Social Isolation' under the International theme of the Day 'Museums for Equality: Diversity and

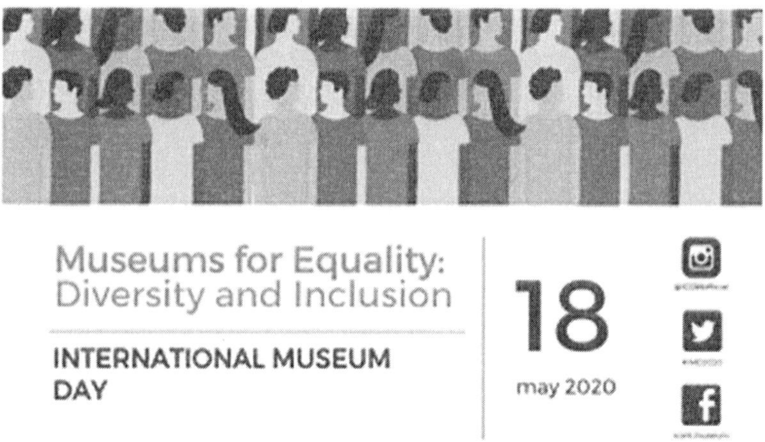

Fig.-21.2: ICOM logo, 2020

Note. ICOM logo, 2020[http://imd.icom.museum/]

Inclusion' [see Figure 2.] *(Delhi & Management, 2020).*

An online panel discussion was organized by Museum of Art and Photography (MAP), an Institutional Member of ICOM India, on the topic 'Taking the Museum to the People' held on 27th May 2020 (Museum of Art & Photography, n.d.). A two days International Web-Conference on 'Museum as Profession: Challenges and Issues' was jointly organised by Department of Museology, Aligarh Muslim University, Uttar Pradesh and Ishan Promote Art, Culture and Improve Society (IPACAIS), Pratapgarh, Uttar Pradesh on 24th-25th August 2020 (Pradesh, *et al.*, 2020). Numerous Museums are now hosting online exhibition and virtual tours. Digitization has given an all-encompassing space where people can connect and access the information. The museums that addressed the situation by switching over to online mode are:

Chhatrapati Shivaji Maharaj Vastu Sangralaya

On their site, they have uploaded selected images of the objects from various galleries in the museum, like sculpture gallery, pre-and protohistory, print and various other sections. They have a theme called 'Object of the Month' in which they take one object and give insights about its history. The object of the current month is 'Chandrashekhar', a sculpture of Shiva.

Further, the museum has exhibited an online collection of *Mewar Ramayan*. They collaborated with Google Art and Culture projects and exhibit the exhibition named Humsafar-The Companion, 15 variations on the Sari: India's Iconic Drape, Animal in Indian Art and Fauna of the Indian subcontinent. We can always have a see to it while visiting their official site i.e. www.csmvs.in.(see Figure 3).

National Museum, New Delhi

They have started a show on Instagram '#Meetourcurators', where curators come up with detail description of a particular object. People can have a peep into the working nature of

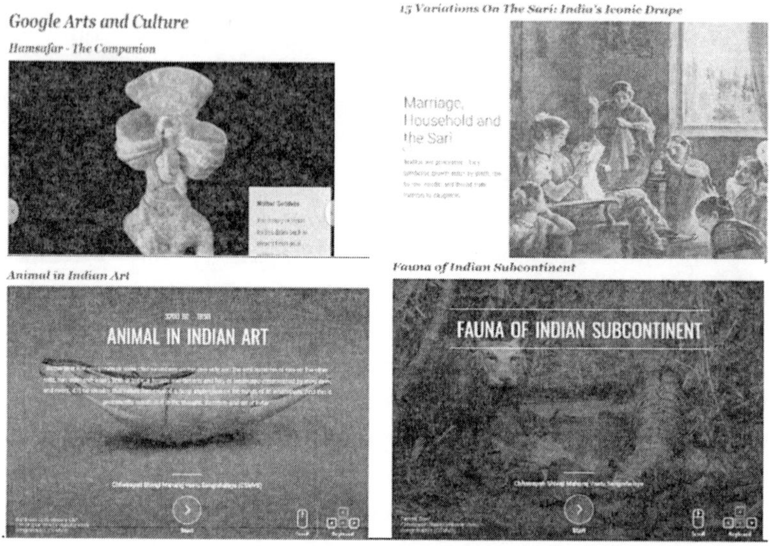

Figure 21.3: Online Exhibition

Source: [https://www.csmvs.in/collection/digital-collections/google-arts-and-culture]

curators. In this stream, they have likewise opened a section on their website named 'museum at home' in which videos related to various objects, and galleries are uploaded namely, North-East traditions, Visual representation of *Ramayana* through Indian miniature paintings and details about the sculptures like *Nataraj*, *Kuber*, *Vishnu*, and many more. They have provided a virtual tour of 360 paranomic views of the sculptures, online exhibition of arms and armour, tribal lifestyle, bronze gallery and many noteworthy exhibitions. They have created accounts on a various social media platform like Facebook, Twitter, Instagram, and YouTube. All the exhibition can be viewed on their official website www.nationalmuseumindia.gov.in. (National Museum, New Delhi, n.d.)

Indian Museum, Kolkata

The Indian Museum created a section named Virtual Gallery in collaboration with Google Art and Culture Project. They organised an online exhibition on the life of Buddha in India, Saktirupena, Ananya and many more, and displayed 306 objects online with a brief description of its history. It includes Textile, Sculpture, Coins and Paintings. For further details visit their website.

Victoria Memorial Hall, Kolkata

They developed a section of virtual tour and exhibition and also worked on the practice of 'object of the month'. The exhibition currently has paintings of Abanindranath Tagore and Gaganendranath Tagore. Additionally, there is a theme exhibition on 'Magnificent Heritage of India as seen by Daniells', 'Virtual Exhibition of 1857—the First spark of Independence in the Museums of India'. This can be viewed on their official website.

Partition Museum, Amritsar

They collaborated with Google Art and Culture project and are working on developing a virtual gallery. With Google Art and National Rail Museum, they organised two exhibitions on the theme 'Trains and the Raj' and 'Railways and Partition'. These exhibitions can be accessed on YouTube and their website. They have a section of Oral histories where people have shared their experience about partition which is noteworthy. It is essential to visit it online. (The Partition Museum, 2018)

Similarly, many museums around India have become accessible for their visitors through digital transformation in which Dr. Bhau Dalji lad Museum, Mumbai, National Gallery of Modern Art, Mumbai and Delhi deserve a special mention. India's own virtual museum building software 'Jatan' has linked all the Archaeological site museums virtually and also museums of National Importance like Allahabad Museum; Salar Jung Museum, Hyderabad; Indira Gandhi Rashtriya Manav Sangrhalaya, Bhopal; Nehru Memorial Museum and Library. This is an initiative by the Ministry of Culture and it is available on their portal. Through digital software like 'Jatan' and 'Google Art and Culture Project', it is possible to access the collection of museums around the globe (Ministry of Culture, Virtual Museums). Indian culture app also needs special mention [see Figure 21.4]. Government considering the need of time positioned itself for the digital future; Indian culture application is one such endeavour by the Ministry of Culture. They have presented the data of cultural relevance from various repositories all over India. This application is created by IIT, Bombay and the data is provided by the Ministry of Culture and curated by Indira Gandhi National Open University. It is available on Google play store or can be visited on their official website.

Even though digitization has given new hope to museums,

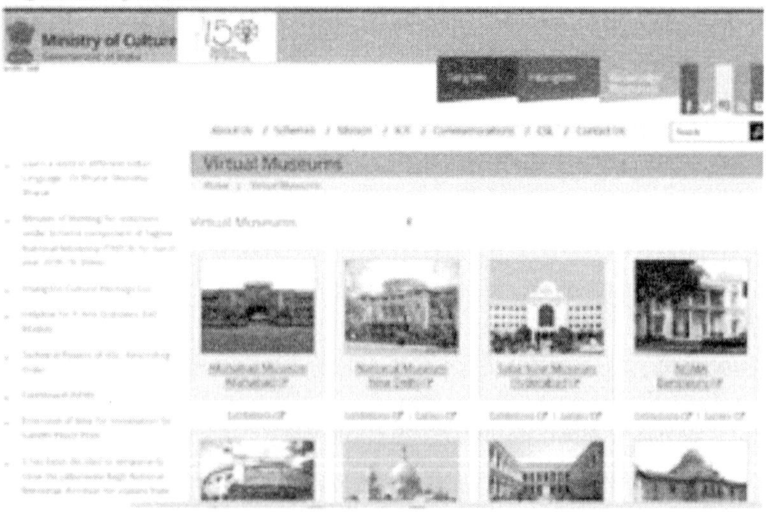

Fig. 21.4: Virtual Museums developed by Jatan

Note. Virtual Museum developed by Jatan.[https://indiaculture.nic.in/virtual-museums]

yet the challenge is half of humanity does not have access to the Internet says International Telecommunication Union. Moreover, data received from the OCED shows, that around 327 million fewer women than men have access to smartphones and the internet. (UNESCO, 2020 p.6) This has additionally heated up the discussion concerning how much access ought to be provided to visitors? Would a virtual exhibition remove the real aspect of museums? Whether that interactive sessions and visitor's participation would come to end and we would follow the old school theory of 'look but don't touch' regardless in today's era where museums emphasise on 'touch and feel' concept like Abhinav Gallery created by National Museum, New Delhi for Specially-Abled people. What might be happening of museum outreach programmes and connecting museum to society? What would happen about the security of collection and its conservation in this situation of the financial crisis? Covid-19 has left with numerous questions and made us cognizant about the loopholes in our system and its practices.

With so many blended messages originating from the national government, media and social media, people are seeing museums to provide a fact-based scientific and humanistic appraisal of the situation. Museums are held with the responsibility of not only creating awareness but also document the period for the coming generation. In the midst of turmoil, Museums are stable, responsible, creative and empathic and rethinking to finding out new ways to define their part in society addressing the situation.

REFERENCES

1. Atkinson, Rebecca. (2020). How Are Museums Collecting during Coronavirus Lockdown? Museums Association, Retrieved October 4, 2020 from www.museumsassociation.org/museums-journal/analysis/2020/04/03042020-how-are-museums-collecting-covid-19/.
2. Azoulay, Audrey. (11 May 2020). UNESCO Launches ResiliArt Movement for Artists and Cultural Professionals in the Face of COVID-19. UNESCO,.

Retrieved October 1, 2020, from https://en.unesco.org/news/unesco-launches-resiliart-movement-artists-and-cultural-professionals-face-covid-19.

3. Chhatrapati Shivaji Maharaj Vastu Sangrahalaya. Retrieved September 17, 2020, from https://www.csmvs.in/
4. Delhi, N., & Management, D. (2020). *REPORT 2019-2020. May 2019*, 1–16.
5. Doshi, P. (2011). La evasiva definiciÛn de la gripe pandÈmica. *Bulletin of the World Health Organization, 89*(7), 532–538. Retrieved from https://doi.org/10.2471/BLT.11.086173
6. Indian Culture. Retrieved September 21, 2020, from https://indianculture.gov.in/
7. Indian Museum Kolkata. Retrieved September 21, 2020 from https://indianmuseumkolkata.org/
8. International Council of Museums. (n.d.). Museums and COVID-19: 8 Steps to Support Community Resilience. Retrieved September 25, 2020, from https://icom.museum/en/news/museums-and-covid-19-8-steps-to-support-community-resilience/.
9. Ministry of Culture, Government of India. Virtual Museums. Retrieved September 21, 2020, from https://indiaculture.nic.in/virtual-museums.
10. Museum of Art & Photography. (n.d.). Taking the Museum to the People. Retrieved September 25, 2020 from https://map-india.org/taking-the-museum-to-the-people/
11. National Museum, New Delhi. Retrieved September 21, 2020, from http://www.nationalmuseumindia.gov.in/en/museum
12. Sholts, Sabrina. (26 Feruary, 2020). How Museums Can Help the Public Make Sense of Pandemics. Smithsonian Institution. Retrieved September 25, 2020, from www.smithsonianmag.com/smithsonian-institution/how-museums-can-help-public-make-sense-pandemics-180974281/.
13. Schwarzer, Marjorie. (23 Apr. 2020). Lessons from History: Museums and Pandemics. *American Alliance of Museums*. Retrieved September 17, 2020 from www.aam-us.org/2020/03/10/lessons-from-history-museums-and-pandemics/.
14. The Partition Museum. (1 Nov. 2018). Railways and Partition - Trains and the Raj. Google Arts & Culture Exhibition Links. Retrieved September 21, 2020, from https://www.partitionmuseum.org/museum/online-exhibition/.
15. UNESCO. (2020). Museums around the world: in the face of Covid-19. *May*, 31.
16. UNESCO. (2 Sept. 2020). UNESCO and ICCROM Analyze Museum Trends during and after the Pandemic. Retrieved October 1, 2020, from https://en.unesco.org/news/unesco-and-iccrom-analyze-museum-

trends-during-and-after-pandemic.

17. UNESCO. (2 June 2020). COVID-19 : UNESCO and ICOM Concerned about the Situation Faced by the World's Museums. Retrieved June 26, 2020, from https://en.unesco.org/news/covid-19-unesco-and-icom-concerned-about-situation-faced-worlds-museums.
18. Victoria and Albert Museum (n.d.). V&A ă Rapid Response Collecting. Retrieved September 25, 2020, from www.vam.ac.uk/collections/rapid-response-collecting.
19. Victoria Memorial. Retrieved September 21, 2020 from http://victoriamemorial-cal.org/home/content/en
20. World Health Organisation. (12 Mar. 2020). What Is a Pandemic? Retrieved September 14, 2020 from www.who.int/csr/disease/swineflu/frequently_asked_questions/pandemic/en/.
21. World Health Organization. (n.d.) WHO Coronavirus Disease (COVID-19) Dashboard. Retrieved September 14, 2020 from https://covid19.who.int/.

22
History of Epidemics and Covid-19: An Analysis

Vibha Singh

ABSTRACT

In India, 8,636,011 confirmed cases and 127,571 confirmed deaths due to COVID-19 were reported as of November 11, 2020, and in the transmission of a cluster of cases. And total confirmed cases globally are 51,251,715 and total deaths are 12,70,930. Due to the absence of a specific vaccine or therapy, non-pharmacological interventions including social distancing, contact tracing are essential to end the worldwide COVID-19. A causal-loop model has been proposed that predicts the dynamics of COVID-19 in overall India. A complete scenario is given to demonstrate the estimated pandemic lifecycle along with the real data or history to date, which in turn divulges the predicted inflection point of the phases of SARS-CoV-2. The proposed model monitors the dynamics of components, namely transmission event, number of infectious people, and risk of transmission per interpersonal contact. It reveals that achieving a reduction in the contact rate between uninfected and infected individuals by quarantined susceptible individuals can effectively reduce the basic reproduction number. The model shows that the elimination of the ongoing SARS-CoV-2 pandemic is possible by combining the restrictive social distancing and contact tracing. The predictions proposed are based on secondary data and reports with reasonable assumptions, whereas the accurate course of epidemic heavily depends on how and when quarantine, isolation, and precautionary measures are enforced.

Keywords: COVID-19, Corona virus, Causal loop, Pandemic

Covid-19 Pandemic spread in the world at an exponential rate. World Health Organization (WHO) declare Covid-19 as an epidemic to pandemic on 11th March, 2020. According to WHO data on 11th November, 2020, 51,251,715 total confirmed cases, 1,270,930 confirmed deaths, and 36,669,404 (97%) (world meter 11/11/2020) recovered throughout the world. Novel corona virus has already beaten the previous records of two life-threatening outbreaks, namely Middle East Respiratory Syndrome Corona virus (MERS-CoV) and Severe Acute Respiratory Syndrome Corona virus (SARS-CoV), posing major threat to the global public health and economy after the second World War. Covid-19 is a group of enveloped non-segmented with a positive-sense, single-stranded RNA viruses that belong to the order of Nidovirales, a family of *Coronaviridae*, and subfamily of Ortho-coronavirinae and widely spread among mammals and humans. In December 2019, a local epidemic of pneumonia was first identified in Wuhan city of Hubei province China, and the mainland China became the epicenter of Covid -19. Most of the initial stages were usually incorporated to the wholesale Wuhan seafood market, which also traded live animals. This communicable corona virus disease has traits like fever, dry cough, sore throat, breathlessness, and fatigue. With human migration through air, the disease has now spread throughout the world as well as the territories of the world, making Europe and USA as new epicenters. Covid-19 is the third zoonotic human-to-human transmission that has arisen globally in the present century, after SARS- CoV, which spread around 37 countries, and the MERS-CoV that spread around 27 countries.

In India, the pandemic Covid-19 was first confirmed in the state Kerala on January 30th, 2020, when a student returned from Wuhan, the province of China. The Govt. of India has incorporated social distancing as a precautionary measure to prevent the possibility of third stage human-to-human transmission that can stimulate the spread of the corona virus diseases. Indian Government also imposed 14 hours voluntary public curfew ('Janata Curfew') on March 22nd, 2020, to make aware the people about the peculiar epidemiological traits compared with the previous two epidemics of SERS-CoV and MERS-CoV. Moreover, the Government of India has declared a 21 days nationwide lockdown from March 25th, 2020, to April 14th, 2020, to prevent the spread of corona virus diseases among humans, affecting India's 1.3 billion population.

In the second phase, the lockdown has been extended up to May 3rd, 2020, to combat against Covid-19 pandemic in India. In the lack of any specific vaccine or therapeutics, social distancing has been recognized as the most commonly utilized preventive measures to control the novel corona virus diseases. The main target of these initiatives was the control of social interactive places, like schools, colleges, theaters, cultural programs, and other public spheres, except for essential public services like hospitals, medicine shops, police, and fire, etc. Indeed the outbreaks of COVID-19 have drastically altered the daily life, health of the public as well the economy. This is one of the main interests for each and everyone how long this situation will continue and when the disease will be under control? When the entire world will return to its earlier situation? (Kapparashetty, 2020).

Table 22.1: Some of the major Pandemics that occurred over time

S.N.	Year	Name	Death toll (millions)	Type/Pre-human host
1	165-180	Antonine plague	5	Believed to be either Smallpox Or Measles
2	541-542	Plague of Justinian	30-35	Rats, fleas, Yersinia pestisbacteria
3	735-737	Japanese smallpox Epidemic	1	Variola virus
4	1347-1351	Black Death (Bubonic Plague)	200	Rats, fleas, Yersinia pestisbacteria
5	1520	Smallpox	56	Variola virus
6	1600	17th-century greatplague	3	Rats, fleas, Yersinia pestisbacteria
7	1700	18th-century greatplague	0.6	Rats, fleas, Yersinia pestisbacteria
8	1817-1923	Cholera 6 outbreak	1+	V. cholera bacteria
9	1855	The Third plague	12	Rats, fleas, Yersinia pestisbacteria
10	Late 1800s	Yellow fever	.100-.150	Virus/ mosquitos
11	1981-present	HIV/AIDS	25-35	
12	1889-1890	Russian flu	1	H2N2 (Avian origin)

13	1918-1919	Spanish flu	40-50	H1N1/Pigs
14	1957-195	Asian flu	1.1	H2N2
15	2002-2003	SARS	0.00077	Corona virus/bats, civets
16	2009	Swine flu	2	H1N1/Pigs
17	2015-present	MERS	0.00085	Corona virus/bats, civets
18	2014-2016	Ebola	0.0113	Ebola virus/bates, camels
19	2019	COVID-19	1.26M	Corona virus/ unknown (possibly bats or pangolins)
			(9.43 AM 11/11/2020)	

Source: LePan, N. (2020). Visual Capitalist

History of Pandemics

Disease and illnesses have plagued humanity since the earliest days, our mortal flaw. However, it was not until the marked shift to agrarian communities that the scale and spread of these diseases increased dramatically. Pandemic is the form of epidemic that spreads through human population affecting large number of people, major part of a nation, entire nation, a continent or a part of the entire world. In a simple way a pandemic is an epidemic with higher magnitude in terms of geographical area, number of cases and days of suffering resulting in disabilities or deaths. A disease or condition is not a pandemic merely because it is widespread or kills many people; it must also be infectious (Swetha, Eashwar & Gopalakrishnan, 2019). For instance, cancer is responsible for many deaths but is not considered a pandemic because the disease is not infectious or contagious. Human population have suffered from many pandemics throughout history be it the earlier form of smallpox or tuberculosis. Widespread trade created new opportunities for human and animal interactions that speed up such epidemics. Malaria, tuberculosis, leprosy, influenza, smallpox and others first appeared during these early years. The more civilized humans became – with larger cities, more exotic trade routes, and increased contact with different animals, and ecosystems – the more likely pandemics would occur.

Very few phenomena throughout human history have shaped our societies and cultures the way outbreaks of infectious diseases have; yet, remarkably little attention has been given to these phenomena in behavioral social science and in branches of medicine that are, at least in part, founded in social studies (e.g., psychiatry). This lack of attention is intriguing, as one of the greatest catastrophes ever, if not the greatest one in the entire history of humankind, was an outbreak of a pandemic. In a long succession throughout history, pandemic outbreaks have decimated societies, determined outcomes of wars, wiped out entire populations, but also, paradoxically, cleared the way for innovations and advances in sciences (including medicine and public health), economy, and political systems (Jordë, Singh & Taylor, 2020). Pandemic outbreaks, or plagues, as they are often referred to, have been closely examined through the lens of humanities in the realm of history, including the history of medicine. Few doubt that major epidemics and pandemics will strike again and few would argue that the world is adequately prepared. Table: 22.1 showing some of the major pandemics that have occurred over time (LePan, 2020)

Pandemic phases

According to the World Health Organization pandemic have several stages and planning and action do according to the phase suggested by the WHO. Characteristics of every phase are as-

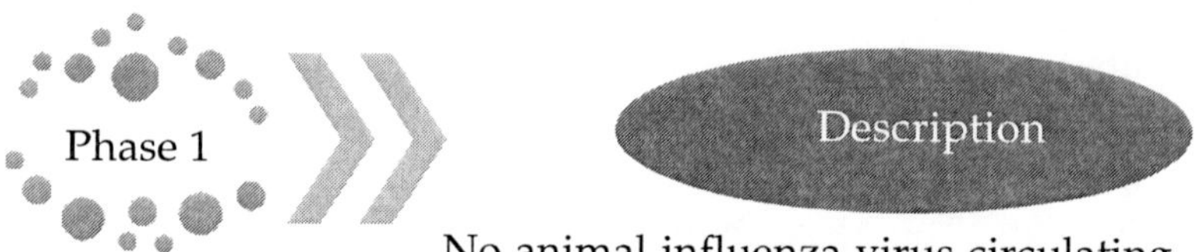

No animal influenza virus circulating among animals have been reported to cause infection in humans.

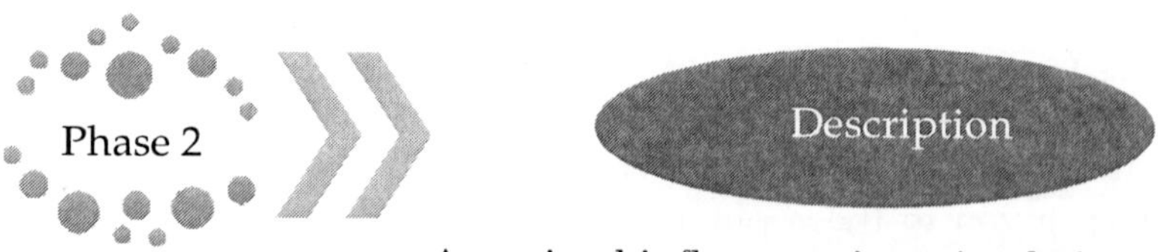

An animal influenza virus circulating in domesticated or wild animals is known to have caused infection in humans and is therefore considered a specific potential pandemic threat.

Phase 3

Description

An animal or human-animal influenza reassortant virus has caused sporadic cases or small clusters of disease in people, but has not resulted in human-to-human transmission sufficient to sustain community level outbreaks.

Phase 4

Description

Human to human transmission of an animal or human-animal influenza reassortant virus able to sustain community level outbreaks has been verified.

Phase 5

Description

The same identified virus has caused sustained community level outbreaks in two or more countries in one WHO region.

Phase 6 — Description

In addition to the criteria defined in the Phase 5, the same virus has caused sustained community level outbreaks in at least one other country in another WHO region.

Post-Peak Period — Description

Level of pandemic influenza in most countries with adequate surveillance have dropped below peak levels.

Post-Pandemic Period — Description

Levels of influenza activity have returned to the levels seen for seasonal influenza in most countries with adequate surveillance.

Source: *World Health Organization (https://www.who.int/influenza/resources/documents/pandemic_phase_descriptions_and_actions.* pdf)

Methodology

System dynamics is basically a modeling tool to understand a complex world problem model. The main contribution to the development process of System Dynamics is by J.W. Forrester.

In the sixties, J.W. Forrester developed System Dynamics as a modeling and simulation techniques for solving complex physical and social problems. J.W. Forrester designed policies for management and change. It provides a perspective and a set of conceptual tools that enable one to frame the structure and dynamics of complex, non-linear, multi-loop feedback systems (Pratap, Singh & Gautam, 2020). In the proposed causal loop diagram model, it is clear that the reinforcing loop is the main cause for the pandemic increases the number of infectious people exponentially. Infectious people increase the risk of transmission per interpersonal contact that further increases the Covid-19 transmission event and it leads to further increase in the number of infectious people and create a reinforcing loop. To balance the reinforcement loop interpersonal contact should be minimized. The role of public performance of protective behavior plays a very crucial role. When public protective behavior performance is high, it reduces the risk of transmission from the environment, environment contamination, and risk of transmission per interpersonal contact. Environmental contamination has a positive relationship with the risk of transmission from the environment and it increases the virus transmission event. Public performance of protective behavior has negative impact on environment contamination and risk of transmission from environment that helps in reducing the Transmission event (Bradley, *et. al.*, 2020).

Transmission events increase the number of susceptible people and it also produces a positive impact on the transmission event, so to balance this loop, respectable people should be quarantined to weaken the reinforcement loop. Due to the nobility of the virus, people have less trust in authority and increase public outrage. Stigma reduces the number of cases detected. Accountability of authority increased the trust and produced the effectiveness of public and health risk communication that help in the public performance of protective behavior and try to reduce the exponential growth of the pandemic. Effectiveness of Public Health Communications and awareness, such as hygiene factors cause disease, people's role, workplace hygiene, personal hygiene, public place rule, and regulations reduce the spread of pandemic (Swetha, Eashwar & Gopalakrishnan, 2019).

The Causal loop diagram (Fig. 22.1) showed the delay in the infected people and became infected people and also in the number of cases detected. The number of infectious people increases the environment cleaning with some delay. Frequency and effectiveness of environment cleaning reduces the environment contamination that in turn also reduces the risk of transmission from environment and reduces the transmission event (He, Peng & Sun 2020). Accountability of the authority plays an important role in building trust that reduces public outrage and that change the public perceived risk. Public awareness produces effect on both public perceived risk and public outrage. Public perceived risk influence public performance on protective behavior. So treating the Covid - 19 effectively makes the authority accountable and trustable. Accountable authority plays an important role. Nobility increased the public outrage that increased the stigma and this reduced the number of cases detected. The impact of stigma on the number of cases defect is reduced by the case finding and contact tracing. A small reinforcement loop is so in our causal loop diagram with the number of susceptible people and transmission events, this reinforcement loop can be balanced by the quarantine of the susceptible people.

Epilogue

Pandemic creates a tough situation in human history and trolls few to millions of death in the world. The first step to reducing the spread of the disease is to maintain the social distance or quarantine the patient. The proposed model reveals that achieving a reduction in the contact rate between uninfected

Fig.22.1: *Causal loop model of integrating component of society responding to the threat of COVID-19*
Source: Bradley et al (2020). A systems approach to preventing and responding to COVID-19

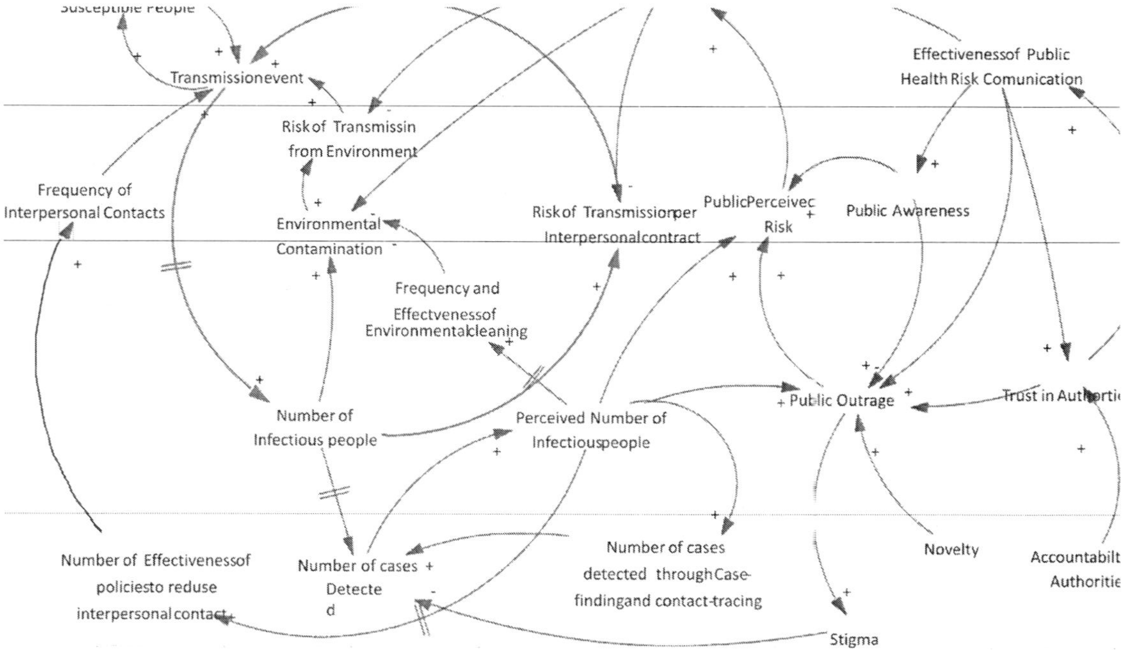

and infected individuals by quarantined susceptible individuals can effectively reduce the basic reproduction number. It is evident that the elimination of the ongoing SARS-CoV-2 pandemic is possible by combining the restrictive social distancing and contact tracing. The predictions made are based on secondary data and report with reasonable assumptions, whereas the accurate course of epidemic heavily depends on how and when quarantine, isolation, and precautionary measures are enforced. In response to the Covid-19 pandemic, lockdown give time to set up the various health infrastructures by breaking the chain of infection. Lockdowns help in maintaining the social distancing but a long span lockdown hurts the economy of the nation and produces stress on the resources of the nation (Jordë, Singh & Taylor, 2020). So the government may work on producing treatment, vaccinations, and effective low-cost treatment.

REFERENCES

1. Bradley, D. T., Mansouri, M. A., Kee, F., & Garcia, L. M. T. (2020). A systems approach to preventing and responding to COVID 19. *EClinical Medicine*, 21. Retrieved from https://doi.org/10.1016/j.eclinm.2020.100325
2. He, S., Peng, Y. & Sun, K. (2020). SEIR modeling of the COVID-19 and its dynamics. *Nonlinear Dynamics*, 1-14.
3. Jordë, •., Singh, S. R., & Taylor, A. M. (2020). *Longer-run economic consequences of pandemics* (No. w26934). National Bureau of Economic Research.
4. Kapparashetty, B. V. (2020). Impact of Covid 19 on Industrial Sector–A Study, *International Journal of Research and Analytical Reviews (IJRAR)*, 7(1), 422-429.
5. LePan, N. (2020). *Visualizing the History of Pandemics.*
6. Pratap, V., Singh, A., & Gautam, A. K. (2020). Determinants of Working Capital: A System Dynamics Approach. *Studies in Indian Place Names*, 40(56), 2015-2023.
7. Samui, P., Mondal, J., & Khajanchi, S. (2020). A mathematical model for COVID-19 transmission dynamics with a case study of India. *Chaos, Solitons & Fractals*, 140, 110173.
8. Sarkar, K., Khajanchi, S., & Nieto, J. J. (2020). Modeling and forecasting the COVID-19 pandemic in India. *Chaos, Solitons & Fractals*, *139*, 110049.

9. Swetha, G., Eashwar, V. M., & Gopalakrishnan, S. (2019). Epidemics and Pandemics in India throughout History: A Review Article." *Indian Journal of Public Health Research & Development, 10*(8), 1570-1576. https://www.who.int/influenza/resources/documents/pandemic_phase_descriptions_ and_actions. pdf
10. Sy, C. et al. (2020). Policy Development for Pandemic Response using System Dynamics: A Case Study on COVID-19. *Process Integration and Optimization for Sustainability*, 1-5.
11. Venkateswaran, J., & Damani, O. (2020). Effectiveness of Testing, Tracing, Social Distancing and Hygiene in Tackling Covid-19 in India: A System Dynamics Model. *arXiv reprint arXiv:2004.08859*.

23

Revisiting Gandhian Ideology as an Alternative Developmental Model in Post-Covid-19 India

Bhimashankar M. Birajdar

ABSTRACT

During the contemporary times due to an outbreak of the COVID-19 pandemic across the world created a global crisis before mankind. It has been adversely influencing on the economies of the almost all developed, developing and under-developing countries. It ruined industries and commerce by worsening the situations of the ever-increasing pace of unemployment and apparent economic emergency. This predicament in the sphere of economy initiated to rethink developmental concerns, agendas before the capitalistic, socialistic models of development across the world. There are uncertainties when India will succeed in overcoming from these precarious situations. Gandhian model of economic development would be an alternative model for the policymakers, rulers in India in the context of 'Aatmnirbhar Bharat Yojna' *(Self-reliant India Scheme) announced by the union government recently. Mahatma Gandhi was believed in development models comprising 'self-sufficiency' and 'village self-rule' (Gram*

Swaraj). He was not against 'industrial revolution' but opposed to modern sophisticated industrial machines because of growth in unemployment. This chapter is a sincere endeavour to bring out salient features of Gandhian economic model—popularly known as ecological economics. As an applied, ideological model of Gandhi should be encouraged, due emphasis should be given in implementation of economic policies for achieving stipulated objectives. On the other hand, there are opportunities to minimise adverse consequences of the western capitalistic model of development, the problem of social inequity, unemployment, rapid urbanization, decentralization of economic administration and participatory democracy.

Keywords: *Aatmnirbhar Bharat Yojna*, Capitalistic, COVID-19, Ecological Economics Socialistic Models of Development, Gandhian Model, *Gram Swaraj*, Industrial Revolution.

We are living in a world wherein science, technology and development have been playing vital roles. However, the notion of development and its models are becoming contentious, controversial issues in developing countries like India. India's economic growth stories have been decelerated due to unprecedented causes. Further, contemporary economic disruption brought by COVID-19 pandemic has worsened the situations and put forth retrospective vision on developmental models, economic theories, means and modes of productions, the problem of unemployment and so on.In fact, the notion of development is quite controversial with many debatable issues. Vandana Shiva, an eminent Indian environment activist argues that 'development is essentially continuance of colonialism'. Gandhi considered the earth as a living organism (Sasikala, 2012, 51-52). Mahatma Gandhi was one of the first political thinkers who portrayed the flaws of modern civilization and capital-centric developmental models. He cautioned that this kind of development could not achieve equitable and just development of society. He firmly believed that modern civilization had been given birth to the capitalist model of development. It extracts, and exploits natural resources on extensive scale, resulting in the land, water and air pollution (Chousalkar, 2006, 285-86). When Gandhi returned to India in 1915 from South Africa, he immediatel ystarted to acquaint himself with genuine socio-economic circumstances of India. Hence, he travelled in the Indian villages and countryside. During peasants' struggles of 1917 and 1918 in the districts of Champaran and Kheda, he confronted with economic exploitative policies of British. His scattered writings from 1920-1940 give us some clues of his visions of development. J. C. Kumarappa, one of his contemporary close disciples, through his writings especially *'Why the Village Movement?'*(1938) and *'The Economy of Permanence'* (1948) had attempted to elaborate, formalize on Gandhian ecological programmes and village-centric economics (Guha, 1998, 67-72). The rulers, policymakers, planners, economists would at least revisit and consider this model as an applied, much needed developmental trajectories for restoring Indian economy by minimizing adverse impacts of social, economic inequities, employment generation, halting ever-increasing urbanization, environmental degradation.

Gandhian Developmental Ideology and Philosophy

Gandhi had opposed to modern capitalism and industrialism. He envisaged that rapid industrialization resulted in exploitation of natural resources in Third World countries by rich western countries. Hence, he was against the western paradigms of development and economic policies and put forth an alternative path of development based on ecological economics. His developmental ideology and philosophy relied on the five principles, namely new philosophy of men, decentralisation in economic development, world peace and resolution of conflicts through peaceful manner, the concept of *'Gram Swaraj'* and *'Satyagraha'*. To minimize the dominance of the state, he recommended *Panchayat* democracy, which enables local grassroots bodies to entrust decision-making rights (Chousalkar, 2006, 292-296). Gandhi's popular dictum, "World has enough for everyone's need, but not enough for everyone's greed"(GOI, 2014-15) shows that his developmental paradigm reiterates close linkages with moralities and welfare ethics (Barua, 2015, 136). Gandhi in a booklet titled *'Hind Swaraj'* (1906), which he wrote while travelling towards England, criticized significantly western developmental models (Tella, 2018, 78). It has claimed to give us an alternative perspective on development while exploring how the present mode of exploitative development is exploiting man by man and nature by man.The production and distribution pattern, system that Gandhien visaged and endeavoured to implement later in India along with the freedom struggle calling it the *'Swadeshi* Movement', was founded on the fund amental principle of eventual moral progress mingled with dignified and healthy physical survival (Iyangar, 2005, 09). The ultimate intention of Gandhian ideology was the *Panchayat* Raj, the economically self-reliant, politically self-ruling and culturally non-violent democratic village (Kumar, 2010, 27). The ethical economic philosophy and ideology of self-sufficiency were disseminated all over India by Gandhi during the British colonial period. He was not an economist but given his socio-economic basically base on developmental discourses quite often resisted against the exploitative policies of British. He was also influenced by the Marxian principle of neutrality, and its emphasis on the "exploitation of labour". He was very much obsessed with Ruskin's unorthodox doctrine that the wealth of a nation consisted not in its production and consumption of goods, but its people. His economic ideology/ philosophy was essentially associated with individual self-esteem and the welfare of poor people (Kaur and Singh, 2015, 116-117).

Gandhian Ecological Economics

Between 1920 and 1947 the struggle for independence against British imperialism was led by Gandhi. The historical origin of his economic ideology had been reflected in the *'SaltSatyagraha'* (1930). He revealed the unjust economic policies of the British by imposing a tax on an essential basic commodity of common masses (Raut, 2019, 24). The economic ideology of Gandhi would be differentiated between conventional economics. It demonstrates close similarities with ecological economics.Ecological economics is relatively a new area or field of studies that came into mainstream economics to overcome the lacunae between economics, environment or ecology. The concept like sustainable development was not widely elaborated, deliberated at the time of Gandhi, but his appropriate, well-known vision acknowledged in almost all over the world is *Sarvodyaya* safeguard the privileged rights of future generations based on the welfare of all human beings. A Gandhian vision of development relied heavily upon his ethical economics (Sasikala, 2012, 58). The following table shows the differences between Conventional and Gandhian Economics.

In Gandhian holistic economics, industrialization and technological development ought to be carried out within its limitations so that natural processes could not be imbalanced. In brief, Gandhian economics is one of the paramount paradigms of development,which demonstrate an ideal synthesis of economy, ethics and morality for the welfare of entire diverse, plural communities (Kumar, 2010, 35-39).He had a special love for the cow. It was not only because the cows provides nourishing milk and milk products for the family but help us in agricultural including for tilling and organic manure (Molokattu, 2010,157).

Table 23.1 : Differences between conventional and Gandhi and Economics

Ideological Strands	Conventional Economics	Gandhian Economics
• Basic Philosophy	• Materialistic	• Spiritual/Ethical/Moral
• World View	• Human-centric	• Eco-centric (considers equal rights of human and non-human beings)
• Macro Aim	• Profit Maximization	• Sustainable Communities through agriculture and constructive programmes.
• Views on Science and Technology	• An inevitable part of human progress	• Science or technology makes modern man slaves of machines.
• Views on Natural Resources	• Maximum benefit out of natural resources	• Limited use of natural resources
• Views on Modes of Production	• Mass production with the aid of modern technology	• Production by the masses
• Nature of Production	• Capital Intensive	• Labour Intensive
• Views on the Market	• Large scale market induced globalization	• Local and National (*Swadeshi*)
• Nature of Power	• The power vested/rested in the industrial nations or the corporate (centralization of power and resources)	• Power belongs to people (Decentralization of power and resources)
• Outcome/Impact	• Urbanisation, environmental crisis, resource depletion and natural calamities.	• Village Swaraj, environmental Sustainability

Source: Sasikala, A.S. (2012): Environmental Thoughts of Gandhi for a Green Future, in *'Gandhi Marg'*, 34(1), p. 60

Technology, Society and Economy: A Gandhian Overview

Gandhi was not simply against western technology but he also visualized an alternative technological scenario which he thought was more appropriate to the real development of our country. The basic notion behind this was the development of largely self-reliant villages. In this context, Gandhi's views on technology have been so far misunderstood and misinterpreted (Kumar, 2010, 60). When the Indian textile industry was being destroyed by the British, Gandhi did not call for the industrialization of Indian textiles. He pulled out a spinning wheel. As he said, "anything that millions can do together, becomes charged with power." (Shiva, 2010, 183). Science and technology would help in individual production and self-reliance (Kumar, 2010, 124). He gave importance to every scientific invention made for the benefit of all the people. However, he criticized inventions for amassing wealth and destructive purposes. His observations and interpretations in the *Hind Swaraj* wherein he remarked:

> "The workers in the mills of Bombay have become slaves of machinery. The condition of the women in the mills is shocking. When there were no mills, there were not starving. If the machinery craze grows in our country, it will become an unhappy land." (Gamdhi, 2014, 85)

He was opposed to the monopolistic nature of technology. Environmental and technological predicaments are becoming major social problems in India. Hence during contemporary times, these could be minimized or perhaps resolved by linking Gandhian vision of development through balancing man, economy and nature. Gandhi focused equitable distribution of income and wealth; resources to encourage social harmony (Kumar, 2010, 63-97). Gandhi proposed to eliminate or evade all the adverse impacts of mass industrialization. He desired to promote small-scale, self-reliant industries especially cottage and other small industries (*Gram Udyog*) that produce and manufacture required products for consumption in the village or to meet the needs of neighbouring villages. The trajectories of modern nations, and states during contemporary times are accompanied by technological progress through rapid industrialization leading towards capital-centric mass production (Kumar, 2010, 26-33). Gandhi is also often regarded as a father of appropriate technology. He promoted small, local, village-based technology that permits its users to associate themselves with what they want to produce, a technology that would not be replaced by human labour (Moolak kattu, 2010,157). In *Hind Swaraj* he writes:

> Observing all this, our ancestors dissuaded us from luxuries and pleasures. We have managed with the same kind of plough as existed thousands of year ago. We have retained the same kind of cottages that we had in former times and our indigenous education remains the same as before. (Gandhi, 2014, 55)

He had objections to the way the new industries and technologies were incorporated into society. He had an idea of peaceful co-existence, where industrialization would go hand in hand with the village handicrafts and human labour (Kolge, N. Sreekumar, 2009, 60). He further stated that (Jan 27, 1939);

> "I do visualize electricity, shipbuilding, ironworks, machine-making, and the like existing side by side with village handcrafts. But the order of dependence will be reversed."

Gandhian Concept of '*Gram Swaraj*'

Mahatma Gandhi was not an academic economist, but he read the '*Das Capital*' of Karl Marx and '*Unto the Last*' of Ruskin. By understanding Indian situations he emphasized on *Khadi, Charakha* (spinning wheel), *Swadeshi* which were assumed to play prominent roles in '*Gram Swaraj*' (Village Self-rule) (Gupta, 2020, 59). He initiated an association, known as the 'All India Spinners Association' in 1925 with an intension of developing hand-spinning, uninterrupted by changes in political opinions and yet as an integral part of the Congress, which claims to represent not only the rich and the middle classes but also the very poorest of the land (Gandhi, 1927, 33). Gandhian self-reliant reflected in his concept of '*Swadeshi*' also has a lot of implications for the formation of a non-exploitative society (Moolakattu, 2010, 155). He incorporated ideas of self-reliance into his broader thesis on *Swaraj* by adopting spinning wheel and *khadi* as means in Indian freedom struggle against British imperialism. His notion of *Swaraj* was evolved as a critique against the modern machine-based mode of production and mechanization (Tella, 2018, 78). His concept of '*Swadeshi*' was fundamental for the village and small scale, cottage industries. He had condemned the destructive methods of economic policies and development of the West because of relying on developing raw materials instead of concentrating upon utilization of manpower. Gandhi had focused on the growth, development of agriculture and handicraft industries (Chousalkar, 2006, 296-97). Gandhian self-reliant village institutions and decentralized small village industries were relied on perpetual human values, the dignity of labour, simple living and non-violence (Gedam, 2010, 24). Gandhi's innovative vision of *Swdeshi, Swaraj, Satygraha* and *Sarvodaya*e ncourages us to build living economics and living democracies. His legacy gives us hope to reconstruct equitable socio-economic and political equilibriums in India (Shiva, 2010, 95).

Gandhian Concept of De-centralization

In order to prevent centralization of power and production, Gandhi had propounded the policy of decentralization based on non-violence. He was conscious that centralization of production would lead towards centralization of power in the hands of few people who exploit them and accumulates maximum profits. In this way, village could be regenerated through the rural, cottage, small scale industries by enhancing rural employability (Chousalkar, 2014, 117-18). Gandhian concept of development is based on socio-economic, political dimensions. His vision is radically different from decentralization and delegation, as being explored these days. Gandhi anticipated every village a component, free and active for the welfare of all people. He considered decentralization as an indispensable social organization. He further believed that efficient decentralization in socio-economic realms depends upon the economic structure. Hence, the rationale behind the decentralization was the conservation of the environment and maintaining the socio-economic local equilibrium. (Kumar, 2010, 102-04). According to Gandhi, economic equality is a master key to achieve self-sufficient, social system and decentralization (Gupta, 2020, 61). He does not find any dichotomy between man and society. He was a practical man who knew that the social conflicts and struggles between capitalistic and labourer classes were not feasible. Hence he suggested another alternative that is the decentralization of the economic system (Kumar, 2010,126-27). We respect Gandhi as the father of the nation, above all he anticipated independent India to be rejuvenated as a land of village republics. But over the last 73 years we have systematically failed to empower rural and poor peoples to control and manage their own destiny (Gadgil and Guha, 1995, 115).

Social Equity: A Gandhian Appraisal

While taking into consideration the rural sector, one of the largest sectors in India, Gandhi's basic rationale of national development was through sustainable practices. He noticed that it was the weakest link in the socio-economic chain in India. He opposed to India's over-dependence on western industrialization with its socio-economic disparities, environmental degradation due to numerous drawbacks (Khoshoo, 2016, 260). The Gandhian vision of economic development relied on ecological principles such as environmental harmony, economic efficiency, conservation of resources and local self-governance equity with social justice (Khoshoo and Moolakkattu, 2017, 64). He reiterated, 'India is in villages, if villages perish, India perishes. Man is not born to live in forests, but to live in a society' (Khoshoo and Moolakkattu, 2017, 141). The prominent schemes of Gandhi, such as the '*Bhoodan* movement' of Vinoba Bhave, which was sought gifts of land for the landless. Although attracted much publicity, it was an attempt to provide more equitable distribution of arable land to the marginalized, subaltern communities (Metcalf and Metcalf, 2006, 245). The poor have been primarily disregarded and required to be brought in the mainstream of development. Poverty and social inequities had been accelerated as consequences of the cumulative impact of environmental degradation on account of excessive resource extraction, ever-increasing economic disparities, rural migration, urban sprawl, biological impoverishment etc. To overcome these problems Gandhi put forth a bio-industrial rural-centric model of development to India. Gandhi said in 1945 that:

> I believe that if India is to attain to freedom and through India and the world as well then sooner or later we will have to live in huts, not in palaces (Khoshoo, 2016, 264-65).

Actually, his notion simple living and emphasis on villages had been underlined. However, in his ethical perspective of development has no scope for social, economic equities and disparities. He asserted that "real economics entails with social justice, it encourages the well-being of all equally the strongest, moderate and weakest strata's of the society". Dr. J. C. Kumarappa, a Gandhian disciple, a follower of ecological economics, urged through comparing with other economic theories and models and appreciated the Gandhian economy as an economy of service comprising *swadeshi*, trusteeship, bread labour etc. attained attention and acceptance from the entire world (Sasikala, 2012, 58).

Epilogue

Gandhi was not an economic theorist but an economic reformer. Today a challenge before India is to make a creative synthesis between the Gandhian model of rural development and Nehruvian model of industrial development. Gandhian ideologies, philosophies concerned with socio-economic, political aspects are debatable and controversial issues. Somebody claims that his developmental paradigms to contemporary times are outdated as it was restricted within traditional and conventional methods. It is indeed challenging task before policymakers, rulers, bureaucrats to implement almost all key elements because of global economic scenarios, waves of liberalization privatization globalization (LPG), neo-liberal economic order and adherence to the capitalistic-centric structure of developmental economics. In fact, this area of study is a multidisciplinary one intersecting conventional academic boundaries. One of the major dilemma or crisis before policymakers, rulers etc. is neither Gandhian developmental paradigms neither abandoned nor refuted nor comprehensively accepted and implemented fully because of limitations in it. Although MGNREGA (Mahatma Gandhi National Rural Employment Guarantee Scheme), *'Swachha*

Bharat Abhiyan' (Clean India Mission) etc. launched by the union government yet there are substantial scopes for need-based implementation of Gandhian ideological programmes. However, the global economic crisis compelled all of us to relook developmental paradigms in the context of '*Aatmnirbhar Bharat Yojna'* ('Self-reliant India Scheme') announced by the union government of India. Hence, it would give fresh insights, alternatives in minimizing adverse consequences and attempts for further improvements. Moreover, it would be an attempt to find pragmatic alternatives in Gandhian economic philosophy, ideology in restoring decelerated pace of development.

REFERENCES

1. Barua, Archana. (2015). Towards a Philosophy of Sustainability: The Gandhian Way in *Sociology and Anthropology*, 3(2), pp. 136-43
2. Chousalkar, Ashok. (2006): Gandhi and Environmentalism, in *Gandhi Marg*, 27 (03 and 04), Oct.-Dec. 2005 and Jan.- Mar. 2006, pp. 285-97
3. —— (2014). Mahatma Gandhi and the Problem of Sustainable Development. In Patil R. B. (Ed.), *Sustainable Development, Local Issues and Global Agendas*, Jaipur, Rawat Publications, pp.111-26.
4. Gadgil, Madhav and Guha,Ramchandra. (1995). *Ecology and Equity: The Use and Abuse of Nature in Contemporary India*. Gurgaon: Penguin India.
5. Gandhi, M.K. (2014) (Reprint of 1909). *Hind Swaraj*. Varanasi: Sarva Seva Sangh Prakashan
6. —— (1927). *Young India* (1924-1926). Madras: S. Ganesan, Current Thought Press.
7. —— (1939, January 27). *Harijan*
8. Gedam, Shankarrao. (Oct. 2010). Mahatma Gandhipranit Panchayatraj (Mahatma Gandhi's Panchayatraj) in *The Lokrajya* Magazines Special Issue on *Mahatma ManuskichiMashal* (Mahatma Torch of Humanity), Directorate, Information and Public Relations Division, Government of Maharashtra (GOM), Mumbai, pp. 24-25.
9. Government of India (GOI) (2014-15). Annual Report, Ministry of Environment, Forests and Climate Change (*MoEF*), New Delhi, India.
10. Guha, Ramchandra. (1998). Mahatma Gandhi and the Environmental Movement in India. In Kalland and Persoon (Eds.), *Environmental Movements in Asia* .Cornwall, Great Britain : Curzon Press, pp.65-82.
11. Gupta,Bajrang Lal. (2020). Gandhiji Ka Arthchintan Aur Arthvyavahar.

In *Sahitya Amrut* (Jan. 2020). Prabhat Prakashan, New Delhi, pp. 57-61.

12. Iyengar, Sudarshan. (2005). Gandhi's Economic Thought and Modern Economic Development: Some Reflections. Working Paper No. 01 (May 2005). Surat: Centre for Social Studies.
13. Kaur, Amandeep and Singh, Bhupinder. (January 2015). Relevance of Gandhian Economic Thought: An Appraisal. In *International Journal of Advanced Research in Management and Social Sciences*, 4(1). Accessed at www.garph.co.uk on 15.09.2020, pp. 115-23.
14. Khoshoo and Moolakkattu. (2017). *Mahatma Gandhi and the Environment*. NewDelhi: The Energy and Resource Institute (TERI) Press.
15. Khoshoo, T. N. (2016). Gandhian Environmentalism, in James George (Ed.), *Ethical Perspectives on Environmental Issues in India*. Delhi: A.P.H. Publishing Corporation.
16. Kolge, Nishikant and Sreekumar, N. (2009). "Gandhi's Criticism of Industrialization and Modernity: An Environmental Perspective. In Joseph Siby, Mahodaya Bharat (Eds.), *Gandhi, Environment and Sustainable Future*. (Selected papers presented in National Seminar on Gandhi, Science and Environment at Institute of Gandhian Studies, Wardha from 14th to 16th March 2009), pp. 57-64.
17. Kumar, S. B. (2010). *Environmental Problems and Gandhian Solutions*. Delhi: Deep and Deep Publications
18. Metcalf, Barbara and Metcalf, Thomas. (2006). *A Concise History of Modern India* (Second Edn).United Kingdom: Cambridge University Press.
19. Moolakattu, John. (2010). Gandhi as a Human Ecologist, in Raj Kamala (ed.), *Journal of Human Ecology*. 29 (3). Delhi, pp. 151-58.
20. Raut, Bharat Kumar. (2019). Arthvicharachi Grahyata (Validation of Economic Thoughts), in *The Lokrajya* Magazines Special Issue *Yugpurush* articles on the occasion of 150 Birth Anniversary of M.K. Gandhi, Oct. Issue, Directorate, Information and Public Relations Division, Government of Maharashtra (GOM), Mumbai, pp.24-26.
21. Sasikala, A.S. (2012). Environmental Thoughts of Gandhi for a Green Future. *Gandhi Marg*, 34(1), pp. 51-66.
22. Shiva,Vandana. (2010).*Earth Democracy: Justice, Sustainability and Peace*. Dehradún: Natraj Publishers.
23. Tella,Ramya. (2018). Climate Justice and Gandhian Morality. *Economic and Political Weekly*, Sept. 22, 2018, 58 (38), pp.74-80.

24
Post-Covid 19: A Time to Pause and Reflect

Samir Banerjee

Seventy years after independence, an Indian labourer in India is branded a migrant. And this labourer and family want to go home because they have not received wages and have very little to eat with no prospect of surviving. Their home, on the face of it is clearly not India. It is some vernacular geography reachable in their WhatsApp; somewhere way away. The place is reachable, but for this they need vehicles and trains. In case they don't get these, they are willing to walk thousands of kilometers to reach **home**. But go they must, and will. The migrant Indian, a new class-caste has only his *gathari* (bundle) to keep or lose. And for them this is not the first time.

No migrant talks like this; I and presumably you too, do. Besides us, the wise politicians, bureaucrats, businessmen and *jholawalla–backpack wala–briefcase wala* sympathetic social worker are also bothered, if not very worried. All of us have a lot to say about the poor luckless migrant who wants to go home. I am pained at what is happening to the poor man and his family. And, of course, a pain cannot be ignored. It has to be deconstructed, decluttered, analyzed and mitigated. I have appropriated the pain of the migrant. I want to and claim that I can relieve the hapless migrant of the pain. But my pain which seems to have acquired a life of its own is reflected pain. Soon, I realize that the migrant's and my pain although similar is not the same; I can book an online railway ticket in the, 'Rajdhani Express', but can the migrant do so in his, 'Shramik Express'? Perhaps the migrant's problem not my pain, needs urgent resolution? This term 'perhaps' allows me a lot of leeway and flexibility particularly as regards to authority and accountability. This perhaps permits me ingenious entrÈe to develop others so as to mitigate their pain, particularly in situation like what we have now. I have my uses; perhaps I should not become cynical!

This is where Gandhi comes in to help us handle this dilemma and give us some noticeable relevance; he refuses to get into the rhetoric of same, similar and perhaps. For him, the ultimate for *raja, fakir* and *sarvahaara* is in self-realization, a realization which is possible only through social work. For Gandhi as a *satyagrahi* his aspiration was to prioritise the social over the personal. He accepts that the process of *satyagraha* requires a lot of rethinking, relinquishing and acquiring of ideas and convictions, of lifestyles and relationships and above all of having to arbitrate the differences between the individual's personal and social. For him *satyagraha* means "striving and living to achieve self-realisation", wherein self-realisation is withering away of the person's individual-in-society. Therefore, for him *satyagraha* becomes self-realisation through social service; a shift which makes the *satyagrahi*, a judge, jury and the measure of social wellbeing. '*Aap he dandi aap he taraju aap he baithe tolta*': the onus is squarely on I/me/we.

For us the question remains: Why did Gandhi insist on serving others as a means of self-realisation? For this, we need to understand not only the notion of 'self-realization through social work' which is a complex process of intention, intervention and involvement. Further among other things it is recognition of the mutuality of me and the migrant in all its ordinary everydayness. Gandhi first a migrant in South Africa and then an itinerant intrepid social worker, a nomad if not a migrant, sought and articulated this ordinary everydayness of the Indian people; an exercise which was at peace with same, similar and perhaps as well as authority and accountability. For Gandhi the understanding of one's identity covers both the spiritual/transcendental and the material/transactional. Therefore, self-understanding becomes self-realization. For the migrant this understanding and realization is a practice of everyday living. For us this is praxis whether one likes it or not, gives life to 'same, similar and perhaps' which in turn gives birth to ideas such as modernisation, develop mentalism, technology dependence, democracy, environment and so on. Soon these ideas tend to convert the urge for self-realisation into self-recognition; who am I is now recognised through the ideas we profess. Social work as self-realization becomes social work as self-recognition; a transition marked by a fear of transparency. This fear of transparency in turn leads to a fear of open politics. Do we not hear the resonance and a conformation of this all around us: Modernization, Westernisation, *Hindutva, Gandhigiri* and so on and so forth?

> But then *'serving'* can be awkward because it can be inundated by issues such as secular, spiritual and moral in addition to the ever present avarice. The importance of service is that it questions the relation between 'I' and 'Mine', thereby clarifying for us our personal potentialities through an underlining of the ambiguity between our individuality and social proclivities. Service with the aid of 'choice' helps us interrogate the notion of freedom. (Banerjee, 2020, 56).

Perhaps this interrogation is possible when we understand the quaint 'give' and 'take' syndrome, a characteristic combination of opinions, emotions, or behaviour. While *satya* is the 'substance of all morality', it is revealed only by praxis at the critical conjunction of theory and practice. *Satya* encourages, ensures and endures. As a moral link between actions, it ensures a continuum and rootedness. By ensuring harmony in purpose as reflected in thought, speech and action, it upholds creativity in *satya-agraha. Satya* by not depending on reciprocity reconfigures the association of the personal and the social. In the process it defines the fundamental discourse of 'give' and 'take'. 'Give' and 'take' manifest 'change and 'continuity': give the change while take is the continuity. Both are governed and influenced by choice, chance and necessity. The social and the personal reflect this, with the social being more accommodative of chance and the personal favoring necessity. An individual's choice of habits, habitat and habitation are a manifestation of this 'give' and 'take' relationship with the larger milieu. The 'give' ensures the relevance of the individual's essential vibrancy, while 'take' delimits because it impinges on the person's self-acclaim by having to proclaim an inadequateness regarding self-sufficiency of the individual being.

For Gandhi 'give and take' was a problematique. The personal within him would have no problems to choose as an individual, but the social has to respond to parameters which are usually changing and ambiguous, particularly since the notion of 'give and take' also comes with the notion of ownership; and ownership means possession and this in turn means power, the harbinger of untruth. Gandhi tried to sort this out through the notion of truth and the morality of social service (Banerjee, 2020, 86).

Our Milieu

The eminent Gandhian Acharya Ramamurthy, from his vast experience, commenting on the primacy of democracy for the Indian milieu, had said, 'the basic problem of this country is democracy; because democracy means that unless people acquire that strength which helps them recognize their rights and that which helps them recognize their duties, then this bureaucratic state will subjugate them. These people in authority will not allow people to do anything. That is why the basic problem is democracy; and all the other work that we do in the name of development should be considered to be relief work only. Such development work will not bring about any basic change. It will not bring any changes in the policies of the state (Banerjee, 2009, 225). Today this anomaly has become a stumbling block.

The tone, tenor and terms of our democracy is evolving into complex and demanding patterns. It is neither a free for all, nor a tightly controlled mediation by either the state or the elite. As for the people, well they are there. It remains an engagement with scope for a wide range of participants with a major theme being access to opportunities, entitlements and endowments. This is what provides space for the NGOs. But this engagement is under stress. Vast sections of our democracy are faced with rampant consumerism, corruption, debunking of traditions and a seeming paradox of fundamentalist exclusivism cohabiting happily with globalization. Most people are frequently finding that their skills, services and products are becoming irrelevant due to changing and monopolistic markets, technologies and elite-biased changes in state policies. It seems that while the question of choice and selection of economic practices has been left to the haloed market forces, social values are up for grabs. In all this, to add spice, cynical political manipulation seems to be the flavour of all seasons.

Our democracy by any reckoning has entered a very volatile phase. While development has become a tool for the elite to consolidate their agenda, equality in terms of access to opportunities has started becoming a cynical slogan for the opportunists. Sadly many NGOs, i.e. those who survive a constant state inspired purge, too seem to be veering away from an intimate relationship with the people and preferring to act as intermediaries, trainer of trainers and managing, controlling and distributing funds, finances and technologies. NGOs seem to prefer to play second fiddle to the state, international finance, and the agenda of multinational corporate, funding Agencies and such others. Most NGOs are fast becoming honest brokers, always chasing "relevant items" for an agenda. Chandi Prasad Bhatt, the eminent Gandhian puts it thus:

> These days' people's participation has become a very common term. It is supposed to mean peoples participation. I want to ask, as to what is this participation? Participation should be yours; the work should be of the people and it should be a people's programme. Today everybody wants to be the owner. The problem is of the people of the village. But the NGOs convert these in such a manner that it becomes their problem and the villagers have to participate in the solving of the same. Participation then reduces to contributing labour. These days there is a lot of confusion about constructive organizations, voluntary organizations and NGOs. Today they are called VOs; the distinction of English and western has remained. They call themselves social workers but look at their honorariums? It goes up to fifty thousand. It takes years for a person to become a professor or a chief engineer. But if I open an NGO, I myself become the director and decide on my salary. But the people are watching very closely. They will not continue to suffer this (Banerjee, 2009, 227).

The people and the community have always respected the intellectuals, the idealists, the students, the professionals and such others. While condoning their eccentricities they have always appreciated the cutting-edge innovativeness and insight of such elements. The only thing the community expects is that such people explicitly associate with the community, abjure opportunism and search for inspirations and incentives from and on the basis of an organic linkage with the community. Simply put the community expects the ethos of social transformation and intervention to neither be an import nor be a tutored engagement of the elite. Effectively it should become multifarious, holistic, transparent and autonomous. From problem solving it should shift to enabling thus making social transformation conspicuously mutual, i.e. the people and we. Intervention should be mutually arrived expectation not borrowed assurances (Banerjee, 2009, 227-8).

Gandhi had counselled, 'one should never be content with our purity of motive alone'. This caution about intentionalities is the wariness, which informs the distinction between wisdom and knowledge, in that wisdom recognizes that one may commit an error in spite of a purity of motive. To understand the pain (if I may) of the migrant we must aspire for this wariness. The following is an extract from my book (Banerjee, 2020). This part discusses Gandhi's understanding of social service. This understanding can perhaps help us initiate a discourse where the migrant could have a role.

Social Service

For Gandhi social service is serving our fellow-beings, "in order that we may see a glimpse of God through them; because they have got the same spirit as we have, and unless we learn that, there is a barrier drawn between God and ourselves; if we want to demolish that barrier, the beginning is made by complete identification with our fellow-beings". Social service is what helps us understand and recognize our level of incompetence and thereby helps push the bar. While separately the terms social and service stand for a configuration and an ethos, together they represent a structured process between provider and beneficiary. It is this structured process of involvement which aids in liberating us from the arduous constraints and contingencies of day-to-day survival.

> This two-way process between provider and beneficiary is not a deal exchange or reciprocation. For Gandhi, "Action is my domain, and what I understand, according to my lights, to be my duty, and what comes my way, I do. All my action is actuated by the spirit of service" (Raghvan and Iyer, 1986, I, 4).

Providence, competence, a sense of commitment and an inner urge, all seem to be behind his desire to not just serve but also use the process to probe and find a meaning for his own 'being'. Gandhi, however, also argued that the renunciation involved in selfless serving is to give up the possessiveness of the individual so as to acquire *moksha*. For him spiritual freedom and longing for *moksha* was an all absorbing goal encompassing everything. This obviously requires self-control and renunciation; "*service of humanity alone could generate the disinterested self-control essential for spiritual emancipation*" (Harijan, 1946 March 3). Freedom he felt lies in A*nasakti*, selfless service, but this is not easily obtained. Gandhi explains, "I am an humble aspirant for perfection. I know my way to it also. But knowing the way is not reaching its end" (Raghvan and Iyer, 1986, I, 4). The path is exacting, one of action and of service to humanity. The nub of Gandhi's world view, the social context of which revolves around *swadeshi, sarvodaya, swaraj,* and construction programme is his commitment to social service or *Anasakti*. While accepting the social processes of transition and transformation, he refuses to be hustled on to some highway of modernization and development. For him social transformation has to be through processes of conscious intervention and involvement. This brings up the characterization of Gandhi as being an intrepid itinerant social worker.

For Gandhi the urge for freedom and *moksha* is generic to human beings and is engrained in our selves. The import of this is that since the urge for freedom is contemporary and in conjunction with society, the ultimate of freedom which is *moksha,* too, has to be a contemporary discourse. Consequently, the grammar of the discourse of *moksha* has to be service to others. "Through the selfless embodiment of ahimsa and satyagraha, Gandhi believed theophilanthropists (friends of God and man) could ameliorate human misery whilst freeing themselves from worldly hopes and fear. Freedom, he felt, lies in anasakti, selfless service" (Raghvan and Iyer, 1986, I, 17). Social service for Gandhi is to come to terms with the distinct notions of 'love' and 'compassion'. You love to give and to take. Love is never one way. When it is one way it is infatuation. Compassion on the other hand is a one way process of giving without expectations. As such when Gandhi uses the term love-force he is suggesting that all such relationships are two-way.

In South Africa, Gandhi was able to illustrate and indicate the legitimacy of *satyagraha* as a potent tool of non-violent resistance and an enabling practice for the attainment of *swaraj*. He emphasised a couple of very insightful qualities. Firstly, *satyagraha* is not a question of transitory win or loss. It is an all-encompassing mission and always a march forward. As such it is an ongoing succession of awareness building events. However, it is essential import is in how it encourages local involvement and participation because it cannot be a transplant sustained by non-local initiatives. Further, to be genuinely awareness building, such participation has to ensure that they are associative-evolutionary in nature and not coercive or mediatory. Secondly, it has to become free from dependency particularly from that of mediation by any individual or even group of leader's. Andrews had pointed out this problematic to Gandhi when he was in South Africa.

Satyagraha to be faithful to self-realization has to acquire a local narrative independent of the individual intervention or agency of individual *satyagrahis*. But contradictorily it has to be initiated and sustained by individuals. The satyagrahi has to march to a more outreaching inclusive call of which their involvement in *satyagraha* is the beginning. This is what can be characterised as the 'dichotomy of the threshold'; the inside has to be sustained while the outside has to be investigated. While the outside is not external and ignorable for the social in an individual, it is not the same for the personal in the same individual. Similarly, while the local community has to be self-sustaining, creating and sustaining its own creativity and crafts-persons, it has to be able to relate, understand, adopt and adjust with the outside world. In all this, the threshold however should not become the site of contention and skirmish. This is a crucial aspect Gandhi was probing because *satya* and *ahimsa* the core of *satyagraha* have to be inclusive and transparently so. Gandhi's discontinuing of action and even withdrawing *satyagraha* is a pointer to the need to be clear about the nature of action in *satyagraha*. The purpose of his narrative is a mutuality of the insider and the outsider. In other words he refuses to surrender to the dichotomy of the threshold along with the notion that 'contesting the other' is vital to action mediating social transformation.

Gandhi recognised the debilitating influence of the brooding challenge of contesting the other and how it impacts the *satyagrahi* and the people. Perhaps, Gandhi could afford to be large hearted and liberal. Can other *satyagrahis* and particularly *satyarthis* involved in *satyagraha* afford to be generous? People find it extremely difficult to comprehend the intrepid and itinerant nature expected of a *satyagrahi*. In particular for them the trouble is with the itinerant nature of the leadership and the fact that while fearlessness has to be acquired through constant honing, it is not in the giving of anybody. This becomes particularly tiring when *satyagraha* and its minimalism considers period of continuity of a *satyagraha* as being flexible. When action prolongs itinerant tends to get confused with 'enforced presence' and intrepid with 'stubbornness'.

Satyagraha has a threefold thrust: intentions, intervention and involvement. Intentions are based on information and a philosophy or worldview which acts as a guiding principle. For Gandhi the worldview articulates around *satya, ahimsa swaraj* and *satyagraha*. While Raj Kumar Shukla gave the initial information about conditions prevailing in Champaran, Gandhi meticulously collected and documented relevant evidence and information (*Harijan*, 1946 March; also see Pouchepadass, J., 1999). He then used this information to arrive at relevant knowledge to be able to plan his actions. On the details as knowledge was based his specific plans and intentions of resisting the planters and the government. The significance of this knowledge is that intentions based on them are transparent.

Intervention on the other hand is the actual conversion of intentions into action (plans). These need clarity about policy, i.e. principle or course of action proposed to be adopted. These are programmes and strategies which depend upon knowledge of the local conditions. Here knowledge is the product of analysing information gathered. Intervention by a *satyagrahi* is accommodative in that it reaches out to everyone; there is no 'other'. Intervention in many ways is akin to a policy decision. However, it is prone to be afflicted by procrastination due to its proclivity to involve everyone.

Involvement on the other hand is the individual's actual practice or application of ideas, beliefs and methods based again on analysis and knowledge not mere information. For the *satyagrahi* this is essentially based on wisdom or distilled knowledge. This essentially refers to a proper understanding by an individual of how the implementation of action plans impact the attitude of those involved. Essentially involvement is inclusive and as a narrative of resistance, a response to the problematic of 'what we want' and 'what we don't want'. As a matter of fact the *satyagrahi* examines, 'do we really know what we want'? Further, she is also conscious of this becoming rhetoric of vested interests? We cannot forget that even after hundred years, the issues of ownership of land, access to education, health, drinking water, sanitation and communal harmony remain as they did when Gandhi went to Champaran to initiate *satyagraha*!

Involvement begins with acknowledging the mutuality and the support one can provide another not in exchange for what the other can or has done, but as a response to the over-all nurture one receives as a package of being. It presupposes a vision and mission for an individual and for society and it also suggests alternatives in accordance with which one could transform society. In Gandhian parlance this vision as well as mission of involvement is *Sarvodaya*. **Therefore, involvement cannot be a sporadic reaction to a situation. It needs preparation and has to be pragmatic and realistic. The preparation indicates choice while pragmatism indicates chance.** Thus, while on the one hand it is resistance to untruth, it nevertheless has to be a constructive effort which should be need–based and not interest or wants based. Thus, involvement as *Sarvodaya* takes *Satyagraha*, *Swaraj* and *Swadeshi* as its practice. Involvement in many ways is a *Sadhana*, the means of accomplishing self-knowledge and as one grows in self–knowledge it becomes a spontaneous and natural expression of one's own self, i.e. of self-realisation. Involvement, therefore, is an engagement with four cardinals: mediating the relationship between the personal, the family and the social; the question of social transformation and the role of the state; the role of non-state forums in social transformation; the means and ends conundrum. A reading of *Swadeshi, Swaraj, Sarvodaya, ahimsa* and *satyagraha* in terms of their process orientation helps us come to grips with all these issues of involvement. To illustrate, why for instance is there an element of apprehension even coercion in the relationship between the individual, the family and society? It is because the relationship is hardly transparent often burdened with hidden agendas. On the other hand, the role of the state is clear, it is coercive.

This in turn means moving from the moral to the more pragmatic issue of participation and conscious intervention which presupposes motives and intentions. Conscious intervention seeks social participation along certain lines. The problem is with selecting the best approach because some argument (and every argument will have some takers) can negate at least some aspects of any and every orientation and worldview. The only thing that cannot be negated is one's own self. Not surprisingly since leadership is a crucial element in intervention, Gandhi focused on the individual and not on some vanguard, elite or proletariat, not even on an exemplar. Participation, therefore, is action-based, i.e. bound by the specifics of time, space and expectations. Participation during the freedom movement had resistance at its core. Accordingly, participation has to be inclusive and a process of construction and confrontation, methods amply demonstrated by Gandhi. For him participation and resistance is not a response to some 'we-they' syndrome.

Gandhian thought gives primacy to action. And action is to be chosen on the basis of its being desirable. The problem is in defining 'desirable'. One way is to describe it at three levels: the first is how inclusive is it in terms of involvement; the second refers to the comprehensiveness of the action in terms of taking into account all factors implicit and explicit that constitute the action; and lastly, how it measures up to the issue of consequences and thereby truth. Above all, the worth of an action should be judged by the goodness of the consequent state of affair. Since all social actions are mediated events which end up as consequences and over a period give scope for further actions, a veritable action event consequence continuum unfolds. Desirable actions are those which establish goodness in the milieu which they influenced and are contingent upon. Social intervention can thus become *satyagraha* with goodness at the core. *Satyagrahis* don't solve problems, they enable people to seize the occasion. Every action has to be a narrative by and of the people. While the *satyagrahis* as interlocutors do write the prologue the epilogue remains dialogical and a narrative of and by the people. The involvement of the *satyagrahi* is necessary, but never sufficient. They can only create the competence to seek adequate justice, but acquiring justice has to be an act of *tyaag* both by the *satyagrahi* and the people; this entails a conscious giving up of something to acquire something else which necessitates a paradigm shift for both. For the *satyagrahi* in terms of social intervention this corresponds to the issue of the professional and the volunteer. It also raises the vital question of the relationship between competence and expectation which generally is one of tense symbiosis because while they coexist they don't depend on similarity of context for their origination and signification. The volunteer looks at these as contingent to aid intervention and participation while the professional looks at them as qualifications in a bargaining engagement. It is generally understood that credibility of a person depends upon a harmonious blend of the two.

Competence is common to both the professional as well as the volunteer. Purity of motive is never enough. The enigma is in the expectations. A volunteer involves in an activity because he wants to. The professional, on the other hand, has a wide spectrum of expectations and is more accommodative as far as project selection and involvement is concerned. A volunteer involves because of his commitment to the activity. This does not mean that he would like to pauperize himself in the process. His commitment is towards a task that calls for creating a vibrant community. Selfsatiations and self-realisation emerges from the involvement leading to a consolidation of his social-centric commitment. On the other hand, for a professional, involvement is a means to 'acquire access' which then delivers tangible self-satiation. The professional is fully involved takes pride in his job. But the job and self-actualization remains distinct leading to personal-centric commitment.

Thus, the professional's skills and competences are available for hire while the volunteers are not. The volunteer is always bothered about the consequence while the professional need not. While a professional is a mercenary, a volunteer will remain critical and selective. Further, since the volunteer remains concerned about consequences, the capacity to use experience to judge outcomes keeps enhancing, changing and sharpening. A synergy emerges between her the volunteer work and the worksite and he develops an organic link with the labouring community. This is crucial for a person aspiring to influence social transformation and interventional activities. By making her himself personally a part of the process of change, her his relationship goes beyond exchange to that of harmonious give and take. Consequently, while expectations and returns go beyond the narrow domain of exchange value, resilience matures beyond the strictly personal to include the social as a necessity.

Thus, the volunteer tries to remain committed to the holistic impact of actions and tries to be inclusive in approach, avoids expediency and meticulously abstains from moral justifications for promoting the self–interest. Moreover, when there is a conflict of interest in terms of the impact of a strategy on the community, the volunteer while enjoining caution, will take a personal stand regarding commitment. The professional, on the other hand, will prefer to remain neutral and preferably abstain from taking value-based social positions, which might necessitate going beyond the requirements of the profession. For Gandhi the norm is clear, "unrestricted individualism is the law of the beast of the Jungle–willing submission to the social restraint for the sake of the well – being of the whole society enriches both the individual and the society of which one is a member"(CWMG, Vol. 69, 258).

Lastly, the volunteer tries to cultivate detachment, i.e. she he makes a sombre appreciation of the link between contribution and returns for the self as distinct from the impact of the intervention on the community. Some of the above might sound very demanding and idealistic, but for a social worker and particularly a Gandhian, the issue is to recognize these and internalise them with '*shradha*' and '*nistha*' that is with respect and a sense of responsibility. The individual in the process of becoming a professional begins by acquiring a skill; mastering the skill gives the individual a profession. This profession soon becomes an adjunct of the individual. For the professional this adjunct then tends to become the medium and the inspiration, which creates a worldview for the individual via professionalism. Very soon this worldview mediates the professional's search for meanings. The adjunct starts dominating and takes over the narrative of social involvement on behalf of the individual. The volunteer, on the contrary, tries to recognize these insidious characteristics of the adjunct. The volunteer tries to distinguish the essential from the incidental in terms of what Gandhi would recognise as truth from the contingent so that something that is added to another thing but not essentially a part of it doesn't end up becoming the driving force. For the volunteer the profession remains just a skill, albeit crucial. It is another matter that a volunteer by making social work a profession can create in social work an adjunct and end up like the professional a slave to the adjunct and in the process misuse the high status society attributes to the social worker. Few are able to handle the strenuous obligations of being a *yogi*, *saint* or *mahatma*! For Gandhi when consciousness is prefixed to work/service it becomes social work/social service. Such a social worker is no more an ordinary *pracharak*.

Travails of a Worldview

Prospecting a worldview is a difficult discourse. As an interface between hope and conviction, doubt always plays a mischievous role. Doubt assumes a category of profoundness because only time can tell about its impact. But then to wait and do nothing is denied to us. However, we do want to decide about 'what we want as alternatives to live a better life'. We know that society is crawling with consequences of events which have tried to fuse hope and conviction. We also know that to understand this progeny of our creativity and action we need both hindsight and foresight. Further, the pressure only increases when circumstances allow very little time for us to contemplate and respond. While history will follow, the problem is how to respond in the immediate present. Gandhi's *swaraj, swadeshi, sarvodaya* and constructive programme via social work help us respond to the demand of the immediate present. He helps at two levels: firstly, at the level of the individual's preoccupation with the personal and the social and secondly, at the level of the interface between the moment and history. Regarding this Gandhi begins with the known immediate given society. Since for him there is no 'Other' he focuses on the neighbour, neighbourhood and neighbourliness. He encourages us to go beyond and preferably try and transcend the restrictions of the threshold which creates an 'other'. This call for sociability and socialness is a call to be creative, critical and inclusive. In economic terms, it means a sharp shift from exchange and surplus orientation to satisfaction of sustainable needs. In political terms, it means transparency in intervention and involvement practices. And in cognitive terms, it means imbibing and applying the *dharma* of self-service and self-realisation foregrounded on *ahimsa* and *satya*. Above all, it excludes longing, particularly of specific mentifact such as beliefs, values, ideas, etc.

Future always seeks solace in memory. While the moment tries to choose from alternatives to articulate itself, memory encroaches with suggestions regarding the right choice, but the moment is distinct from memory. Memory actually is dead recall. Moment while articulating itself has no memory of itself because it is ceaselessly in the creation mode with no interlude for memory. Since the moment cannot afford to have a memory of its own, under the tutelage of the prevailing hegemony, it tends to adopt an annotation or justification of memory. Further, through such elucidation the moment can either be creative, or mystify memory to suit its ambitions, thereby manoeuvring participants in an event. For instance, a past can be dissected to separate content from context wherein a leader is debunked as a stooge. Again when people fall in love the moment pervades; only latter when marriage is contemplate that we find memory coming in with religion etc. Moment as bearer of memory in unfolding of events tends to encourage anthropomorphism. At times even Gandhi faltered. The curbing of a river which Gandhi uses as illustration in his articles on *'sarvodaya'* is illustrative of this. Gandhi argues, *"But the flow of wealth, like the course of a river, can be regulated. Most of the rivers run out their courses unregulated, their marshy banks poisoning the wind. If dams are built across the rivers to direct the water flow as required, they will irrigate the soil and keep the atmosphere pure"*. (CWMG, Vol. 8, 419). This regulating comes as a double edged sword which can cleave both ways and on either side. Should it cleave on the side of surplus or scarcity, labour or leisure, wants or needs? *Sarvodaya* comes with its clutch of problems. For instance the problem of hegemony of the local, consensus, conservation, reification and, of course, that of development and concern about the future. The last is particularly pertinent because under the garb of concern for others, euphemistically termed as 'serving others', concern often allows service to transform into authority and then power. The preacher-server soon progresses into a leader and then into 'the leader'. Soon his discourse becomes one of heads I win tails you lose, wherein the social as defined by the leader becomes the over-riding paradigm as also the measure of all intervention and involvement in processes of social transformation. Soon all relationship between nature, labour and product, those between the personal and the social and those between scarcity and abundance, labour and leisure, self-help and sharing are all evaluated against performance an ambiguous criteria whose definition remains the exclusive preserve of the leader. Perhaps, this is why Gandhi chooses to remain an intrepid itinerant social worker, always incisively interrogating claims, be they economic, political or socio-cultural. He remained constantly vigilant and cautious about the delusion of freedom and choice, particularly when made under ambiguous definitions of development, faith, involvement and leisure. For him freedom and choice had to correspond effortlessly with the often conflicting notions of wants and needs, ends and means, rights and duties and give and take. While analysing necessity and compulsion Gandhi would urge caution because compulsions emerge as crisis and remain susceptible to manipulation. Perhaps this is why for him *sarvodaya* is not *antodaya*. A*ntodaya* as service has this inclination of becoming leader sensitive. Gandhi sought to separate the action from the potential selfishness inherent in the endeavour.

Accordingly *swadeshi* for Gandhi was not just a question of consuming or not consuming Indian products. It was more an idea of recovering the idea of India as local, sans the parochialism of region, religion or nation. The twentieth century Indian milieu for all practical purpose was a moth eaten frayed brittle social formation albeit with a resilient core. Split at many levels it was certainly seeking cohesiveness and a vigorous identity. Taking his que from earlier thinkers

Gandhi sought to find such an idea through a bold combination of ambition or motivation and empathy or responsiveness. *Swadeshi* was one such strategy. By inserting the qualities of conscious thinking, being and purpose, Gandhi converted *swadeshi* into a conviction regarding the local which while eschewing antagonism towards any country avoided chauvinism. *Swadeshi* by denouncing the prevailing order and renouncing any association with that, which is unacceptable to the local, is an announcement of praxis of rural-mindedness and sociability of the neighbourhood. This in many ways was also a strategy to help the local re-appropriate its body, soul and uniqueness. Similarly *Hind Swaraj* was not to appropriate a house the British build.

For Gandhi *swadeshi* was not a question of the efficacy of the quality of proximity within a social milieu, nor was it an issue of egoism or altruism. It was a question of sustainable cohesiveness which did not depend on external forces for its actuality. Given the trauma of colonial rule the moot question was one of necessity, choice and acts of determinism which influence the local milieu. Thus, "when you demand swaraj, you do not want swaraj for yourself alone but for your neighbour too" (Harijan, 1935, March 1, 1935; *CWMG*, Vol. 60, 254) is how Gandhi understood. *Swadeshi* by questioning the hegemony of the overarching market system designed by the imperial power, sought to address not just some of the splits in the polity but also inculcate an element of patriotism to reclaim a sense of identity for the people. While encouraging certain restrictions it did not deny any necessity. Its stress was on discretion while choosing. Encouraging entitlement and endowment, swadeshi "was not the universality of the use of an article which goes under the name of swadeshi but the universality of participation in the production or manufacturing of such articles". (Young India, 1926, June 17). *Swadeshi* thus embodies service as self-help and self-realization. To conclude, for Gandhi conscious involvement in social transformation processes is a linkage between social service, civil society and the individual around a few fundamentals such as *anasakti,* love and compassion, *satyagraha* and its three fold thrust, choice and pragmatism and lastly the issue of the diversity of the vernacular vis-ë-vis the state.

REFERENCES

1. Banerjee, Samir. *Notes from Gandhigram: Challenges to Gandhian Praxis.* New Delhi: Orient BlackSwan, 2009.
2. *Tracing Gandhi: Satyarthi to Satyagrahi.* London and New York, 2020.
3. *The Collected Works of Mahatma Gandhi.* (1999). Concerned volumes. New Delhi: Publication Division, Government of India.
4. *Harijan.* Ahmedabad, India, 1933-1948.
5. Pouchepedass, Jacques.*Champaran and Gandhi: Planters, Peasants and Gandhian Politics.* New Delhi: Oxford University Press, 1999.
6. Raghavan and Iyer, N. (eds.) (1986). *The Moral and Political Writings of Mahatma Gandhi, (MPWMG).* Vol. I, II & III. Oxford Clarendon Press.
7. *Young India.* Ahmedabad, India, 1919-1932.

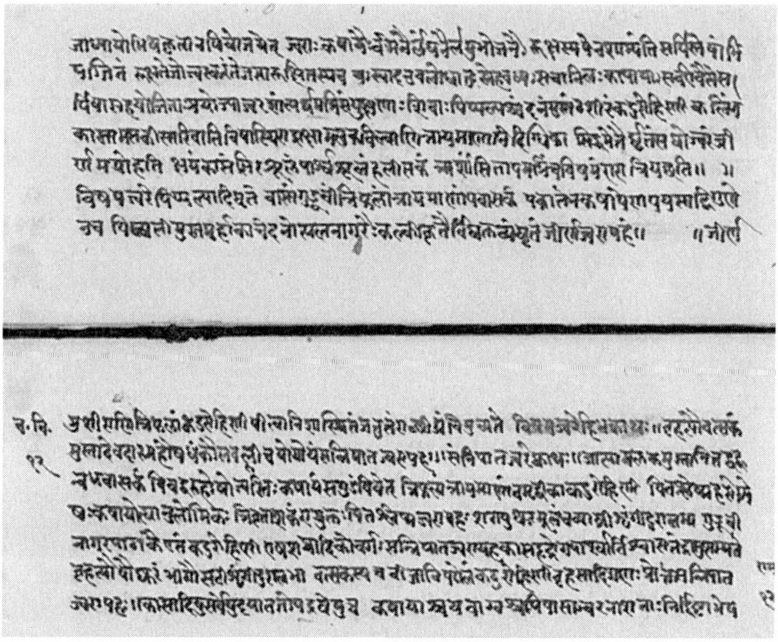

A Section of Ancient Indian text on Medicine:
The *Carakasamhita – Sutrasthana*

Source: Wikipedia, CC-BY 4.0

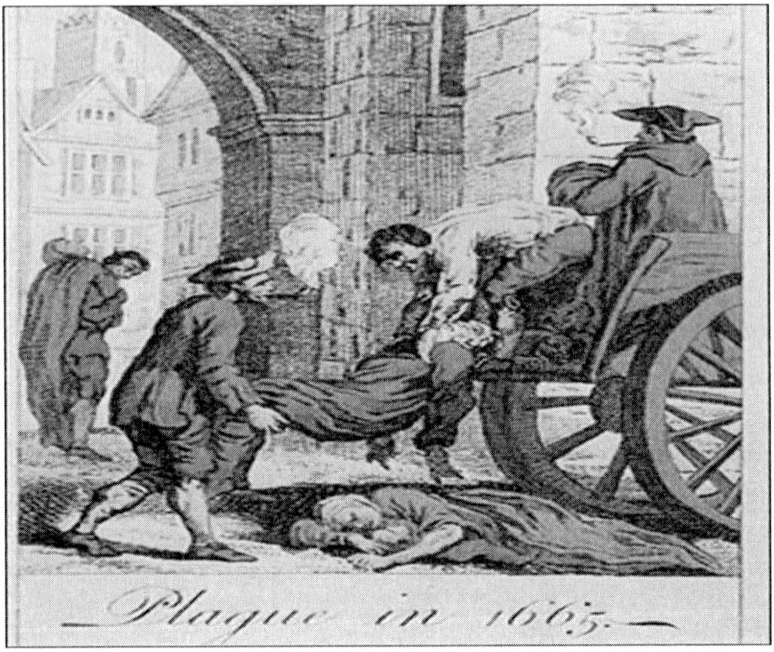

The Great Plague of London, 1665
Source: Wikimedia Commons

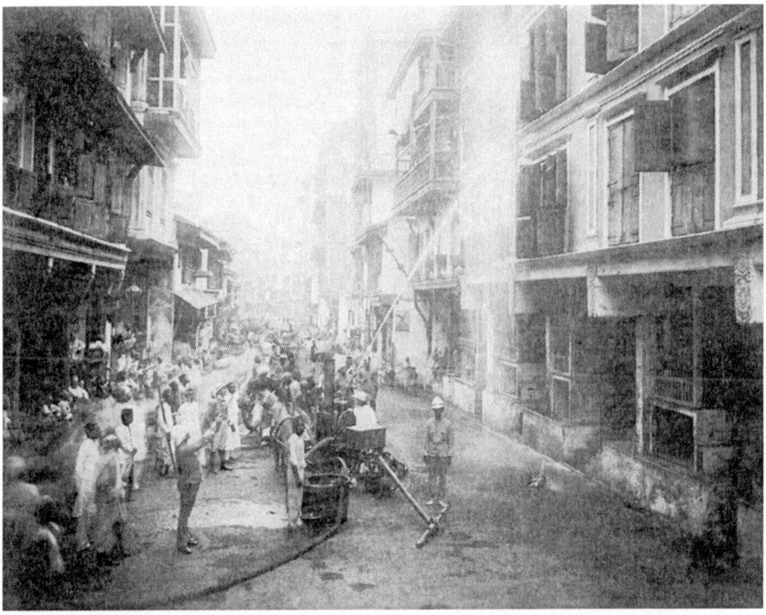

Disinfecting plague houses with a flushing engine, 1897
Source: Photo by Cap. C. Moss, 1897
National Army Museum, https://collection.nam.ac.uk/detail.php?acc=1992-08-74-108

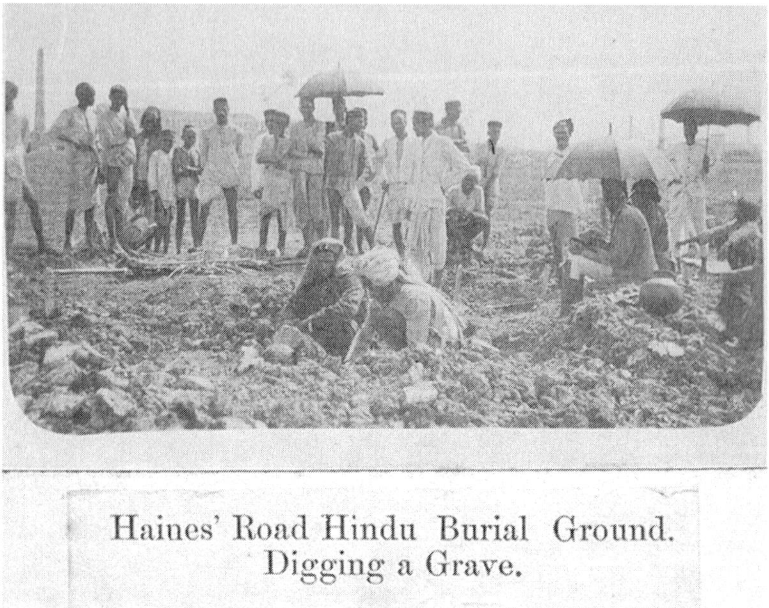

Digging the grave in the Hindu Burial Ground, Haines Road, Bombay, 1897

Source: Photo by Cap. C. Moss, 1897

National Army Museum, https://collection.nam.ac.uk/detail.php?acc=1992-08-74-71

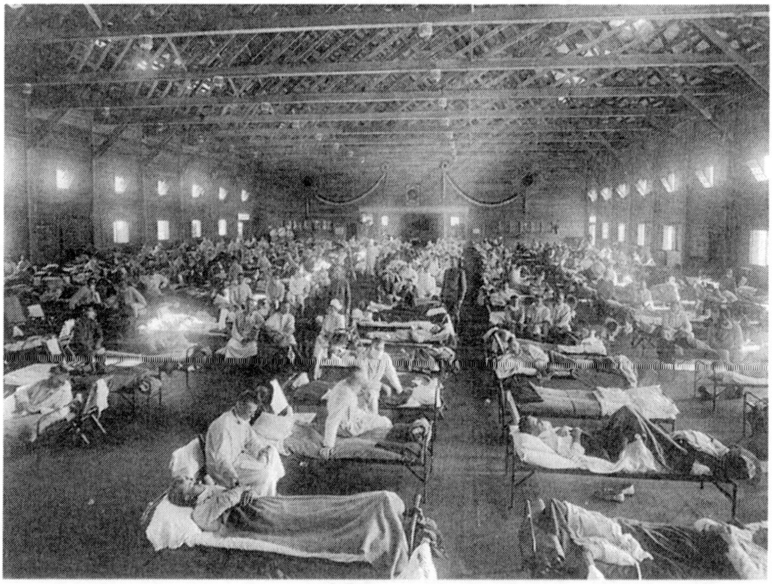

Emergency hospital during Influenza epidemic 1918: Soldiers from Fort Riley,

infected by Spanish flu at Camp Funston, Kansas

Source: Wikimedia Commons, https://en.wikipedia.org/wiki/Spanish_flu#/media/File:Emergency_hospital_during_Influenza_epidemic,_Camp_Funston,_Kansas_-_NCP_1603.jpg

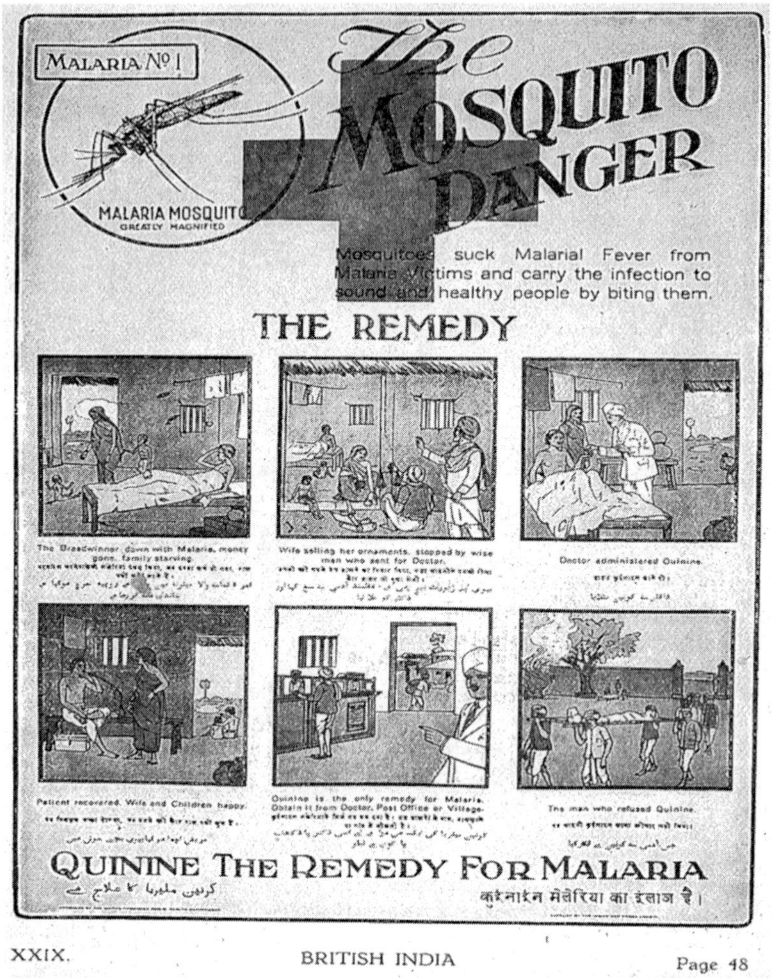
MALARIA Nº I
MALARIA MOSQUITO
GREATLY MAGNIFIED
The MOSQUITO DANGER
Mosquitoes suck Malarial Fever from Malaria Victims and carry the infection to sound and healthy people by biting them.
THE REMEDY
The Breadwinner down with Malaria, money gone, family starving.
Wife selling her ornaments, stopped by wise man who sent for Doctor.
Doctor administered Quinine.
Patient recovered. Wife and Children happy.
Quinine is the only remedy for Malaria. Obtain it from Doctor, Post Office or Village.
The man who refused Quinine.
QUININE THE REMEDY FOR MALARIA
XXIX.
BRITISH INDIA
Page 48

An advertisement for quinine as a malaria treatment from 1927
Source: Wikipedia CC BY 4.0

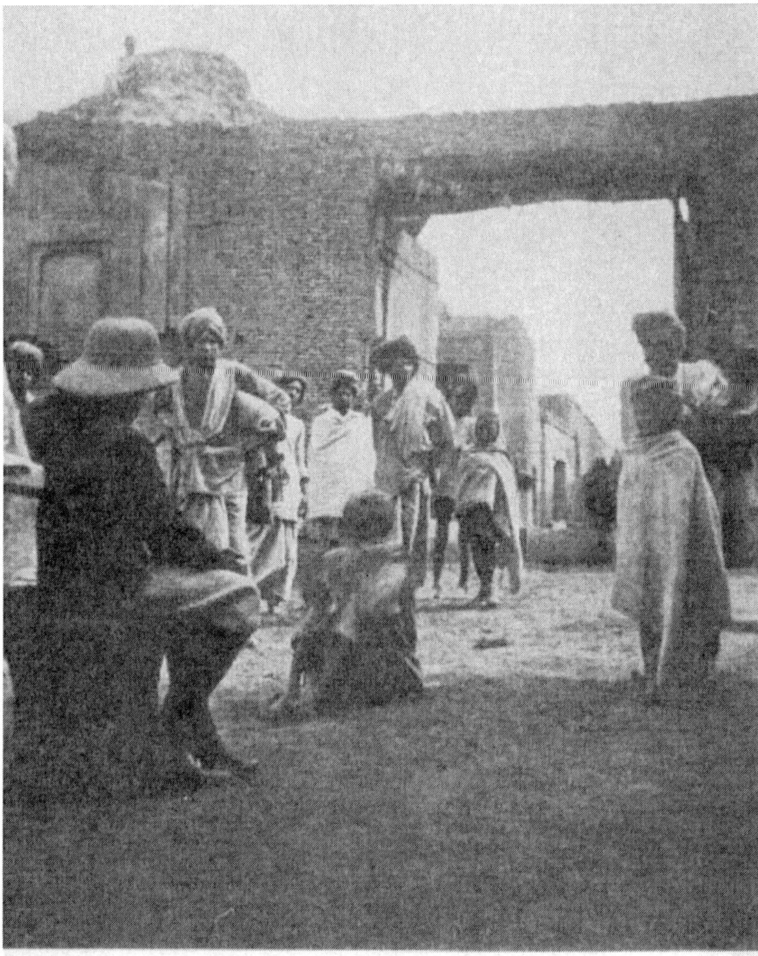

PREACHING INOCULATION

Outside a Small, Plague-stricken Town in the Punjâb.

The preacher is a missionary, and the picture illustrates two vital principles—that the essence of health-promotion is education of the public, and that the chief agents must be those most in touch with its daily life.)

Preaching Inoculation outside a plague stricken town in Punjab (Source: Fremantle Francis, A Traveller's Study of Health and Empire, London, 1911)